JONES' CLINICAL PAEDIATRIC SURGERY
DIAGNOSIS AND MANAGEMENT

D1330208

JONES' CLINICAL PAEDIATRIC SURGERY
DIAGNOSIS AND MANAGEMENT

By the Staff of the Royal Children's Hospital
Melbourne, Australia

Edited by

John M. Hutson
MB, BS(Monash), MD(Melb), FRACS
Senior Lecturer, Department of Paediatrics
Deputy Chairman, Department of General Surgery

Spencer W. Beasley
MB, ChB(Otago), MS(Melb), FRACS
Senior Lecturer, Department of Paediatrics
Surgeon, Royal Children's Hospital

Alan A. Woodward
MB, BS, FRCS, FRACS
Surgeon, Royal Children's Hospital

FOURTH EDITION

MELBOURNE
Blackwell Scientific Publications
OXFORD LONDON EDINBURGH
BOSTON PARIS BERLIN VIENNA

© 1992 by
Blackwell Scientific Publications
Editorial Offices:
54 University Street, Carlton
    Victoria 3053, Australia
Osney Mead, Oxford OX2 0EL
25 John Street, London WC1N 2BL
23 Ainslie Place, Edinburgh EH3 6AJ
3 Cambridge Center, Cambridge
    Massachusetts 02142, USA

Other Editorial Offices:
Librairie Arnette SA
2, rue Casimir-Delavigne
75006 Paris
France

Blackwell Wissenschafts-Verlag
Meinekestrasse 4
D-1000 Berlin 15
Germany

Blackwell MZV
Feldgasse 13
A-1238 Wien
Austria

First published 1992

Set by Semantic Graphics Services, Singapore
Printed in Singapore

DISTRIBUTORS

Australia
    Blackwell Scientific Publications Pty Ltd
    54 University Street
    Carlton, Victoria 3053
    (*Orders*: Tel: 03 347 5552
            Fax: 03 347 5001)

UK and Europe
    Marston Book Services Ltd
    PO Box 87
    Oxford OX2 0DT
    (*Orders*: Tel: 0865 791155
            Fax: 0865 791927
            Telex: 837515)

USA
    Blackwell Scientific Publications, Inc.
    3 Cambridge Center
    Cambridge, MA 02142
    (*Orders*: Tel: 800 759-6102
            617 225-0401)
Canada
    Times Mirror Professional Publishing, Ltd
    5240 Finch Avenue East
    Scarborough, Ontario M1S 5A2
    (*Orders*: Tel: 800 268-4178
            416 298-1588)

Cataloguing in Publication Data

Jones' clinical paediatric surgery.

    4th ed.
    Includes bibliographies and index.
    ISBN 0 86793 169 8.

    1. Children—Surgery. I. Royal Children's Hospital
    (Melbourne, Vic.) II. Jones, Peter G. (Peter Griffith).
    III. Woodward, Alan A. (Alan Arthur). IV. Hutson,
    John M. V. Beasley, Spencer W. IV. Title: Clinical
    paediatric surgery.

    617.98

Contents

Contributors

Staff members of the Royal Children's Hospital, Melbourne, Victoria

A. W. Auldist, FRACS
Chairman, Department of General Surgery
Chapters 23, 26

A. Bankier, FRACP
Clinical geneticist
Chapter (1)

S. W. Beasley, MS, FRACS
Senior Lecturer, University of Melbourne
General Surgeon
Chapters 2, 4, 5, 6, 18, 19, 20, 29, 38, 40, 41, 50, 51,
(14), (23), (24), (26), (36), (39)

W. G. Cole, MSc PhD FRACS
Professor of Orthopaedics,
University of Melbourne,
Chief Orthopaedic Surgeon
Chapters 43, 44, 45, 46, 47, 48

D. Courtemanche, MD
Clinical Research Fellow,
Dept of Plastic Surgery
Chapters 15, 52, 53

P. M. Davidson, MRCP FRCS FRACS
Lecturer, University of Melbourne
Chapters 16, 25

R. V. Dickens, FRACS
Deputy, Division of Surgery,
Head, Clinical Dept of Orthopaedics
Chapter 39

J. M. Hutson, MD FRACS
Senior Lecturer, University of Melbourne
Deputy, Department of General Surgery
Chapters 3, 8, 9, 11, 17, 27, 28, 35, 49, (12), (13), (14),
(15), (25), (31), (33), (37), (43), (44), (45), (46), (47),
(48), (52), (53)

G. L. Klug, FRACS
Senior Neurosurgeon
Chapters 12, 37

B. Lansdell, FRACS
Ophthalmologist
Chapter 13

M. B. Menelaus, MD FRCS FRACS
Senior Orthopaedic Surgeon
Chapter (10)

J. R. Solomon, FRCS FRACS
Surgeon-in-Charge, Burns Unit;
General Surgeon
Chapter 42

K. B. Stokes, FRACS
General Surgeon
Chapter 24

H. L. Tan, FRACS
General Surgeon
Chapters 31, 33

R. G. Taylor, FRACS
General Surgeon
Chapter 36

J. Vorrath, FRACS
Senior Otolaryngologist
Chapter 14

A. A. Woodward, FRCS FRACS
General Surgeon
Chapters 1, 7, 10, 21, 22, 30, 32, 34, (16), (42)

Foreword to the First Edition

The progressive increase in the body of information relative to the surgical specialties has come to present a vexing problem in the instruction of medical students. There is not time in the medical curriculum to present everything about everything to them and in textbook material one is reduced either to synoptic sections in textbooks of surgery, or to complete and authoritative textbooks in the specialty too detailed for the student or the non-specialist.

There has long been a need for a book of modest size dealing with paediatric surgery in a way suited to the requirements of the medical student, general practitioner and paediatrician. Peter G. Jones and his associates from the distinguished and productive group at the Royal Children's Hospital in Melbourne have succeeded brilliantly in meeting this need. The book could have been entitled 'Surgical Conditions in Infancy and Childhood', for it deals with the child and his afflictions, their symptoms, diagnosis and treatment rather than the surgery as such. The reader is told when and how urgently an operation is required, and enough about the nature of the procedure to understand its risks and appreciate its results. This is what students need to know and what paediatricians and general practitioners need to be refreshed on.

Many of the chapters are novel, in that they deal not with categorical diseases but with the conditions which give rise to a specific symptom; thus: Vomiting in the First Month of Life, The Jaundiced Newborn Baby, Surgical Causes of Failure to Thrive. The chapter on genetic counselling is a model of information and good sense.

The book is systematic and thorough. A clean style, logical sequential discussions and avoidance of esoterica allow the presentation of substantial information over the entire field of paediatric surgery in this comfortable-sized volume with well chosen illustrations and carefully selected bibliography. Many charts and tables, original in conception, enhance the clear presentation.

No other book so satisfactorily meets the needs of the student for broad and authoritative coverage in a modest compass. The paediatric house officer (in whose hospital more than 50 per cent of the patients are, after all, surgical) will be serviced equally well. Paediatric surgeons will find between these covers an account of the attitudes, practices and results of one of the world's great paediatric surgical centres. The book comes as a fitting tribute to the 100th Anniversary of the Royal Children's Hospital.

MARK M. RAVITCH
Professor of Pediatric Surgery
University of Pennsylvania

Preface to the Fourth Edition

The objective that prompted the first edition of this book was to bring together information on surgical conditions in infancy and childhood for the use of senior medical students and resident hospital staff. It has been a source of great satisfaction to the contributors to find that the book has successfully fulfilled this aim and that a fourth edition has now been required. Family doctors, paediatricians, and a wide spectrum of those concerned with the welfare of children have also, it seems, found it helpful.

A knowledgeable medical publisher once commented to Peter Jones that this is not a book about surgery but about paediatrics, and perhaps that is what it should be, given the omission of almost all details of operative surgery, that is, the 'what', while concentrating on the 'why' and 'when'.

The plan used for the first three editions has been changed somewhat, with the chapters now grouped according to particular areas of interest. This should allow readers to find quickly the subject they require. All the chapters have been completely rewritten, with some chapters amalgamated into different sections. Paediatric surgery has continued to advance rapidly, and many of the diagnostic aids described in the third edition have been replaced with ultrasonography or other modern radiological techniques.

Many of the contributors to the fourth edition are making their first appearance by updating or rewriting completely the chapters provided by their predecessors on the staff. This has ensured that the style and content remain as up-to-date as possible.

Mr Peter Jones has now retired, and it was a daunting task for the new editors to follow his example. We believe it is a fitting tribute that the publishers have sought to rename the book in his honour. Despite being extensively rewritten with almost a complete set of new illustrations, the book nevertheless retains its original flavour. The printing of this edition in a larger format than previous editions and the aggressive editing which we have undertaken to shorten many of the chapters, should make this book popular with students. We hope that it remains as useful and useable as its predecessors.

J. M. H.
S. W. B.
A. A. W.

October 1991

Acknowledgements

Many members of the Royal Children's Hospital community have made valuable contributions to this fourth edition.

We are indebted to Dr David Boldt, Director of Radiology, for allowing us to update the radiographs from the teaching collection. We thank the staff of the Education and Resource Centre for the quality of their art work and photography, which continues at a very high standard. The secretarial staff of the Department of Surgery, Mrs Elizabeth Vorrath, Mrs Veronica Bello and Mrs Judith Hayes, are thanked sincerely for their untiring effort.

Finally we express our gratitude to Mark Robertson and Aileen Boyd-Squires of Blackwell Scientific Publications (Australia) for bringing this edition to fruition.

1

Antenatal Diagnosis and Genetic Counselling

ANTENATAL DIAGNOSIS

The widespread use of ultrasound diagnosis in pregnancy has uncovered many fetal abnormalities which previously presented to the surgeon after birth. At first, it was expected that the antenatal diagnosis of fetal problems would lead to better treatment and an improved outcome. Unfortunately, this expectation has not been fulfilled because antenatal diagnosis has opened a Pandora's box of lethal, complex anomalies which in the past never survived the pregnancy, and were recorded in statistics of fetal death *in utero* and stillbirth. However, there is no doubt that in the less severe anomalies perinatal treatment is improved by foreknowledge of the problems.

Indications and timing for antenatal ultrasound

At present, the indications for ultrasound are usually obstetric in nature, and fetal anomalies are diagnosed in a serendipitous fashion. The list of fetal anomalies diagnosed on ultrasound is expanding rapidly with the increasing sophistication and use of this examination (Fig. 1.1). Careful examination of the fetus has become an important part of the ultrasound examination and is just as important as the obstetric evaluation. If there is a previous history of fetal anomalies, for example spina bifida, an ultrasound examination in early pregnancy will be of great value, as there is a significant risk of spina bifida in subsequent pregnancies.

Seventeen weeks is regarded as the best time for the early detection of fetal anomalies. If a problem is diagnosed at this stage, the ultrasound may be repeated at suitable intervals throughout the pregnancy to observe progress of the abnormality. More invasive tests, such as amniocentesis and fetal blood sampling, may be indicated (see below).

NATURAL HISTORY OF FETAL ANOMALIES

Before the advent of ultrasound, paediatric surgeons saw only a selected group of infants with congenital anomalies. These babies had survived the pregnancy and lived long enough after birth to reach surgical attention. Thus the babies coming to surgical treatment were already a selected group, mostly with a good prognosis.

Antenatal diagnosis has brought paediatric surgeons into contact with a new group of conditions with a poor prognosis, and at last the full spectrum of pathology is coming to surgical attention. For example, posterior urethral valves causing obstruction of the urinary tract were thought to be rare with an incidence of 1 : 5000 male births; most cases did well with postnatal valve resection. It is now known that the true incidence of urethral valves is 1 : 2500 male births and these additional cases did not come to surgical attention as they were severe examples of intrauterine renal failure with either fetal death *in utero* or early neonatal death from the respiratory problems of Potter's syndrome. It was thought that antenatal diagnosis would improve the outcome of such congenital anomalies, but the overall results have appeared to become worse with these severe 'new' cases being included.

There are similar problems with the antenatal diagnosis of diaphragmatic hernia (Fig. 1.2). Congenital

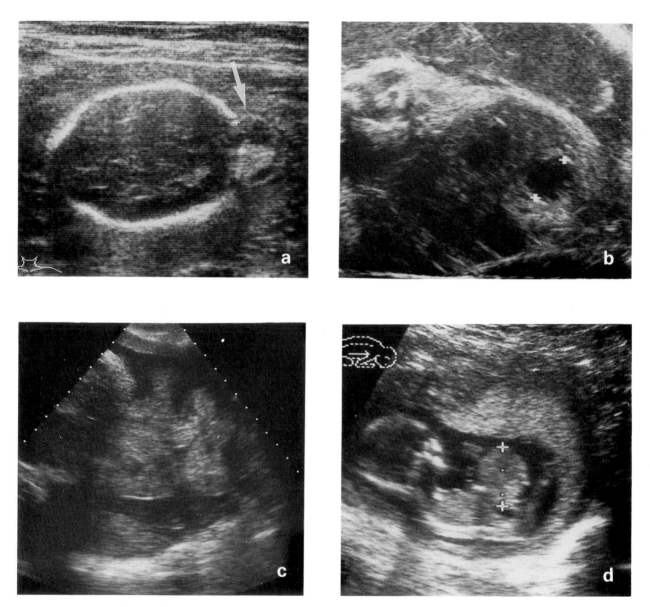

Fig. 1.1 (a) Encephalocele shown in a cross-section of the fetal head. The sac protruding through the posterior skull defect is arrowed. (b) Bilateral hydronephrosis shown in an upper abdominal section. The dilated renal pelvis containing clear fluid is marked. (c) The irregular outline of the free-floating bowel in the amniotic cavity of a term baby with gastroschisis. (d) A longitudinal section through a 14 week fetus showing a large exomphalos. The head is seen to the left of the picture. The large sac (marked) is seen between blurred images of the arms and legs.

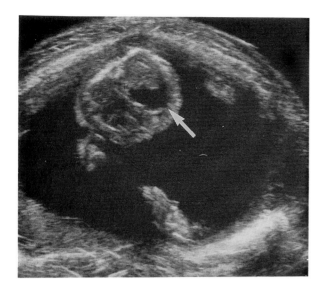

Fig. 1.2 Cross-section of a uterus with marked polyhydramnios. The fetal chest is seen in cross-section within the uterus. The fluid-filled cavity within the left side of the chest is the stomach protruding through a diaphragmatic hernia (arrow).

diaphragmatic hernia was not associated with multiple congenital anomalies when cases presented after birth. Now, antenatal diagnosis of diaphragmatic hernia has uncovered a more severe subgroup with associated chromosomal and multiple developmental anomalies. It would seem that the earlier the diaphragmatic hernia is diagnosed, the worse is the outcome.

Despite these problems, there are many advantages in antenatal diagnosis. The outcome of many conditions is improved by the prior knowledge of 'congenital' anomalies.

MANAGEMENT FOLLOWING ANTENATAL DIAGNOSIS

Mode of delivery

The fetal anomaly itself usually does not dictate the mode of delivery: this decision is made on obstetric criteria. An exception to this rule may be spina bifida, where there is some evidence that nerve function is preserved better after Caesarean section. The timing of delivery may be influenced by evidence of fetal deterioration in the last trimester, such that delivery may be induced to prevent further damage to the fetus. In gastroschisis the gut may be mobile and healthy in early pregnancy only to become progressively thickened and adherent in the last weeks before delivery. This deterioration may be prevented by inducing labour early, for example at 36 weeks. The place of delivery is also important. If a diagnosis of gastroschisis is made on antenatal ultrasound the delivery should be at a major maternity centre with full neonatal resuscitation services. For management purposes cases diagnosed on antenatal ultrasound may be classified into three groups.

Good prognosis

In these cases, for example cleft lip or talipes equinovarus, the condition allows normal progress of the pregnancy and no specific treatment is required until after birth. In some cases, for example vesicoureteric reflux, antenatal diagnosis is helpful as it allows prophylactic antibiotics to be commenced immediately after birth; these children need never have a serious urinary tract infection. The parents are counselled to prepare them for the infant's problems. Antenatal diagnosis gives parents time to come to terms with these problems before delivery and helps them cope with the realities of the abnormality after birth.

Poor prognosis

Anencephaly or diaphragmatic hernia with severe chromosomal anomalies would be two examples of conditions with a poor prognosis. These are lethal problems and the outcome of the pregnancy is predetermined by the time the diagnosis is made.

Late deterioration

Initial assessment of the fetal anomaly indicates a good prognosis with no reason for interference, but later in gestation the fetus deteriorates and some action must be undertaken to prevent a lethal outcome. An example would be the lower urinary tract obstruction seen in posterior urethral valves. Loss of liquor with oligo-hydramnios is a sign of intrauterine renal failure. There are several ways to treat this problem. If the gestation is at a viable stage, for example 36 weeks, labour could be induced and the urethral valves treated after birth. If the risks of premature delivery are higher, for example 28 weeks gestation, temporary relief may be obtained by using percutaneous transuterine techniques to place a shunt catheter from the fetal bladder into the amniotic cavity. These catheters tend to become dislodged by fetal activity. A more definitive approach to drain the urinary tract is intrauterine surgery to perform a vesi-costomy and allow the pregnancy to continue. This procedure has been performed with success in a few cases of posterior urethral valves. These patients are highly selected and there are very few centres in the world performing intrauterine surgery. At present this surgery is regarded as experimental and reserved for rare situations, but this may not always be the case.

Antenatal ultrasound has become the most important means of diagnosing fetal anomalies and has given us a valuable means of understanding the natural history of developmental abnormalities.

GENETIC COUNSELLING

When a child is born with birth defects, there is inevitably shock and confusion until the diagnosis is clarified and the family begin to assimilate and accept the information given to them and make plans for the future. Acceptance depends both on the nature of the problem and the parents' perception of its significance. Some achieve resolution in days; others may take months or years. Given the opportunity, parents raise questions such as: 'Why did this happen?'; 'Why did it happen to us?'; 'What will now happen to our child?'; 'Did I cause this problem by something I did (or failed to do) during the pregnancy?'; 'Could this happen next time?'

All parents have the right to accurate information and the opportunity to express their feelings. Information should include formal genetic counselling, but does not necessarily involve a geneticist. When the diagnosis and aetiology are clear, the counselling is best done by the managing surgeon or specialist physician. Counsel-lors should ensure that they are equipped with up-to-date information.

Requirements for genetic counselling

Knowledge of the precise diagnosis

Any counselling is only as good as the information on which it is based. Knowledge of genetic heterogeneity and the possible differential diagnoses is necessary, so that by careful observation, similar patterns of birth defects can be distinguished. For example, pits in the lower lip associated with cleft lip/palate distinguish the dominantly inherited clefts (1 : 2 recurrence risk in offspring) from the common cleft lip/palate which has a much lower recurrence risk (1 : 25). When the child looks unusual or when multiple birth defects are present, a syndrome diagnosis should be considered. Some conditions may be inherited in different ways and examination of close relatives may be necessary.

Detailed family history

In order to clarify patterns of inheritance, one needs to document a three-generation pedigree, including con-sanguinity, fetal losses and any deaths. Direct questioning for birth defects and minor features of the condition may reveal other affected members. It is desirable that a positive history should be confirmed by examination of the family member or from medical records.

Knowledge of birth defects

Information should include the natural history of the condition, likely length and quality of life, potential complications and the availability of treatment and its likely outcome. Knowledge of the relevant medical and genetic literature is important.

Antenatal diagnosis for subsequent pregnancies

For many conditions, antenatal diagnosis now is available, giving families the option of not continuing the pregnancy of a fetus with birth defects. The technology and expertise are advancing so rapidly that one needs to have up-to-date knowledge of which conditions can be tested for, the technique used, its complications and the laboratory facilities available. The techniques are selected on the basis of the problem in question and the attitude of the couple to first and second trimester termination of pregnancy, and are balanced against the risks of the procedure.

As mentioned previously, ultrasound examination at 17 weeks can detect many structural abnormalities; although the accuracy of the examination depends on the skill of the operator, knowledge of fetal development and experience with birth defects.

Chorion villous sampling (CVS) is performed at 10 weeks of pregnancy for the detection of chromosome abnormalities and biochemical disorders. Genetic engineering methods can diagnose an increasing number of disorders. Sufficient tissue can be obtained by CVS for DNA studies. Most results are available within 2 weeks. This procedure carries a higher risk of spontaneous abortion (1 : 50) than the procedure of amniocentesis (1 : 200).

Amniocentesis is performed at 16 weeks of pregnancy and can uncover the range of problems detected by CVS. In addition, measurement of substances in the amniotic fluid can be performed, for example α-fetoprotein estimation to detect neural tube defects. Most results take 3–4 weeks. Interruption of pregnancy at this stage of gestation involves induction of labour.

Transabdominal tissue sampling is another method used when fetal tissue is needed, for example examination of fetal skin for detection of lethal epidermolysis bullosa.

Knowledge of genetic principles

Once the diagnosis is made, the recurrence risk for single gene defects can be calculated from the known pattern of inheritance (autosomal recessive, autosomal dominant, X-linked). Empirical recurrence of risk estimations are available from pedigree studies for many conditions of multifactorial inheritance or unknown aetiology. It is important to put the risk in perspective by comparing it with the background risk of birth defects in any pregnancy (this being 1 : 50–1 : 25 [2–4%]) and to emphasize that the risk applies to every subsequent pregnancy.

Communication skills

It is necessary to have an understanding of people and their reactions to situations of stress, grief and loss, as well as a knowledge of the psychological effects of genetic diseases on self-image and life. It is essential to listen to what the couple ask and to be aware of their discomfort and areas which they avoid. A grieving couple may not be ready for detailed factual information initially, in which case it is better left to a later session.

The role of the counsellor is to inform and to educate. The information should be presented simply in an unbiased and non-directive manner. When people consider alternatives of antenatal diagnosis and pregnancy, the counsellor should challenge the couple to consider all aspects of their situation. The final decision is made by the couple and ideally should be in line with their beliefs and needs.

FURTHER READING

Antonarakis S. E. (1989) Medical progress, diagnosis of genetic disorders at the DNA level. *N. Engl. J. Med.* **320**: 153–163.

Brock D. J. H. (1982) Current Review in Obstetrics and Gynaecology, Vol. 2. *Early Diagnosis of Fetal Defects.* Churchill Livingstone.

Clayton P. T. & Thompson E. (1988) Dysmorphic syndromes with demonstrable biochemical abnormalities. *J. Med. Genet.* **25**: 463–472.

Emery A. E. H. & Pullen I. M. (1984) *Psychological Aspects of Genetic Counselling.* Academic Press.

Harper P. S. (1988) *Practical Genetic Counselling*, 3rd edn. John Wright, Bristol.

Jones K. L. (1988) *Smith's Recognisable Patterns of Human Malformation*, 4th edn. W. B. Saunders.

Kessler S. (1979) *Genetic Counselling: Psychological Dimensions.* Academic Press Inc.

Kingston H. M. (1989) ABC of clinical genetics. Dysmorphology and teratogenesis. *Brit. Med. J.* **298**: 1235–1239.

Najmaldin A. S., Burge D. M. & Atwell J. D. (1990) Antenatally diagnosed urological abnormalities: where do we stand? *Pediatr. Surg. Int.* **5**: 195–197.

Scott J. (1986) Introduction to recombinant DNA. *J. Inher. Metab. Dis.* **9** (Suppl. I): 3–16.

Scott J. E. S. & Renwick M. (1990) Northern Region Fetal Abnormality Survey Results 1987. *J. Pediatr. Surg.* **25**: 394–397.

2

The Care and Transport
of the Newborn

The newborn infant with a major surgical condition should be transported and treated in a neonatal unit with paediatric surgical facilities. It is only in such a unit that the specialized surgical, anaesthetic and nursing expertise and facilities necessary for neonatal surgery will be found.

A detailed pre-operative assessment is necessary to detect associated or coexistent developmental anomalies. Vital disturbances which should be corrected before operation and predictable complications should be anticipated and recognized early.

RESPIRATORY CARE

The aims of respiratory care are: (i) to maintain a clear airway; (ii) prevent abdominal distension and aspiration of gastric contents; (iii) provide supplementary oxygen if necessary. Assessment of gestational age and weight will identify the premature infant who is susceptible to respiratory distress syndrome and apnoeic episodes. Small-for-dates babies are more likely to suffer asphyxia at birth, meconium aspiration and pneumothorax. An emergency tray with oral airways, face mask and bag, laryngoscope, endotracheal and suction tubes should be readily available.

Placing the baby in the prone position improves the airways and reduces gastro-oesophageal reflux and aspiration of gastric contents.

Suction of the pharyngeal secretions maintains a clear airway, especially in the premature infant with poorly developed laryngeal reflexes and in the infant with oesophageal atresia.

A nasogastric tube, size 8 French, will prevent life-threatening aspiration of vomitus, provided the tube is kept patent and allowed to drain freely with additional aspiration at frequent intervals. It will also reduce abdominal distension and improve pulmonary ventilation in patients with intestinal obstruction or diaphragmatic hernia.

Oxygen therapy, endotracheal intubation and ventilation will be required in the pre-operative resuscitation of some neonates with conditions such as diaphragmatic hernia.

CIRCULATING BLOOD VOLUME

Conditions which diminish the circulating volume include neonatal bowel obstruction and gastroschisis. The fluid is lost from vomiting, ileus and evaporation.

Blood loss in the neonatal period may be due to birth trauma, haemorrhagic disease from Vitamin K deficiency or clotting defects associated with sepsis. The blood volume of a full term infant is 80 mL/kg. Blood loss of 30 mL in a neonate is equivalent to losing 500 mL in an adult.

Fresh whole blood is cross-matched for major operations in the neonatal period. Blood loss during the operation is kept to a minimum and measured by weighing all swabs and packs used. The haemoglobin concentration in the first few days of life is about 19 g/dL and the haematocrit 50–70%. Blood viscosity is relatively high, and blood loss in this circumstance may be replaced in part with blood and in part with a crystalloid solution, which lowers the viscosity of the blood.

Diminished blood volume in a sick neonate with a bowel obstruction will lead to poor peripheral circulation. The baby will be lethargic and pale, with cool limbs, venoconstriction and cyanosis. Acidosis becomes a complicating factor. In this situation a 'bolus infusion' of a crystalloid solution such as Hartmann's solution over 15 min at 10 mL/kg is used for resuscitation. Where this is effective the peripheral circulation will improve dramatically. If this initial infusion is not adequate, further bolus infusions of crystalloid at 10 mL/kg may be given and the clinical response monitored.

CONTROL OF BODY TEMPERATURE

The sick neonate with a surgical condition is prone to hypothermia, defined as a core body temperature of less than 36°C. In hypothermia, heat production is stimulated above normal metabolic requirements and may be boosted by thermogenesis from increased metabolism of brown fat deposits. However, if heat loss exceeds heat production the body temperature will continue to fall, leading to acidosis and depression of respiratory, cardiac and nervous function.

All metabolic functions are altered by hypothermia. Newborn infants, especially the premature, are at risk of excessive heat loss because of the relatively large surface area to volume ratio and the lack of subcutaneous insulating fat.

Heat loss occurs from the body surface to the environment by radiation, conduction, convection and the evaporation of water. Excessive heat loss during transport, assessment and operation must be avoided, particularly in conditions such as gastroschisis where the eviscerated bowel provides a very large surface area for evaporation. Heat loss is controlled once the bowel is wrapped in domestic clear plastic wrap. The baby then is placed in the warm environment of a humidicrib.

Radiant overhead heaters are of particular value during procedures such as the insertion of intravenous cannulae or the induction of anaesthesia because they allow unimpeded access to the infant. Wet packs should never be applied to a neonate as they will accelerate evaporative and conductive heat losses.

FLUIDS, ELECTROLYTES AND NUTRITION

Many infants with a surgical condition cannot be fed in the perioperative period. Intravenous fluids provide daily maintenance requirements and prevent dehydration. The total volume of fluid given must supply maintenance requirements, restore fluid and electrolyte deficits and replace ongoing losses.
Maintenance water requirements are:
60–80 mL/kg on day 1 of life
80–100 mL/kg on day 2
100–150 mL/kg on day 3 and thereafter.
Maintenance electrolyte requirements are:
Sodium: 3 mmol/kg per day
Chloride: 3 mmol/kg per day
Potassium: 2 mmol/kg per day.
Maintenance joule requirements are:
100–140 kJ/kg per day.

These maintenance requirements can be provided in the first week by a solution made up of 5% dextrose in 0.225% sodium chloride (sodium: 35 mmol/L) with the addition of potassium chloride at 20 mmol/L. However, this solution is inadequate for long-term maintenance of body functions as it has many deficiencies, especially in kJ.

Replacement of fluid and electrolyte deficiencies often will be necessary in surgical patients, such as those with neonatal bowel obstruction. Before birth, the placenta maintains fluid and electrolyte balance. At birth, electrolyte levels are normal despite long-standing bowel obstruction, and extracellular water levels are relatively high. Persistent vomiting after birth soon will cause dehydration and electrolyte imbalance. The degree of dehydration can be measured by the clinical parameters of tissue turgor, the state of peripheral circulation, depression of the fontanelle, dryness of the mouth and urine output. Bodyweight loss also gives an approximation of water loss.

The rule of thumb for estimating water loss is that a body mass loss of 5% or less has few clinical manifestations: 5–8% shows moderate clinical signs of dehydration; 10% shows severe signs and poor peripheral circulation. Thus a 3000 g infant who has been vomiting and has a diminished urine output but shows no overt signs of dehydration, will have lost approximately 5% of body mass and will require 3000 × 5% mL = 150 mL fluid replacement to correct the deficit. Maintenance requirement must be administered also.

Electrolyte deficiency can be measured by electrolyte estimations. This will give a good guide for electrolytes that are distributed mainly in the extracellular fluid, for example sodium. It will not be as reliable for electrolytes that are found mainly in the intracellular space, for example potassium. Fluid and electrolyte deficiency due to vomiting will need to be replaced with a crystalloid solution which contains adequate levels of sodium, for example 0.9% sodium chloride (sodium: 150 mmol/L).

Continuing losses of fluid and electrolytes need to be measured and replaced. Losses may arise from nasogastric tube aspirates in bowel obstruction, diarrhoea from an ileostomy, and the excessive urinary losses which may occur after the relief of urinary obstruction, for example posterior urethral valves. When the losses are high they are best measured and replaced with an intravenous infusion of electrolytes equivalent to the fluid being lost.

Intravenous nutrition will be required when the period of starvation extends beyond 4–5 days. Common indications for intravenous nutrition in the neonatal period include necrotizing enterocolitis, extensive gut resection and gastroschisis. The aim of intravenous nutrition is to provide all substances necessary for normal growth and development. Intravenous nutrition may be maintained for weeks or months as required. Complications of prolonged nutrition include sepsis and obstructive jaundice.

Oral nutrition is preferred where possible and breast feeding is best. Surgery to the alimentary tract may make oral feeding impossible for a variable period: gut enzyme function may be poor and various substrates in the feeds may not be absorbed. Lactose intolerance is seen commonly and leads to diarrhoea with the passage of acidic fluid stools. Other malabsorptive problems relate to sugars, protein, fat and the osmolarity of the feeds. These can be handled by altering the conformation of the feeds or, in severe cases, by a period of intravenous nutrition to allow the gut enzymes time to recover.

BIOCHEMICAL ABNORMALITIES

Important problems include metabolic acidosis, hypoglycaemia and hypocalcaemia. These are corrected before operation because they may adversely influence the infant's response to anaesthetic agents.

Metabolic acidosis

Metabolic acidosis, which may result from hypovolaemia, dehydration, cold stress, renal failure or hypoxia, increases pulmonary vascular resistance and impairs cardiac output. Acidosis is corrected by giving a dose of sodium bicarbonate, which is calculated from the estimated base deficit, using the formula:

Base deficit × weight (kg) × 0.3 = dose of sodium bicarbonate (mmol)

Hypoglycaemia

Hypoglycaemia occurs in the sick newborn, especially if premature. Liver stores of glycogen are small, as are fat stores. Starvation and stress will use up liver glycogen rapidly and there will be a switch to fatty acid metabolism to maintain blood glucose levels, with consequent ketoacidosis. Gluconeogenesis from amino acids or pyruvate is slow to develop in the newborn, due to the relative inactivity of liver enzymes. A point is soon reached where blood glucose levels cannot be maintained and severe hypoglycaemia will result, causing apnoea, convulsions and cerebral damage. These may be prevented by intravenous dextrose infusions in the sick infant. Young babies should not be starved for longer than 4 h before surgery.

Hypocalcaemia

Hypocalcaemia may occur in infants with respiratory distress. The ionized calcium level in the blood maintains cell membrane activity. Hypocalcaemia may cause twitching and convulsions and can be corrected by slow infusion of calcium gluconate.

PREVENTION OF INFECTION

The poorly developed immune defences of the newborn infant predispose to the development of infection with Gram positive and Gram negative organisms. Any infection spreads rapidly, with resulting septicaemia. The signs of infection in the neonate include hypothermia, pallor and lethargy.

Early recognition and treatment of infection is aided by bacteriological cultures from the infant's nose, throat, umbilicus and rectum, both on admission to hospital and subsequently on a regular basis. This is important in picking up 'marker organisms' such as multiple antibiotic-resistant *Staphylococcus aureus*. When infection is suspected, a 'septic workup' is performed, taking specimens of CSF, urine and blood for culture and starting appropriate intravenous antibiotics immediately.

Infants undergoing surgery are at special risk of infection, and care must be taken not to introduce pathogenic organisms: this applies particularly to cross-infection in the neonatal ward. A short course of prophylactic antibiotics may be indicated to cover major surgery.

PARENTS

An important part of the care for neonates undergoing surgery is the reassurance and support of the infant's anxious parents. The mother often is confined in a maternity hospital while her baby is separated from her and undergoing major surgery in another institution. Close communication is important in this situation, and the mother and the baby should be brought together as soon as possible. That the parents should handle and fondle the baby is important for bonding and for the infant's general welfare. With goodwill, gentle contact between infant and mother can be achieved even in difficult circumstances.

GENERAL PRINCIPLES OF NEONATAL TRANSPORT

Transport of a critically ill neonate is a precarious undertaking, and the following principles should be followed:

(1) The infant's condition should be stabilized before embarkation

(2) The most experienced/qualified personnel available should accompany the patient

(3) Specialized 'retrieval' services should be used

(4) Transport should be as rapid as possible, but without causing further deterioration or incurring unnecessary risks to patient or transporting personnel

(5) Transport should be undertaken early rather than late

(6) Equipment should be checked before setting out

(7) The receiving institution should be notified early so that additional staff and equipment can be prepared for arrival.

TRANSPORT OF NEONATAL EMERGENCIES

A list of the more common emergencies is given in Table 2.1. Most infants with these conditions should have transport arranged as soon as the diagnosis is apparent or suspected.

Some developmental anomalies do not require transportation, and specialist consultation at the hospital of birth may suffice (e. g. cleft lip and palate, orthopaedic anomalies). Where doubt exists concerning

Table 2.1 Neonatal surgical conditions requiring transportation

Obvious malformations	Exomphalos/gastroschisis
	Myelomeningocele/ encephalocele
	Imperforate anus
Respiratory distress	
Upper airways obstruction	Choanal atresia
Pulmonary disease	Pierre-Robin syndrome
Lung compression	Emphysematous lobe
	Pulmonary cyst(s)
	Pneumothorax
	Diaphragmatic hernia
Congenital heart disease	
Acute alimentary or abdominal emergencies	Oesophageal atresia
	Intestinal obstruction
	Necrotizing enterocolitis
	Haematemesis and/or melaena

the advisability or timing of transportation, specialist advice should be sought.

Choice of vehicle

The choice between road ambulance, helicopter or fixed-wing aircraft will depend on distance, availability of vehicle, time of day, traffic conditions, airport facilities and weather conditions. In general, fixed-wing aircraft offer no time advantage for transfers of under 160 km (100 miles).

Patients with entrapped gas, for example pneumothorax or significant abdominal distension, should not travel by air; if air travel is mandatory, special provision must be made to fly at low levels if the aircraft is unpressurized, to avoid expansion of the trapped gases with decrease in ambient atmospheric pressure.

Communication

In transporting infants and older children, communication can be crucial to survival and expedites treatment.

Any change in the patient's condition should be reported to the receiving unit in advance of arrival. Detailed documentation of the history and written permission for treatment, including surgery, should be sent with the infant. In addition, neonates require 10 mL of maternal blood to accompany them, as well as cord blood and the placenta if available.

Details of stabilization procedures can be discussed with the headquarters of the transport team if difficulties arise while awaiting the arrival of the transport team.

Written permission for transport is required. A full explanation of what has been arranged and why, and an accurate prognosis should be given to the parents who should be allowed as much access as possible to the infant or child prior to transport. The parents should be given a 'Polaroid' photograph of the infant, taken before departure or at admission to hospital, if they are to be separated from the infant.

Equipment required

If a specialized retrieval team is not available, the following basic equipment is required.

Newborn infants require a portable incubator which operates from the ambulance battery or a self-contained source. A thermometer or temperature probe is essential to monitor temperature; protection against cold stress can be aided by the use of plain plastic wrap or baby blankets.

An adequate supply of oxygen must be taken; cylinders must be immobilized carefully in the transporting vehicle, and the volume required is calculated from the flow rate and the estimated time of transport (+50% for unexpected delays) (Table 2.2).

Suction for clearing secretions is required; care is needed with the suction provided for adult transport in ambulance vehicles, and low suction pressures should be used, especially for neonates. Controlled suction can be provided by the use of an oral mucus extractor.

A bag and mask of suitable size for emergency hand ventilation should be carried for any patient at even remote risk of respiratory failure.

A battery-operated infusion pump (peristaltic or syringe-type) is required for a patient who has an intravenous infusion line. In the absence of a mechanical pump, controlled rates can be provided by the use of a three-way tap and syringe to give an intermittent bolus at 1 min intervals.

Restraining devices immobilize the stretcher, incubator and other equipment and control the patient safely.

Drugs vary with the requirements of the individual patient, but may include analgesics, vasopressors and hydrocortisone.

STABILIZATION OF NEONATES PRIOR TO TRANSFER

In neonates, associated medical conditions (Table 2.3) require careful attention.

Table 2.2 Oxygen cylinders

Size	Volume (L)	Duration of supply (h)		
		2 L/min	5 L/min	10 L/min
B	220	1.75	0.75	0.33
C	440	3.25	1.5	0.75
D	1500	12.25	5.0	2.5

Table 2.3 Neonatal medical conditions requiring stabilization before transport

(1) Prematurity
(2) Temperature control problems
(3) Respiratory distress causing hypoxia and/or respiratory failure
(4) Metabolic derangements
—hypoglycaemia
—metabolic acidosis
—hypocalcaemia
(4) Shock
(5) Convulsions

Table 2.4 Incubator temperature

Baby's weight (g)	Incubator temperature (°C)
<1000	35–37
1000–1500	34–36
1500–2000	33–35
2000–2500	32–34
>2500	31–33

Temperature control

An incubator or radiant warmer is required; recommended incubator temperatures are shown in Table 2.4. The infant should be covered except for parts required for observation or access. Axillary or rectal temperatures should be taken half hourly (quarter hourly if under a radiant warmer).

Respiratory distress

Oxygen requirements

Enough oxygen should be given to abolish cyanosis. If measurements of blood gases are available, an arterial P_{O_2} of 50–80 mmHg is desirable. Although an excessively high P_{O_2} is liable to initiate retinopathy of prematurity, a short period of hyperoxia is less likely to be detrimental than a similarly short period of hypoxia.

Respiratory failure

Infants in severe respiratory failure (clinical or $P_{CO_2} >$ 70 mmHg) or those with apnoea may require endotracheal intubation and intermittent positive pressure ventilation.

Metabolic derangements

Hypoglycaemia should be corrected by intravenous infusion of glucose. Monitoring of babies at risk should be done with Dextrostix. Intravenous infusion may be by the umbilical or a peripheral route.

Acid–base balance should be estimated if facilities are available. Otherwise, a small volume of sodium bicarbonate (3 mEq/kg, slowly i.v.) may be given to an infant who has been asphyxiated severely, has had recurrent hypoxia or shows signs of poor peripheral circulation.

An infusion of blood or plasma expander (SPPS) at 10–20 mL/kg, i.v. over 0.5–1 h may be required to correct shock.

Convulsions should be controlled with phenobarbitone (10–15 mg/kg, i.v. or orally) or diphenylhydantoin (15 mg, i.v. or orally).

Specialist advice regarding management of specific conditions should be sought from the transporting agency. For example, in gastroschisis and exomphalos, the exposed viscera should be wrapped in clean plastic wrap to prevent heat loss; moist packs or gauze should never be used. A nasogastric tube with continuous drainage is required for patients with diaphragmatic hernia (Chapter 5), bowel obstruction (Chapter 7) or exomphalos (Chapter 9). In oesophageal atresia frequent aspiration of the blind upper pouch, at 10–15 min intervals, is essential to avoid aspiration (Chapter 6).

FURTHER READING

Ferrara A. & Harin A. (1980) *Emergency Transfer of the High-Risk Neonate*. C. V. Mosby, St Louis.

Lane J. C. & Jarosch G. (1983) Mercy flights. *Med. J. Aust.* **2**: 311–314.

Owen H. & Duncan A. W. (1983) Towards safer transport of sick and injured children. *Anaesth. Intensive Care* **11**: 113–117.

Roy R. N. D. (1977) Neonatal transport. *Med. J. Aust.* **2**: 862–864.

Roy R. N. D. & Brown M. F. (1983) *Stabilization and Transport of Newborn Infants*. Newborn Emergency Transport Service Publication.

3

The Child in Hospital

Great effort should be made to minimize psychological disturbances in children undergoing surgery. The important factors to consider are: the age and temperament of the child; the site, nature and extent of the surgical procedure; the degree and duration of discomfort after operation; and the time spent in hospital.

Children between 1 and 3 years old are the most vulnerable, and procedures which can be safely deferred should be postponed until 4 or 6 years of age, when the child can comprehend and cooperate better.

The temperament and ability to cope with stress are infinitely variable; the trust which the child is prepared to grant those who care for him is a measure of the confidence he has in his own family circle. Major disturbances within the family may affect the patient's equanimity and the ability of the parents to give him support, and for these reasons elective surgery may be deferred after the birth of a sibling or the death of a close relative.

PREPARATION FOR ADMISSION

Preparation for elective admission is important for children over 4 or 5 years of age and, whether assisted by a booklet (see Further Reading) or advice, is largely in the hands of the mother, whose acceptance of the situation is its endorsement in the child's eyes.

The child needs a brief and simple description of the operation, and if something is to be removed, it should be made clear that it is dispensable. Children should also be told that they will be asleep while the operation is performed, that it will be over when they wake, that they will be 'stiff' and a little 'sore' for a day or so, and when they will be able to go home. It is pointless to say that it will not hurt at all, for honesty is essential to preserve trust.

How the child's questions are handled is just as important as the factual content of the answers; possible sources of fear should be dealt with, and the pleasant aspects suitably emphasized. The amount of information must be adjusted to the child's age and particular needs; more details will be expected by older children.

EFFECT OF SITE OF SURGERY

Operations on the genitalia or the body's orifices, including circumcision after the age of 2 years, are more likely to cause emotional upset than other operations of the same magnitude. The correction of a hypospadias is potentially one of the most disturbing, for in addition to the site and the age (1–4 years), it may require about a week confined to bed, and the use of the unfamiliar bed pan. One or both parents should visit as much and as long as possible, and suitable occupational therapy is of considerable value.

Anal and oesophageal surgery should be completed in infancy and subsequent dilatations performed under anaesthesia wherever possible. Many boys who have experienced both operations would prefer, in retrospect, bilateral orchidopexy to tonsillectomy by even the gentlest hands.

DAY SURGERY

Time spent in hospital should be as short as possible. 'Day surgery', with admission, operation and discharge on the same day, is cost-effective, convenient and suitable for at least 30–50% of elective paediatric surgery.

The greatest advantage is minimizing the psychological impact on the child, which is magnified by sleeping away from home for even one night. There are many other obvious advantages, including minimal disturbance of breast feeding and reduced travelling by parents.

Although surgical technique is important (haemostasis, secure dressings), day surgery has been made safer and more acceptable by improved anaesthetic techniques: timing and choice of premedication and anaesthetic agents, minimal trauma during intubation, quick recovery, and long-acting local anaesthetic blocks or caudal analgesia in lieu of the usual postoperative injections of narcotics.

In the most vulnerable 1–3 year age group, day surgery has reduced the likelihood of behavioural disturbances. Suitable operations for day surgery depend on parental attitudes, logistics and careful selection of individual patients.

WARD ATMOSPHERE AND PROCEDURES

Unlimited visiting by parents, living-in quarters for mothers and a more understanding approach by all who care for children, have led to a less formal and more friendly atmosphere in hospital.

The procedures necessary for investigation or in preparation for operation should be scrutinized carefully to see whether they are necessary. Blood tests or X-rays are rarely required for elective day surgery.

The introduction of anaesthesia is an important source of fear and distress. Effective premedication, skilful intravenous induction and the prompt administration of hypnotics and analgesics after operation keep discomfort to the absolute minimum.

Even after major abdominal surgery, some toddlers will be walking within 48 h. They might just as well be playing on the floor or sitting at a table, and today that is where they are, with no subsequent ill effects. The play room is not required for most postoperative patients, since once they can walk to the toilet and play room they can be discharged home. The child usually sets the pace of his convalescence, and as a general rule will show no desire to move when he should rest, for example, during a period of paralytic ileus.

Play materials, a day room, television and bright surroundings act as constant stimuli to those who are well enough to be 'up and doing'.

A single, absorbable subcuticular stitch can be used to close almost all incisions, and avoids the anxiety and time spent in removing sutures.

PARENTAL SUPPORT

The parents always require consideration, especially when a first-born baby is transferred to a children's hospital on the first day of life. The baby may stay there for several weeks, at precisely the time when the mother's emotions are in turmoil and normally she would be establishing a new and unique relationship. Feelings of guilt at producing an infant with a congenital abnormality or inadequacy following removal of the infant from her care and the lack of close physical contact, may lead her to reject the baby and to exaggeration of the usual puerperal emotional instability. To help overcome this when separation is unavoidable the mother should be given a Polaroid photograph of her baby, should see the baby again as soon as possible and care for him as much as the illness permits (Chapter 2).

Reassurance by frequent supportive interviews, help from the family doctor, the husband, a particular friend or a medical social worker, are all important in overcoming anxieties and establishing the infant in the family picture. The mother should live in, and be assisted to express breast milk for her infant if this is feasible, and eventually to resume breast feeding.

RESPONSE OF THE CHILD

The average child's natural optimism, freedom from unfounded anxiety, remarkable powers of recuperation, and apparently short memory for unpleasant experiences can make even major surgery a relatively short and simple matter; most patients are out of bed in 2–3 days and active for much of the day or already at home by 3–6 days.

Even when minor surgery has been uneventfully concluded, the child may show some disturbances for up to 2 months after leaving hospital, and the parents should be made aware of this possibility. Signs of insecurity, increased dependency, and disturbed sleep are not uncommon but fortunately are of short duration when met with warm affection, reassurance and understanding by the parents.

The undesirable psychological effects of surgery must be put in proper perspective by mentioning the beneficial effects which so often follow operation: the well-being after removal of an uncomfortable hernia, the freely expressed satisfaction at the excision of an unsightly lump or blemish.

Finally, in older children there is, not infrequently, a detectable increase in confidence and poise which comes from facing and coping adequately with an operation, often the first occasion on which the child has been away from home and, metaphorically at least, standing on his or her own two feet.

THE TIMING OF SURGICAL PROCEDURES

Surgical conditions in infancy and childhood can be classified according to the degree of urgency with which treatment should be carried out. Three categories can be distinguished.

(1) The immediate group, that is conditions where immediate investigation and/or definitive operation is required

(2) The intermediate group, where treatment is not urgent but should be undertaken without undue delay

(3) The elective group, where operation is performed at an optimum age determined by one or more factors which affect the patient's best interests.

The immediate group

Trauma, acute infections, abdominal emergencies and acute scrotal conditions naturally fall into this category. No attempt will be made to itemize them all, for in most cases the needs of the patient are obvious or well known.

A particularly important subgroup is neonatal emergencies. Most of these are the result of develop-

mental abnormalities causing disorders of function which threaten life. The best prognosis depends upon early diagnosis, speedy transport to a hospital where appropriate skills and equipment are available, and effective surgical management (see Chapters 4–11).

The intermediate group

Inguinal hernias are prone to strangulation, especially in the first year of life. For this reason, herniotomy should be performed within a few days of diagnosis in those less than 1 year of age.

Investigation of swellings or masses suspected to be malignant should be undertaken within a day or two of their discovery.

The elective group

Factors favouring deferment of operation

Factors which favour deferment of operation and hence may determine an optimum age include:

(1) The possibility of spontaneous correction or cure. In infants, scrotal hydroceles, encysted hydroceles of the cord, true umbilical hernias and sternomastoid tumours all show a strong tendency to spontaneous resolution.

(2) Strawberry naevi (intracutaneous capillary haemangiomas), although they may progress and enlarge in the first year of life, usually involute and fade spontaneously in the ensuing 2–4 years (Chapter 53). In general they should be left alone to do so, for surgical measures are required rarely.

(3) The difficulties posed by minute and delicate structures can be avoided by postponing operation until they are more robust, although this is seldom the sole reason for deferring operation; for example, an undescended testis can be repaired more easily in a 12 month old boy than shortly after birth.

(4) The supposedly greater capacity of older children to tolerate major operations is now much less important. With modern methods of anaesthesia and adequate resuscitation, including immediate replacement of blood loss, major operations can be performed on very young infants.

(5) The development of cooperation and comprehension with age. Voluntary exercises are important after some operations and it may be desirable to defer them until the necessary degree of cooperation is forthcoming.

(6) The effects of growth are important in some instances. The excision of a coarctation of the aorta is deferred until the patient is 5–6 years old, because at this age the diameter of the aorta is approximately five-sevenths the normal adult aorta. The anastomosis obtained after adequate excision of the narrowed segment at this stage is therefore unlikely to cause any significant obstruction even if subsequent growth at the suture line is limited. Chest wall deformities are corrected at adolescence, once chest wall growth is almost complete.

(7) Coexistent anomalies and intercurrent diseases, for example infections, will affect the timing of operations. The situation in each patient should be assessed to establish the order of priorities when there are multiple abnormalities, and to determine whether the treatment of non-urgent conditions should be deferred temporarily.

Factors favouring early operation

Factors which favour early operation rather than deferred treatment include capacity for healing and adaptation in the very young. For example, a fracture of a long bone at birth causes such an exuberant growth of callus that clinical union occurs in 7–10 days, and the subsequent moulding will remove any residual bony deformities.

(1) Stimulation of development by early treatment occurs in infants with a congenital dislocation of the hip. When splinting is commenced in the first week of life, this will prevent the secondary dysplasia of the acetabulum and femur, which in the past was thought to be the primary cause of the dislocation.

(2) Malleability of infantile tissues is an advantage for example in talipes, in which the best results are obtained when treatment is commenced in the first few days after birth.

(3) Avoidance of undesirable psychological effects. Often these can be prevented by completing treatment, including repetitive painful procedures, before the memory of things past is established or before the child goes to school, where obvious deformities or disabilities are likely to attract attention.

(4) Effect on the parents. The family as a whole should be considered and when it is not disadvantageous to the child, early operation may resolve parental anxiety and prevent rejection of the child.

FURTHER READING

Bar-Maor J. A., Tadmore C. S., Birkhan J. & Shoshany G. (1989) Effective psychological and/or 'pharmacological' preparation for elective pediatric surgery can reduce stress. *Pediatr. Surg. Int.* **4**: 273–276.

Cloud D. T., Reed W. A. *et al.* (1972) The surgicenter: a fresh concept in outpatient pediatric surgery. *J. Pediatr. Surg.* **7**: 206–212.

Cohen D., Keneally J. *et al.* (1980) Experience with 'day-stay' surgery. *J. Pediatr. Surg.* **15**: 21–25.

Corkery J. J. & Cole A. E. (1974) Some nursing implications of a 5 day surgical ward. *J. Pediatr. Surg.* **9**: 7–11.

Ludman L., Spitz L. & Lansdown R. (1990) Developmental progress of newborns undergoing neonatal surgery. *J. Pediatr. Surg.* **25**: 469–471.

McCollum A. T. (1975) *Coping with Prolonged Health Impairment in Your Child.* Little Brown, Boston.

Shandling B. & Steward D. J. (1980) Regional anaesthesia for postoperative pain in pediatric outpatient surgery. *J. Pediatr. Surg.* **15**: 477–480.

Suruga K., Miyazawa R., Kimura K. & Miyano T. (1990) A study on more than 20 years of postoperative follow-up in pediatric surgical cases. *J. Pediatr. Surg.* **25**: 731–736.

4

Respiratory Distress in the Newborn

When a newborn baby breathes more rapidly than normal, respiratory distress is present. The degree of distress may be slight initially, but progressive deterioration may culminate in irreversible respiratory failure.

Neonatal respiratory distress usually is not the province of the paediatric surgeon, but may occur in a specific group of neonatal patients in whom the causes are amenable to surgical correction. Respiratory failure may have developed already when the baby presents, and prompt action can save life and regain the opportunity for corrective surgery. Those concerned with the care of the newborn must be able to recognize respiratory distress, and the paediatric surgeon must be familiar with the causes and principles of management in this age group.

In only a few cases can a firm diagnosis be made solely on clinical grounds, and X-rays of the thorax and abdomen should be obtained as soon as possible.

RECOGNITION OF RESPIRATORY DISTRESS

The most important clinical feature is a raised respiratory rate.

Tachycardia is almost invariably present, but if the rate is more than 200/min the situation is serious. On the other hand, bradycardia is a dangerous sign and often portends imminent complete respiratory failure.

Other cardiovascular signs, such as the presence of 'dextrocardia', and the nature of the peripheral pulses, will provide further clues.

The abdomen frequently is scaphoid in babies with a diaphragmatic hernia, but can be distended when there is a pulmonary cause for the respiratory distress. Intestinal obstruction and neonatal peritonitis also can cause abdominal distension and respiratory embarrassment.

While pulmonary signs may help localize pulmonary lesions the mechanics of respiration also should be assessed; thus respiration may be 'laboured' or associated with deformity of the chest wall or may exhibit inspiratory retraction indicative of obstruction of the airways.

A surgical cause is only present in a proportion of babies with respiratory distress, and the surgeon must be familiar with other conditions which enter into the differential diagnosis, for example the 'respiratory distress syndrome' and cerebral birth injuries (Table 4.1).

To determine the cause of tachypnoea, all the clinical evidence must be assessed, including the obstetrical details and any abnormal physical signs which may be present. For example, a baby who is pale and cyanosed and improves following the administration of oxygen may have a diaphragmatic hernia (Chapter 5). A scaphoid abdomen and barrelled chest with the heart sounds best heard on the right are suggestive physical signs and a chest X-ray will confirm the diagnosis. By contrast, an infant with cyanosis and respiratory distress which is relieved by crying may have choanal atresia (Chapter 14).

THE PRINCIPLES OF MANAGEMENT

When respiratory failure is present already, urgent treatment is required, regardless of the underlying cause.

An accurate diagnosis of the cause is made on the clinical signs and the results of investigation, usually radiology.

The degree of respiratory or metabolic acidosis must be determined as a guide to the resuscitation required.

Where applicable, surgery is undertaken to correct the cause, usually after correction of the physiological disturbances.

Table 4.1 Causes of neonatal respiratory distress

Type of obstruction	Examples
Upper respiratory tract obstruction	
Nasal	Choanal atresia
Pharyngeal	Pierre-Robin syndrome
	Hamartoma of tongue
Laryngeal	'Infantile larynx'
	Vocal cord palsy
	Subglottic haemangioma
	Laryngeal web/cyst
Tracheal	Tracheomalacia
	Massive cystic hygroma
	Vascular ring
Lower airways obstruction	Meconium aspiration
	Aspiration of gastric contents
	Lobar emphysema
Alveolar disease	Hyaline membrane disease
	Pneumonia
	Congenital heart disease
	Pulmonary oedema
	Diaphragmatic hernia
Pulmonary compression	Pneumothorax
	Diaphragmatic hernia
	Repaired exomphalos or gastroschisis
	Congenital lobar emphysema
	Congenital lung cysts
	Duplication cysts
	Abdominal distension
Neurological disease	Birth asphyxia
	Apnoea of prematurity
	Intracranial haemorrhage
	Convulsions

SPECIFIC CONDITIONS

One of the important aspects of neonatal respiratory distress is that many of the causes have a wide clinical spectrum: for example, one diaphragmatic hernia may produce a direct threat to life within minutes of birth, while another of identical size may cause no distress in the neonatal period and give rise to symptoms only after several weeks (Chapter 5).

Choanal atresia is discussed in Chapter 14 and oesophageal atresia in Chapter 6.

Pulmonary dysplasia

Malformations of part or all of one lung causing respiratory distress in the newborn are: congenital lobar emphysema and congenital cysts of the lung, either solitary or multiple. The physical signs are never diagnostic and X-rays are required to make the diagnosis. Again there are considerable variations in the clinical picture, and when there is obvious respiratory distress, surgery is indicated. Resection of the affected segment of lung not only removes functionless pulmonary tissue in which there is little or no gaseous exchange, but also allows expansion of the normal areas which have been compressed by the overdistended segment, lobe or lobes.

Congenital lobar emphysema

The underlying abnormality is due to bronchomalacia from congenital deficiency of the cartilage, and results in expiratory obstruction and trapping of air in the affected lobe.

The cardinal symptom is tachypnoea amounting to dyspnoea, most noticeable when the baby is being fed. Not infrequently there is a dry cough and stridor. Cyanosis is usually an indication for urgent treatment. The mediastinum is displaced and the chest wall over the affected area is prominent and relatively immobile; breath sounds are diminished and the percussion note typically is hyper-resonant.

X-rays show an area of increased radiolucency in which there are some bronchovascular markings. There is also downward displacement of the diaphragm on the affected side, and the overdistended lung may herniate across the midline (Fig. 4.1).

The lobes most commonly affected are the left upper lobe or the right middle lobe and the treatment is lobectomy.

Congenital cystic lung

The clinical features are similar to those of lobar emphysema in that respiratory distress occurs early, but usually it is more urgent and severe. X-rays show a large

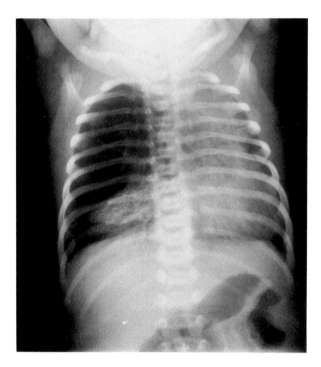

Fig. 4.1 Congenital lobar emphysema of the right upper lobe which is overdistended and herniating across the midline.

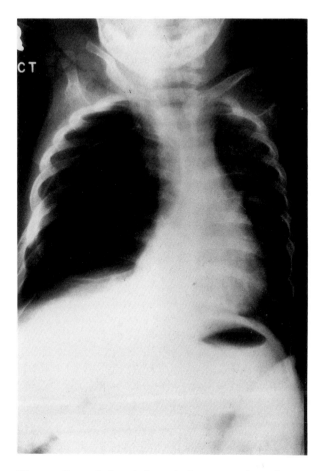

Fig. 4.2 Congenital cystic lung. A giant cyst replaces the right lower lobe, compresses the remainder of the right lung, and herniates across the midline to displace the heart and compress the left lung.

cyst with a sharply defined border (Fig. 4.2) or an extensive multicystic area; the findings are otherwise similar to those of lobar emphysema, namely, compression and collapse of unaffected areas of the lungs and displacement of the mediastinum.

The aim of surgery is to remove the portion of the lung that is not only functionless but also interfering with the function of the remainder. The distribution of disease determines the area to be removed and segmental resection, lobectomy or even pneumonectomy may be required.

Pulmonary sequestration

Pulmonary sequestration is an uncommon malformation in which there is non-functioning lung tissue which has no connection with the normal bronchial tree, and a blood supply which arises from an anomalous systemic artery, often the aorta (Fig. 4.3). It usually occurs on the left side and may be either intralobar or extralobar, depending on whether it shares visceral pleura with the normal lung. It may present as a pulmonary infection, because of its space-occupying effect, or be found incidentally on chest X-ray.

Mediastinal conditions

Very rarely, large cystic teratomas and duplication cysts cause respiratory distress and should be removed. In the neonate, oesophageal duplication cysts present with increasing respiratory distress.

Pulmonary interstitial emphysema

This is the condition of extreme prematurity where assisted ventilation is required for severe respiratory distress syndrome. High ventilatory pressures force air into the lung interstitium, which tracks along peribronchial spaces, producing interstitial cysts which have a characteristic appearance on X-ray (Fig. 4.4). Treatment is directed at reducing the ventilatory pressures. In severe and progressive cases, thoracotomy may be required to deflate the cysts.

Pleural conditions

Neonatal pneumothorax

Pneumothorax may be due to diffuse pulmonary disease or to a minimal localized abnormality such as a subpleural emphysematous bleb. The pneumothorax may be suspected on clinical grounds by sudden deterioration in condition, displacement of the trachea or apex beat, and a hyper-resonant percussion note, but X-rays are required to confirm the diagnosis.

In neonates, the severity of the symptoms frequently is out of proportion to the size of the pneumothorax. Even a small pneumothorax may be associated with severe respiratory distress when there is pre-existing parenchymatous lung disease. Intercostal drainage is urgent.

Empyema

Empyema occasionally occurs in the early days of life and is usually staphylococcal, but may be caused by a Gram-negative organism. An early diagnostic paracentesis is helpful to identify the organism and to determine its sensitivities. Drainage of the pleural cavity by an intercostal catheter usually is necessary, and when the pus is thick or loculated, open thoracotomy for drainage may be required.

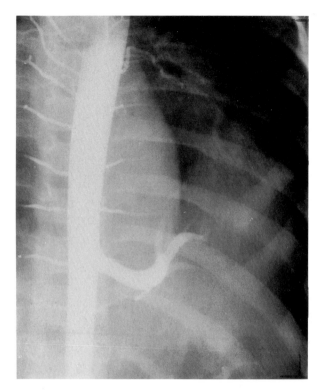

Fig. 4.3 Anomalous blood supply from the aorta to a left pulmonary sequestration.

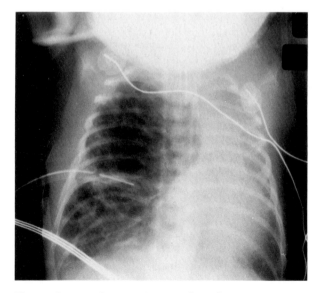

Fig. 4.4 Severe pulmonary interstitial emphysema.

Haemothorax

Haemothorax is an infrequent complication of haemorrhagic disease of the newborn and may produce an alarming clinical picture; this is due to mechanical factors which interfere with respiration, and to the reduction of the circulating blood volume. Pleural paracentesis and blood transfusion are required.

THE MEDICAL MANAGEMENT OF ACUTE RESPIRATORY FAILURE

Acute respiratory failure occurs when oxygenation and/or ventilation are impaired sufficiently to be an immediate threat to life.

Causes of respiratory failure

Acute respiratory failure in neonates is usually the result of asphyxia due to:
(1)   Birth asphyxia
(2)   Injuries sustained during birth
(3)   Developmental anomalies, including congenital heart disease
(4)   Immaturity of the pulmonary system (part of prematurity)
(5)   Increased susceptibility to infection.
The factors in infants which predispose to respiratory failure are summarized in Table 4.2.

Signs of respiratory failure

In the neonate, especially the premature, acute hypoxia causes pallor, apnoea, bradycardia, hypotension and lethargy. The clinical signs of hypercapnia—sweating, tachycardia and hypertension—are seen rarely, but pulmonary haemorrhage, cerebral haemorrhage, severe hyperkalaemia and hypoglycaemia all may occur as the result of hypoxia.

Treatment

General management of respiratory failure is dictated by

Table 4.2 Factors predisposing infants to respiratory failure

Factor	Comment
Metabolic rate	Metabolism per kg is twice that of adults
Respiratory rate	Lung surface area per kg is about the same as for an adult; so the infant has much less respiratory reserve
Compliance	The chest wall of the infant is less able to adjust to a reduction in lung compliance or an increase in airways resistance
Airways calibre	Relatively larger total airways resistance than in older children or adults
Airways obstruction	The narrow airways are more prone to obstruction by oedema and secretions
Temperature control	Temperature regulation is poor in the newborn, especially in the premature. In a cold environment, oxygen consumption may increase two- or three-fold. With limited respiratory reserve, respiratory failure can occur rapidly

the clinical features, supported by serial estimations of the blood gases.

Nursing care

An infant with incipient respiratory failure requires close observation at all times. Neonates should be nursed in an isolette or under a radiant heater so that the temperature is controlled and observation unimpeded.

Handling should be kept to a minimum, for it can increase oxygen consumption dramatically.

The position most favourable in nursing neonates is prone, with hips and knees flexed, and the head turned regularly and frequently from one side to the other. This reduces apnoeic episodes, shortens gastric emptying time and reduces the risk of regurgitation and aspiration. The supine position is preferred if bag and mask ventilation or resuscitation are needed.

Oxygen

The method of delivery of oxygen depends upon the age and oxygen concentration required, for example isolette, head box, mask, nasal catheter(s), oxygen cot or tent. The concentration required depends on the disease process.

All patients having prolonged oxygen therapy should have arterial blood gas estimations and adjustment of inspired oxygen concentrations to ensure adequate arterial saturation. Premature infants receiving oxygen therapy are at risk of retinopathy of prematurity and frequent blood gases are necessary to maintain the arterial P_{O_2} in the range of 6.6–10.6 kPa (50–80 mmHg). Dependence on hypoxia for 'ventilatory drive' is extremely rare in children and so is pulmonary oxygen toxicity; neither should be considered as reasons for restricting oxygen therapy.

Fluids and feeding

Oral feeding should be suspended in children with severe dyspnoea, and nasogastric feeding should be substituted. If abdominal distension occurs, feeding must be discontinued to avoid regurgitation and aspiration, and to prevent restriction of descent of the diaphragm: all potential causes of additional respiratory embarrassment.

Nasogastric feeding can be recommenced once artificial (mechanical) ventilation has been instituted.

Intravenous fluids are required to prevent dehydration and supply parenteral nutrition, but fluids may need to be restricted in some patients with pulmonary disease.

Sodium bicarbonate may be required to correct metabolic acidosis (Chapter 2). Regular biochemical monitoring and an accurate fluid balance are the key to fluid management.

Temperature control

Seriously ill neonates are particularly vulnerable to cold stress, and maintenance of body temperature is of vital importance before, during and after operation (Chapter 2).

The neonate has a narrow 'thermoneutral' range in which oxygen consumption is minimal and optimal: abdominal wall skin temperature is optimal between 36° and 36.5°C. Exposure to an environmental temperature of 20°–25°C increases oxygen consumption threefold and may precipitate cardiorespiratory failure.

For reasons of access, critically ill neonates should be nursed in open cots with servocontrolled radiant heat. Insensible water loss may be increased, particularly in infants of very low birthweight, but this can be taken into account when planning fluid requirements.

Respiratory physiotherapy

In the newborn, gentle suction is performed at intervals to remove pooled secretions and to stimulate coughing. However, pharyngeal and endotracheal suction may cause a sudden fall in Pa_{O_2}, that necessitates an increase in the concentration of oxygen in the inspired gases.

Monitoring

Respiratory and cardiovascular signs should be monitored, along with the oxygen concentration in the inspired air. Blood for gas analysis is obtained by percutaneous puncture or, more accurately, in samples from an indwelling catheter in a peripheral artery, which also can be used for a continuous record of the arterial pressure. Continuous transcutaneous monitoring of oxygen and carbon dioxide levels is now available in most centres.

Ventilatory support

In neonates, nasotracheal intubation is the preferred type of artificial airway (Table 4.3). Tubes of appropriate size and composition can be left *in situ* for long periods with minimal adverse effects or complications.

Humidification of dry inspired gases is necessary to avoid viscid and retained sputum, atelectasis, blockage of the endotracheal tube with inspissated secretions, and to preserve mucociliary function.

Table 4.3 Use of nasotracheal tube in neonates

Advantages	Disadvantages
Protects or ensures uninterrupted airway	Narrows the upper airways
Overcomes upper airway obstruction	Bypasses natural humidification, heating and filtering of inspired gases
Allows precise tracheo-bronchial toilet and suction	Prevents coughing and expectoration of secretions
Facilitates continuous positive airway pressure	May cause subglottic irritation and stenosis: a risk which can be minimized by using a tube of the correct size allowing a small air leak during positive pressure ventilation
Enables mechanical ventilation	

Inspired gases should be delivered to the trachea at 37°C, fully saturated with water vapour, using a safe, servocontrolled humidifier. This is an important contribution to maintenance of body temperature and to reduce insensible fluid losses from the airways.

Suction of the trachea is necessary to stimulate coughing and to remove accumulated secretions, usually once an hour, but in some cases more frequently. Suction can cause hypoxia and atelectasis and may introduce infection, and techniques are used to avoid these risks. Gentle 'bagging' with an oxygen-rich mixture is used before and after suction to reduce hypoxia and re-expand the lung. In infants at risk of retinopathy of prematurity, the oxygen concentration in the 'bag' should not be more than 10% higher than the mixture used for ventilation. In older children 100% oxygen can be used.

Continuous positive airways pressure

This is a technique that employs a distending pressure (5–10 cmH$_2$O) applied to the airways of a patient who is breathing spontaneously. It is used in pulmonary conditions causing hypoxaemia due to atelectasis, alveolar instability and intrapulmonary shunting. Continuous positive airways pressure (CPAP) increases functional residual capacity and compliance, re-expands areas of atelectasis, decreases intrapulmonary shunting and increases arterial P_{O_2}. In premature infants, CPAP often will improve the regularity of respiratory movements and decrease apnoeic episodes. The technique requires careful control to avoid reduced cardiac output, retention of fluids, rupture of alveoli and pneumothorax.

Intermittent positive pressure ventilation

Intermittent positive pressure ventilation (IPPV) is used to correct hypoventilation, and sometimes (e.g. raised intracranial pressure, pulmonary hypertension) to produce hyperventilation and to lower Pa_{CO_2}. Mechanical ventilators have been designed specifically for neonatal and paediatric use. IPPV is often combined with positive end-expiratory pressure (PEEP). PEEP is used for the same reasons as CPAP, that is as a means of improving oxygenation. The hazards of IPPV are greater than those of CPAP and related directly to the level of pressure applied. Barotrauma to immature lungs may result in a chronic lung disease in neonates known as bronchopulmonary dysplasia.

Intermittent mandatory ventilation (IMV) is a technique of mechanical ventilation in which a predetermined minute volume is guaranteed, while, in addition, the patient breathes independently from the ventilator. With infant ventilators, a constant flow is provided during the expiratory phase from which the infant can breathe. It is a technique useful for weaning from mechanical ventilation and as a means of minimizing barotrauma.

Controlled ventilation involves the use of relaxants and sedatives which paralyse respiratory movements, to completely abolish the work of breathing and improve gas exchange. The technique is useful in critically ill neonates and those with difficult ventilatory problems, but it should only be employed where expert surveillance and sophisticated monitoring are available. Inappropriate pressure settings can cause a pneumothorax with sudden deterioration, and inadvertent disconnection rapidly results in potentially fatal hypoxia.

FURTHER READING

Gregory G. A. (1981) Respiratory failure in the child. *Clinics in Critical Care Medicine*. Churchill Livingstone, London.

Kellnar S. & Trammer A. (1990) Therapy of neonatal chylothorax. *Pediatr. Surg. Int.* **5**: 216–217.

Levin D. L. (1984) *A Practical Guide to Pediatric Intensive Care*. S. V. Losby, St Louis.

Oh T. E. (1985) *Intensive Care Manual*, Chapters 79–81. Butterworths, Sydney.

Ryckman F. & Rodgers B. M. (1985) Obstructive airway disease in infants and children. *Surg. Clin. North Amer.* 1663.

Stark J., Roesler M. *et al.* (1985) The diagnosis of airway obstruction in children. *J. Pediatr. Surg.* **20**: 113–117.

Wensley D. F., Goh T. H., Menahem S., Edis B., Venables A. W. & Robertson C. F. (1989) Management of pulmonary sequestration and scimitar syndrome presenting in infancy. *Pediatr. Surg. Int.* **4**: 381–415.

5

Diaphragmatic Hernia

EMBRYOLOGY

The diaphragm develops largely from three structures: (i) the pleuroperitoneal membrane; (ii) the septum transversum; (iii) marginal ingrowths from the muscles of the body wall.

Congenital diaphragmatic hernia results from failure of formation of part of the diaphragm, failure of fusion of one part with another or failure of its muscular components to form. Whereas failures of formation or fusion result in a defect and a hernia, failure of 'muscularization' produces a thin, weak diaphragm with an upward bulge of part or all of one or other leaf. This is referred to as an eventration and may be difficult to distinguish clinically from a variant in which there is a diaphragmatic hernia with a sac.

PATHOLOGY

The Bochdalek type is the commonest type of congenital diaphragmatic hernia (1 : 5000 live births) and results from a defect in the posterolateral part of the diaphragm (Fig. 5.1). During intrauterine development, the small bowel, stomach, spleen and left lobe of the liver pass through the defect to the chest, limiting the space available for the developing lung. This causes lung hypoplasia, which in many infants is severe enough to produce severe respiratory distress within minutes of birth, and may not be compatible with life.

The Morgagni-type hernia is rare and results from a defect close to the anterior midline, between the costal and sternal attachments of the diaphragm, and the sac usually contains part of the colon or small bowel and, less commonly, part of the liver.

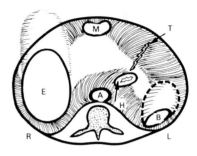

Fig. 5.1 Diaphragmatic hernias. Diaphragm as seen from below, showing: (B) Bochdalek left posterolateral defect; (M) anterior or Morgagni type; (H) hiatus for oesophagus and hiatus hernia; (E) large eventration in the tendinous portion of the right cupola; (T) a tear which causes a post-traumatic hernia (A: aorta).

Occasionally, a hernia may occur through the apex of the cupola or at the periphery adjacent to the costal margin. The rarity of these types means that there is no typical pattern of symptoms, but the possibility of an unusual type of diaphragmatic hernia must be borne in mind. Oesophageal hiatal hernias also occur and usually produce symptoms caused by gastro-oesophageal reflux (Chapter 18).

PRESENTATION

Congenital diaphragmatic hernias may be seen at any age and have a wide variety of symptoms and signs, depending on the type and size of the hernia, the severity of lung hypoplasia, and the presence of associated anomalies. Most congenital posterolateral hernias are large and present shortly after birth with cardiorespiratory symptoms. In severe cases the infant becomes cyanosed with severe respiratory distress within minutes of birth. In other patients, there is a tachypnoea, increased respiratory effort, hyperinflated chest, scaphoid abdomen and heart sounds are on the right side. This is because 85% of posterolateral hernias involve the left hemi-diaphragm. The remainder are right-sided (12%) or bilateral (3%).

Unlike posterolateral hernias most anterior hernias are symptomless until strangulation occurs; that is except in the rare event that the hernia protrudes into the pericardial cavity rather than into the inferior mediastinum and causes cardiac tamponade, presenting as cardiorespiratory distress in the neonatal period.

Diaphragmatic hernias are being diagnosed on antenatal ultrasound with increasing frequency (Chapter 1).

INVESTIGATION

Diagnosis of a posterolateral hernia is confirmed by a chest X-ray (Fig. 5.2). Loops of bowel can be seen in the left chest. The heart is deviated to the contralateral side (usually the right). Little room is reserved for the lungs, particularly the left lung which is compressed and may be difficult to see on X-ray. There is often little bowel gas in the abdomen. Occasionally, it may be difficult to distinguish a diaphragmatic hernia from lung cysts, in which case a repeat chest X-ray is performed after a nasogastric tube is inserted (the tip of which can be seen in the chest) or by doing a barium study, which will show bowel within the thoracic cavity when a hernia is present.

TREATMENT

Posterolateral hernias

The early treatment involves intensive cardiorespiratory support and decompression of the bowel by insertion of a nasogastric tube to prevent bowel dilatation within the chest. Care must be taken to avoid hyperinflation and barotrauma of the small hypoplastic lungs. Ventilation with a face mask (bagging) should be avoided as this forces air into the stomach, increasing its volume at the expense of the already compromised lungs. Vigorous endotracheal ventilation also should be

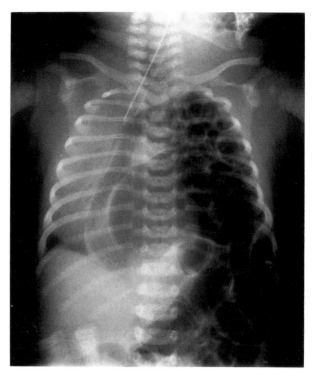

Fig. 5.2 X-ray of congenital diaphragmatic hernia (Bochdalek type). Multiple bowel loops fill the left pleural cavity and the heart is displaced to the right.

avoided because of the risk of causing a tension pneumothorax, which can lead to rapid demise of the infant. Sudden deterioration of the infant's condition during initial resuscitation or during transport suggests the development of a tension pneumothorax, and this may require prompt drainage by needle aspiration or intercostal intubation. The infant should be transferred to a tertiary neonatal intensive care unit.

Surgery to return the bowel to the abdominal cavity and to repair the defect in the diaphragm is performed when the infant's condition is stable. This may be between 12 h and 7 or more days after birth. In left-sided defects a left transverse or subcostal abdominal incision is used. The management of the infant with severe hypoplastic lungs is difficult and may involve extracorporeal membrane oxygenation or even, in the future, heart–lung transplantation. The major cause of death remains pulmonary hypoplasia. The combined lung weight in infants dying with this condition is often less than one-third of normal.

Anterior hernias

In some cases the diagnosis is made on incidental X-rays of the chest in a symptomless patient, but repair is advisable because of the risk of strangulation, which can be achieved by direct suture through an abdominal approach.

Eventration of the diaphragm

When there is an extensive eventration or deficiency in the muscle layer, symptoms probably will occur in the neonatal period, and if respiratory distress is present, an operation will be required. The diaphragm is plicated.

FURTHER READING

Anderson K. D. (1986) Congenital diaphragmatic hernia. In: Welch K. J., Randolph J. G., Ravitch M. M., O'Neill J. A. & Rowe M. I. (eds), *Pediatric Surgery*, 4th edn. p. 589. Year Book Medical, Chicago.

Ein S. M. & Barker G. (1987) The pharmacological treatment of newborn diaphragmatic hernia—update 1987. *Pediatr. Surg. Int.* **2**: 341–345.

Harrison M. R., Langer J. C., Adzick S. N. *et al.* (1990) Correction of congenital diaphragmatic hernia *in utero*, V initial clinical experience. *J. Pediatr. Surg.* **25**: 47–57.

Kluth D., Peterson C. & Zimmerman H. (1987) The developmental anatomy of congenital diaphragmatic hernia. *Pediatr. Surg. Int.* **2**: 322–326.

Pokorny W. J., McGill C. W. & Harberg F. J. (1984) Morgagni hernias during infancy: presentation and associated anomalies. *J. Pediatr. Surg.* **19**: 394–397.

Puri P. & Gorman W. A. (1987) Natural history of congenital diaphragmatic hernia: implication for management. *Pediatr. Surg. Int.* **2**: 327–330.

6

Oesophageal Atresia and Tracheo-oesophageal Fistula

Oesophageal atresia is a congenital anomaly in which there is complete interruption of the lumen of the oesophagus in the form of a blind upper pouch, and a lower oesophageal segment which usually communicates with the trachea via a distal tracheo-oesophageal fistula. Less common variations of the abnormality occur also (Fig. 6.1).

Coexistent congenital anomalies affecting other systems are common and include urinary, intestinal (duodenal atresia, anorectal abnormalities) and skeletal abnormalities (hemivertebra, absent radius).

Maternal polyhydramnios is common in oesophageal atresia, particularly if there is no distal tracheo-oesophageal fistula. About 40% of infants with oesophageal atresia are born prematurely.

PATHOPHYSIOLOGY

The effect of oesophageal atresia on the infant is that saliva, or milk if the infant has been fed, accumulates in the upper oesophageal pouch and spills over into the

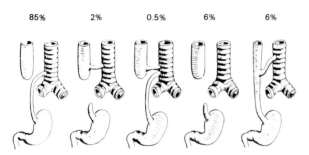

85%   2%   0.5%   6%   6%

Fig. 6.1 The anatomical variants of oesophageal atresia and/or tracheo-oesophageal fistula. The percentage frequency of each variant is shown.

trachea, causing choking and cyanosis, and soilage of the lungs. Gastric contents may be aspirated through the distal tracheo-oesophageal fistula into the bronchial tree. Pulmonary complications follow, initially atelectasis, followed by pneumonia. Abdominal distension from air passing down the fistula into the stomach may elevate and splint the diaphragm, adversely affecting the infant's ability to ventilate adequately.

EARLY DIAGNOSIS

Oesophageal atresia should be recognized as soon after birth as possible, for delay leads to progressive pulmonary complications. The diagnosis is made when a catheter cannot be passed through the oesophagus into the stomach (see below).

Maternal polyhydramnios

The association with polyhydramnios is sufficiently common that in every baby born to a mother with polyhydramnios, a firm rubber catheter, size no. 10, that is 6–7 mm in diameter, should be introduced through the mouth and passed carefully down the oesophagus; if it becomes arrested at about 10 cm from the lips, the diagnosis of oesophageal atresia has been established. A small catheter will curl up in the upper oesophagus and give a false impression of oesophageal continuity (Fig. 6.2).

Symptoms soon after birth

Oesophageal atresia should be suspected when a newborn infant has been resuscitated at birth by adequate

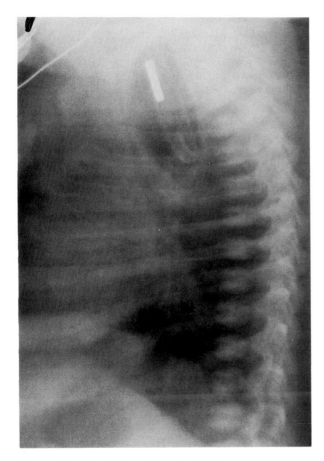

Fig. 6.2 A small catheter will curl up in the upper oesophageal pouch and give a false impression of oesophageal continuity. Therefore, a wide-bore catheter, for example no. 10 gauge, should be used.

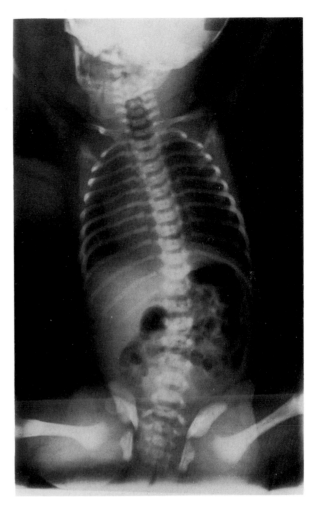

Fig. 6.3 Plain X-ray of the chest and abdomen shows air in the stomach and small bowel, indicating that there is a distal tracheo-oesophageal fistula.

aspiration of mucus with a catheter, and then within the next few hours develops rattling respirations, tachypnoea or fine frothy white bubbles of mucus in the nostrils or on the lips.

Diagnosis before feeding

Oesophageal atresia should be diagnosed before the infant is fed, because feeding causes an acute episode of spluttering, coughing and cyanosis, with aspiration of milk into the lungs.

PRE-OPERATIVE INVESTIGATION

X-ray

An X-ray of the thorax and abdomen is taken to demonstrate the presence of air in the stomach and small bowel, which indicates that there is a fistula between the trachea and the lower segment of the oesophagus (Fig. 6.3). The X-ray also provides information on the state of the lungs and the presence of vertebral and rib anomalies. It may show evidence of a right-sided aortic arch.

Echocardiography

Nearly 25% of infants with oesophageal atresia have congenital heart disease. It is important to identify cardiac lesions pre-operatively because a prostaglandin E_1 infusion will need to be commenced before repair of the oesophagus if the lesion is 'duct-dependent'. In most babies the cardiac defect does not delay the oesophageal surgery, and oesophageal repair takes precedence over surgery to the heart. An echocardiograph may identify a right aortic arch and influence the surgical approach to the oesophagus.

Renal ultrasound

If the infant has not passed urine, a renal ultrasound must be performed to exclude bilateral renal agenesis. If the infant has no kidneys or has severely dysplastic kidneys, as occurs in 3%, no surgery is justified.

Genetic consultation

If the infant has dysmorphic facies and other features suggestive of a major chromosomal abnormality, early consultation with a geneticist is mandatory. There are a number of chromosomal aberrations, for example trisomy 18 and 21, and other associations, such as VATER and CHARGE, which are well known to occur with oesophageal atresia. In some cases, treatment may be delayed until after chromosomal analysis.

TREATMENT

The condition is treated by early complete correction. In preparation for surgery, the upper pouch should be kept empty by frequent suction. The infant should be placed in an incubator or under an overhead heater to avoid excessive heat loss. Vitamin K is given intramuscularly and intravenous fluids commenced. Antibiotics are given during surgery.

The operation is performed usually within 12 h of admission to hospital. Through a right posterolateral extrapleural thoracotomy, the fistula is divided and closed, and a direct end-to-end anastomosis of the upper and lower segments of the oesophagus is constructed. Postoperatively, oral feeds can be commenced on days 3 or 4.

ANATOMICAL VARIATIONS

Oesophageal atresia without a fistula

In this situation, the gap between the two segments of the oesophagus may be so great that a primary anastomosis is impossible at birth. On the initial X-ray, these babies have no gas below the diaphragm (Fig. 6.4). A gastrostomy is fashioned to allow enteral feeding and the overflow of saliva from the upper pouch is controlled by frequent suction. At about 6 weeks, an oesophageal anastomosis is performed. Occasionally this fails and oesophageal replacement is required at 6–12 months of age.

'H' fistula

Sometimes the oesophagus is intact but there is a communication between the trachea and oesophagus, usually at the level of C7 or T1. These infants present in the first week or so of life with episodes of coughing, cyanosis during feeding, and pulmonary complications. Sometimes they present later with a history of recurrent pulmonary infections or abdominal distension mimicking a bowel obstruction. The diagnosis is made by performing a barium swallow or mid-oesophageal contrast study, and observing the contrast pass through the fistula into the trachea. Treatment is by operative division of the fistula through a cervical approach.

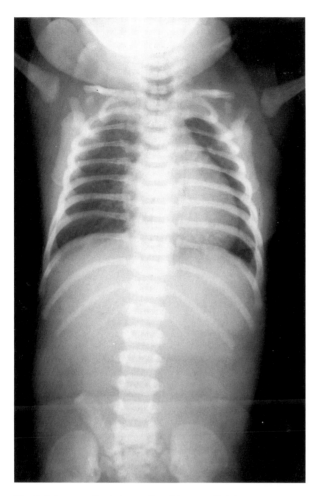

Fig. 6.4 In oesophageal atresia without a distal tracheo-oesophageal fistula there is no air below the diaphragm. Most of these infants have no fistula, while a few have a proximal tracheo-oesophageal fistula.

SPECIAL PROBLEMS

Effect of prematurity

Prematurity is common in these infants. Provided facilities are available, they should have their oesophageal atresia repaired early, before the expected respiratory distress of hyaline membrane disease becomes severe. Failure to divide the tracheo-oesophageal fistula early in these babies leads to severe problems with ventilation because air escapes preferentially through the fistula into the stomach.

Gastro-oesophageal reflux

Gastro-oesophageal reflux is common with oesophageal atresia and may contribute to the development of an oesophageal stricture. If this occurs, a fundoplication is required.

Tracheomalacia

Tracheomalacia is a structural weakness of the trachea and commonly occurs in association with oesophageal atresia. It is responsible for the 'seal bark' brassy cough characteristic of oesophageal atresia patients. It tends to improve with time but in the neonatal period may cause breathing difficulties. Occasionally, splinting of the trachea (tracheopexy, aortopexy) to prevent collapse of the airways is required.

COMPLICATIONS OF SURGERY

There are three main complications: (i) leak from the oesophageal anastomosis; (ii) oesophageal stricture; (iii) recurrent tracheo-oesophageal fistula. The majority of anastomotic leaks are minor and should be treated by withholding oral feeds, antibiotics and total parenteral nutrition. They usually seal spontaneously and surgery is required only if uncontrolled mediastinitis or empyema develop. Oesophageal stricture may present with dysphagia or choking on feeds. Gastro-oesophageal reflux as a contributing factor should be excluded and treatment involves fundoplication if gastro-oesophageal reflux is present, or oesophageal dilatation. A recurrent tracheo-oesophageal fistula rarely closes spontaneously and requires re-exploration and division.

PROGNOSIS

In the absence of associated congenital abnormalities or severe prematurity, survival in oesophageal atresia virtually is assured.

FURTHER READING

Beasley S. W., Auldist A. W. & Myers N. A. (1989) Current surgical management of oesophageal atresia and/or tracheo-oesophageal fistula. *Aust. NZ J. Surg.* **59**: 707–712.

Beasley S. W., Myers N. A. & Auldist A. W. (1991) *Oesophageal Atresia.* Chapman & Hall, London.

Chetcuti P., Myers N. A., Phelan P. D. *et al.* (1988) Adults who survived repair of congenital oesophageal atresia and tracheo-oesophageal fistula. *Br. Med. J.* **297**: 344–346.

Chittmittrapap S., Spitz L., Keily E. M. & Brereton R. J. (1989) Oesophageal atresia and associated anomalies. *Arch. Dis. Child* **64**: 364–368.

Louhimo I. & Lindahl H. (1984) Esophageal atresia: primary results of 500 consecutively treated patients. *J. Pediatr. Surg.* **18**: 217–229.

Myers N. A. & Egami K. (1987) Congenital tracheo-oesophageal fistula: 'H' or 'N' fistula. *Pediatr. Surg. Int.* **2**: 198–211.

7

Neonatal Bowel Obstruction

Neonatal bowel obstruction presents with the triad of bile-stained vomiting, abdominal distension and failure to pass meconium. It is caused by a group of congenital anomalies which have many features in common, both in terms of diagnosis and for the metabolic consequences for the neonate.

ANTENATAL DIAGNOSIS

Maternal polyhydramnios may indicate fetal bowel obstruction or the obstruction may be diagnosed serendipitously when ultrasonography is performed for obstetric reasons. Dilated fluid-filled loops of gut are seen on ultrasound. Usually the diagnosis is non-specific, but sometimes a characteristic pattern is seen, for example the 'double bubble' of duodenal atresia. Antenatal diagnosis is of particular importance if there is a family history of cystic fibrosis or Hirschsprung's disease.

POSTNATAL DIAGNOSIS

Bile-stained vomiting in the neonatal period always is significant and must be evaluated carefully as it is indicative of bowel obstruction.

Abdominal distension is a less specific feature as gaseous distension may occur without bowel obstruction. Furthermore, some high bowel obstructions, for example malrotation with volvulus or duodenal atresia may not have abdominal distension.

The normal neonate passes meconium within 24 h. Neonates with bowel obstructions do not pass meconium, with three notable exceptions: (i) babies with Hirschsprung's disease may pass meconium, especially after rectal examination; (ii) some sticky meconium

pellets may be passed in meconium ileus; (iii) onset of symptoms in malrotation with volvulus may be delayed for some time after birth.

Investigations

The plain X-ray (erect and supine) is the most important test and will show distension of the gut with fluid levels. The level of the obstruction may be related to the number of fluid levels, for example a double bubble in duodenal atresia, three or four fluid levels in upper jejunal atresia and many fluid levels in ileal atresia or Hirschsprung's disease. Fine calcification indicates prenatal gut perforation with meconium peritonitis. Free gas in the peritoneal cavity is seen when perforation occurs after birth.

Contrast studies are useful in some patients. Incomplete high obstructions are assessed with a barium meal, which will demonstrate a malrotation with volvulus or a duodenal web. A barium enema is a suitable test for low obstructions, such as Hirschsprung's disease or meconium ileus.

COMPLICATIONS OF OBSTRUCTION

Fluid losses from lack of fluid intake, vomiting and sequestration of fluid in the bowel and peritoneum are a major problem.

Metabolic acidosis is due to anaerobic metabolism from poor tissue perfusion and a lack of glucose for energy production.

Hypothermia results from inadequate warming during examination and resuscitation of the sick neonate, who already has poor thermoregulation.

Respiratory distress is seen in many babies with bowel obstruction from abdominal distension limiting the diaphragm's excursion during inspiration. Inhalation of vomitus may produce a pneumonitis and atelectasis.

Sepsis from gut organisms is due to migration of organisms through ischaemic gut wall or more obviously through a gut perforation. Septicaemia with virulent gut organisms may lead to the rapid demise of the neonate.

GENERAL TREATMENT

Nasogastric tube

The passage of a nasogastric tube to aspirate gut content relieves respiratory distress from abdominal distension and helps to measure the fluid losses. It is mandatory in all cases of bowel obstruction.

Resuscitation

As surgical correction is imminent, the resuscitation must be rapid and the time scale is measured in hours. Fluid boluses of Hartmann's solution are given at 10 mL/kg. A maintenance glucose infusion is continued during resuscitation and sodium bicarbonate is given to correct acidosis. An overhead heater maintains body temperature during resuscitation and respiratory support with oxygen and occasionally ventilation is given. Some degree of sepsis is assumed and antibiotics are given after cultures are taken. Surgical correction of the underlying cause should not be unduly delayed or further complications such as gut perforation may ensue.

HIRSCHSPRUNG'S DISEASE

In 1887, Hirschsprung described two infants who died with gross abdominal distension and a hugely dilated colon containing masses of faeces. This functional obstruction became known as 'Hirschsprung's syndrome', and in 1948, Zuelzer and Wilson noted that there were no ganglion cells in the affected parts of the bowel. This

established a histological basis for Hirschsprung's disease, which is now recognized as the commonest cause of intestinal obstruction in the newborn.

Hirschsprung's disease occurs in 1 : 5000 births, and genetically there are two types:

(1) A larger group, in which males are affected five times as often as females, and there is a relatively short aganglionic segment, usually involving the sigmoid colon, rectum and anal canal

(2) A smaller group with a long aganglionic segment, equally common in boys and girls, with a higher degree of 'penetrance', and more likely to affect subsequent siblings.

The affected segment begins at the anus and extends proximally for a variable distance—in most cases as far as the sigmoid colon, but sometimes as high as the ascending colon. In a few cases, the affected segment extends into the small bowel, and in rare instances the entire alimentary canal is devoid of ganglia, excluding hope of survival.

All degrees of obstruction are seen in neonates, for example complete within 24 h of birth; episodes of partial obstruction for several weeks before the diagnosis is made; or with no symptoms at all in the first month of life.

The three classic signs are: (i) delay in the passage of meconium; (ii) vomitus containing bile; (iii) abdominal distension.

On rectal examination with the little finger, the anus and rectum may feel tight and 'conical', consistent with the unused nature of the distal bowel. Plain X-rays show multiple fluid levels in the small bowel. If a contrast enema is performed it may show a transitional zone usually in the sigmoid colon or rectum (Fig. 7.1), or a 'microcolon'. 'Microcolon' describes the narrow empty colon (Fig. 7.2) and is found in any fetal alimentary abnormality which prevents meconium reaching the rectum. In all except those with Hirschsprung's disease, there is nothing basically wrong with the structure of this unused colon.

Palliation of partial obstruction by enemas as a long-term plan is unsuccessful, although it may provide temporary relief and the opportunity to obtain a rectal biopsy (by mucosal suction biopsy) to confirm the diagnosis before laparotomy.

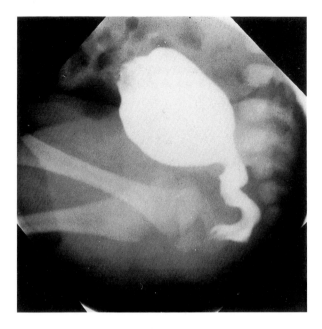

Fig. 7.1 Transition zone between dilated proximal colon and narrow distal bowel as seen on barium enema.

Treatment

Treatment can be planned once a suction rectal biopsy has confirmed the diagnosis. In neonates, a one-stage definitive operation without a preliminary colostomy is feasible, but most surgeons employ the following protocol:

(1)   An initial colostomy placed in normal bowel above the cone of transition, as confirmed by frozen sections taken from the colon at laparotomy

(2)   Excision of the aganglionic bowel at 3–6 months when the patient is in optimal condition; usually with removal of the colostomy at the same time

(3)   Closure of the colostomy 1–2 weeks later, if not already closed in the course of the definitive resection.

MECONIUM ILEUS

In cystic fibrosis of the pancreas, the alimentary canal is affected *in utero* and there is a change in the physical

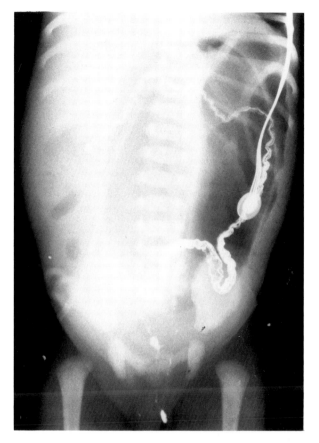

Fig. 7.2 'Microcolon'. The unexpanded but otherwise normal bowel distal to any complete intestinal obstruction *in utero*.

properties of the meconium; it becomes excessively sticky and tenacious causing a mechanical obstruction.

Typically, there are grey–white globular pellets in the lower ileum just distal to a segment containing impacted tenacious black–green meconium. Proximal to this again, there are several loops of hypertrophied bowel distended with fluid. The bowel distal to the obstruction is narrow and empty, no meconium is passed and abdominal distension and vomiting appear soon after birth.

Plain abdominal X-rays reveal fluid levels and in some cases a foamy pattern of air bubbles trapped around the impacted meconium. A contrast enema shows a microcolon.

Treatment

Treatment is based on the assumption that these infants have cystic fibrosis. Antibiotics are commenced at once, and dehydration, which would make secretions even more tenacious, must be prevented.

The obstructing meconium is removed by one of several methods: in uncomplicated cases (i.e. no meconium peritonitis or localized volvulus) a gastrografin enema controlled by fluoroscopy may relieve the obstruction; if this fails intra-operative evacuation, resection, temporary enterostomy to inject chemical solvents or enterotomy without resection is required. The prognosis is fair, for there is no constant relationship between meconium ileus and the severity of the cystic fibrosis, which can be diagnosed conclusively by a 'sweat test' at about 2 weeks of age.

VOLVULUS NEONATORUM

The fetal alimentary canal returns from the extraembryonic coelom into the abdomen at 8–10 weeks, and the bowel undergoes rotation and fixation at certain points by the attachment of its mesentery to the posterior abdominal wall.

When the process is incomplete or deviates from the normal plan, the result is malfixation or malrotation.

Commonly the normal oblique attachment of the mesentery from the duodenojejunal flexure to the caecum is absent, and the small bowel is attached to the posterior abdominal wall by a narrow stalk based around the superior mesenteric vessels. The caecum is undescended, that is, situated in the right hypochondrium and abnormally fixed by peritoneal bands running laterally across the second part of the duodenum.

The poorly attached small bowel undergoes volvulus around the axis of the 'universal mesentery', which is twisted so that the flow of blood is cut off, producing a strangulating obstruction of the small bowel. This typically occurs in the newborn, hence the term 'volvulus neonatorum'. The terminal ileum and caecum are drawn into the volvulus and are wrapped around the stalk of the mesentery in two or three tight coils.

Clinical features

Bile-stained vomiting associated with a soft nondistended abdomen is the early feature of volvulus. The diagnosis should be made at this early stage before widespread ischaemic gut damage occurs.

No obstruction may occur in the first day or two after birth and meconium may be passed normally; then, with variable suddenness, bowel actions cease with the onset of obstruction.

In some cases the symptoms are recurrent, a feature which is very suggestive of volvulus neonatorum, for there are few causes of intestinal obstruction in the newborn, except perhaps Hirschsprung's disease, which produce episodic obstruction.

The signs vary, depending on the tightness of the volvulus and whether the extrinsic bands across the duodenum are tighter than the volvulus. When strangulation occurs, there are signs of shock, especially pallor, and a vague mass of congested bowel may be palpable in the centre of the abdomen. Blood or blood-tinged mucus may be passed rectally. Distension is variable and often absent or confined to the epigastrium when the duodenum is obstructed, for a large vomit can empty the short length of bowel proximal to the obstruction.

Investigations

A plain X-ray of the abdomen is not helpful in the early stage of volvulus. The most reliable radiological confirmation of malfixation is a barium meal with fluoroscopy, which will show that the duodenojejunal flexure is located at a lower level than (i.e. caudal to) the second part of the duodenum. The contrast may then show the spiral twist of the volvulus as well (Fig. 7.3).

Treatment

Laparotomy is urgent to limit gut ischaemia. The volvulus is untwisted, and it often requires three full rotations to release the caecum. The narrow root of the small bowel mesentery is broadened by dissection which separates the caecum from the duodenum. The

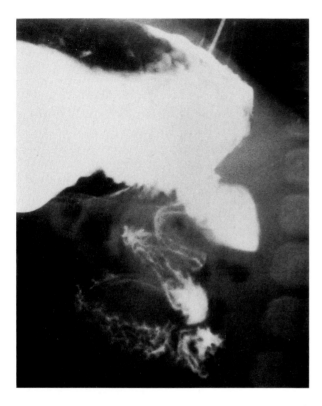

Fig. 7.3 Volvulus neonatorum. Barium meal shows a spiral twist of the bowel below the mid-duodenum.

small bowel is placed to the right and the colon to the left. The appendix is removed.

There is no need to fix the intestines for, surprisingly, there are virtually no recurrences once all the areas of malfixation are freed. Rarely, the greater part of the small bowel is gangrenous, resection is inescapable and consequent malabsorption is likely if there are only a few centimetres of viable bowel between the duodenum and the colon.

DUODENAL OBSTRUCTION

Duodenal obstruction is caused by duodenal atresia, or by stenosis due to a septum or membrane with a small hole in it. Still less commonly, an annular pancreas may be wrapped around the duodenum, but usually this is

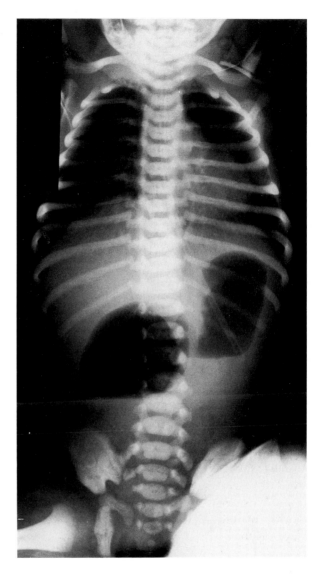

Fig. 7.4 Duodenal atresia. Plain X-ray shows a 'double bubble', one in the stomach and the other in the dilated proximal duodenum.

accompanied by severe stenosis or atresia of the duodenum at the site of envelopment.

Atresia of the duodenum occurs most commonly in the second part and is associated with Down syndrome in about 30%.

Acute obstruction develops in the neonatal period, but signs may be delayed for a day or so while the secretions accumulate in the distended stomach and proximal duodenum.

X-rays of the abdomen show a 'double bubble' pattern: two large loops each with a fluid level and no aeration of the more distal bowel (Fig. 7.4).

A duodenal septum or membrane is a form of obstruction which may be incomplete in the neonate, for example the small hole in the septum permits the passage of air and some fluid; the diagnosis may be missed if symptoms are mild or transient. It may present in children of 2–3 years of age. The membrane is pushed onwards by peristalsis so that it may bulge far along the duodenum, stretching its mucosal attachment. X-rays show some dilatation of the duodenum but the typical radiographic signs of complete obstruction are absent, and the diagnosis can best be demonstrated by a contrast meal and fluoroscopy.

Treatment

In atresia of the duodenum, with or without an annular pancreas, the obstruction is circumvented by duodeno-duodenostomy. The surgical treatment for duodenal septum is duodenoplasty, but the bile ducts may pose a special problem because they open very close to or actually into the edge of the septum.

SMALL BOWEL ATRESIA

Atresia of the bowel can occur at any point (Fig. 7.5), most frequently in the distal ileum (Fig. 7.6), but is rare in the colon. There is often only one atresia, although there may be several close together or widely scattered.

The cause may be interruption of the mesenteric arcades by a vascular accident *in utero*, a theory supported by experimental surgery on fetal animals.

The form of the atresia may be a very tight stenosis with no functional orifice, or a thick septum with the bowel in continuity or a missing segment with a gap of a centimetre or more between the closed ends. The adjacent vascular arcades are distorted and their termi-

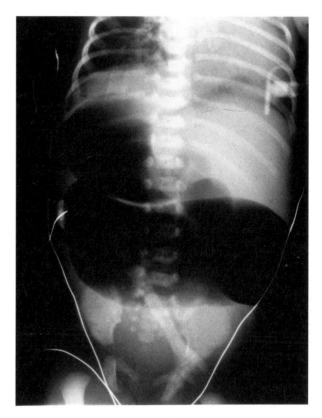

Fig. 7.5 Intestinal atresia: plain X-ray showing obstruction of the jejunum. Infant also has situs inversus.

nal branches may be very small or absent. All the bowel distal to the atresia, including the colon and rectum, is unused and unexpanded, that is microcolon, which can be demonstrated by a contrast enema.

Treatment involves enteroenterostomy to re-establish bowel continuity.

DUPLICATIONS OF THE ALIMENTARY TRACT

These are rare developmental anomalies in which a length of bowel is duplicated in such a way that the two segments share the same blood supply and a common wall, while the mucosal linings are separate. They can arise at any point from the mouth to the anus, and involve any length from 1–2 cm to the whole length of

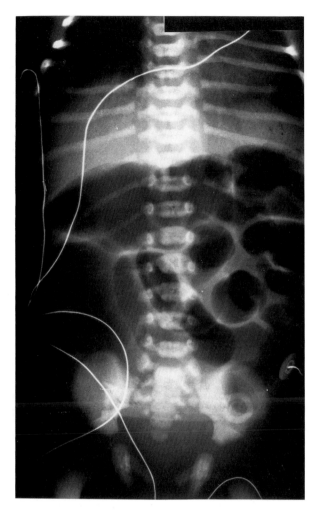

Fig. 7.6 Ileal atresia.

the large bowel. A duplication may or may not communicate with the main alimentary channel.

There are two basic types:

(1) Short closed cystic segments. The segment forms a cyst which bulges into the lumen or compresses and angulates the adjoining small bowel, causing obstruction. A small intraluminal cyst may cause obstruction in the neonatal period, but larger ones less intimately connected with the common wall usually cause progressive obstruction later in infancy or in early childhood.

Occasionally a large tense cyst is palpable as a very mobile mass in a child without obstructive symptoms.

(2) Long tubular communicating duplications are much less common and more likely to be lined by ectopic (gastric) mucosa, which may cause a peptic ulcer (Chapter 23). If the diagnosis of a duplication containing ectopic gastric mucosa is suspected, it may be demonstrable by means of a technetium ^{99m} scan. The resection of a long duplication involves the removal of an equivalent length of bowel, and when this is unacceptable because of the inadequate length of bowel remaining, a practical alternative is to remove the lining alone.

NEONATAL NECROTIZING ENTEROCOLITIS

Necrotizing enterocolitis is a disease with combined ischaemia and infection of the bowel wall. Although not strictly a 'cause' of intestinal obstruction, it typically produces abdominal distension and bile-stained vomiting, resembling obstruction, but distinguishable by features such as passage of blood and a characteristic radiological picture. A greater awareness of the entity may have contributed to the increased incidence in recent years, but there has been an absolute increase in the number of cases reported throughout the 'Western' world.

Predisposing factors

Some of these are 'observed associations', and it is still uncertain which really contribute to the development of the condition (Table 7.1). However, necrotizing enterocolitis can occur in infants previously regarded as normal, in whom none of the above conditions can be found.

Aetiology

The mechanism has not been elucidated fully. The most widely held theory to explain the intestinal ischaemia is that in a stressed, hypoxic state, blood is preferentially distributed to the heart and brain, at the expense of the splanchnic circulation, skin and muscle.

(39)

Table 7.1 Predisposing factors and observed associations in neonatal necrotizing enterocolitis

Prematurity
Respiratory distress:
atelectasis
hyaline membrane disease
Birth asphyxia
Fetal distress during labour
Prolonged antepartum rupture of membranes
Twins
Caesarean section
Congenital heart disease
Jaundice
Catheterization of the umbilical vessels
Hyperosmolar feeds
Sepsis

Local vascular changes have been implicated, for example a catheter in the umbilical vein, if badly positioned, alters the portal haemodynamics; a catheter in the umbilical artery may have a similar effect on the arterial supply if advanced too far up the aorta, and also has the potential to produce emboli.

Certain bacteria appear to be important; *Klebsiella* species resistant to the commonly used antibiotics are found in a significant number of infants who develop necrotizing enterocolitis. Other enteropathogens (e.g. *Escherichia coli*, *Clostridia difficile* and *Streptococcus faecalis*) and *Pseudomonas* species also have been isolated.

The type of feed and when it is commenced may have some relevance, for example the disease appears to occur more frequently in infants who were fed early with artificial milk formulae. Breast milk may afford some protection against the disease in the 'at risk' infant, but this is not certain.

Pathology

Necrotizing enterocolitis may be generalized and involve most of the small and large intestine or be segmental in distribution, in which case the ileum and colon commonly are affected. There is histological evidence of impaired perfusion, resulting in tissue anoxia and necrosis. The mucosa is affected most, because of a shunting mechanism, but the process may involve the entire thickness of the bowel wall.

When the mucosa is damaged, production of mucus is impaired and bacteria normally present in the lumen can invade the intestinal wall, further damaging the bowel and entering the bloodstream to produce bacteraemia or septicaemia. The damaged mucosa bleeds into the lumen, and gas collects in the bowel wall (pneumatosis intestinalis) due to the activity of gas-forming organisms or by diffusion of intraluminal gas through breaches in the damaged mucosa.

The consequent pathological course varies: perforation with generalized peritonitis or local abscess formation follows transmural necrosis; healing with restoration of normal function occurs in less-affected bowel; and fibrosis with the formation of a stricture may be the result of healing in a severely involved segment.

Clinical picture

The onset of symptoms is between 2 and 14 days after birth. The infant is ill, lethargic, febrile and not interested in feeds. Abdominal distension and bile-stained vomiting occur, and there may be passage of loose stools containing a variable amount of blood.

When complicated by peritonitis, the anterior abdominal wall becomes oedematous and red, with dilated veins, and palpation causes pain. A mass may be palpable if a localized intraperitoneal abscess has formed or if there is a persistent dilated loop of bowel.

Investigations

The radiological findings are typical. Plain films of the abdomen show dilated loops of bowel in which there are intramural bubbles of gas (pneumatosis intestinalis; Fig. 7.7). Gas outlining the portal vein and/or its radicles may be visible. Free gas in the peritoneal cavity, best seen under the diaphragm, is present if the intestine has perforated. Separation of adjacent loops of bowel suggests appreciable amounts of intraperitoneal exudate, an indication of peritonitis, with or without a perforation.

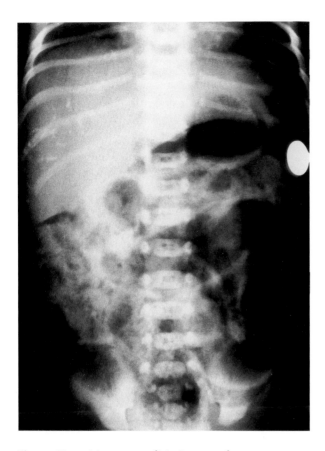

Fig. 7.7 Necrotizing enterocolitis. Intramural gas.

Bacteriological specimens, for example blood culture and rectal swabs, should be taken before antibiotics are commenced or altered. The nose, throat and umbilicus also are swabbed.

Biochemistry, haematology, electrolytes, acid–base and bilirubin are monitored. The haemoglobin level may fall progressively as a result of sepsis and haemorrhage and serial measurements are required. The platelet and white cell counts are depressed in severe disease. The infants are acidotic.

Management

Initially this consists of stopping oral feeds, decompression of the intestine by suction via a wide bore nasogastric tube and parenteral administration of fluids and appropriate antibiotics (penicillin and gentamicin).

Intensive measures listed in the section on the pre- and postoperative care of the neonate and adequate respiratory management also may be required. Acidosis is corrected.

Frequent clinical and radiological reassessment is essential, for it may show the need for surgery.

The indications for operation are continued clinical deterioration despite intensive and appropriate resuscitation; or the development of a complication suggesting the presence of full-thickness bowel necrosis, such as perforation or intra-abdominal abscess. Features which are useful in determining the need for operation include free gas on X-ray, progressive signs of peritonitis (distended red and tender abdomen), persistent acidosis despite attempted correction, and a sudden and profound fall in the platelet count.

Operation is confined to the resection of perforated or necrotic bowel and drainage of any intraperitoneal abscesses. The mortality rate until recently was high, but with earlier diagnosis and more effective treatment this is diminishing.

FURTHER READING

Beasley S. W. & de Campo J. F. (1987) Pitfalls in the diagnosis of malrotation. *Austr. Radiol.* **31**: 376–383.

Beasley S. W., Auldist A. W., Ramanujan T. M. & Campbell N. T. (1986) The surgical management of neonatal necrotizing enterocolitis 1975–1984. *Pediatr. Surg. Int.* **1**: 210–217.

Boulton J. E., Ein S. H., Reilly B. J., Smith B. T. & Paper K. E. (1989) Necrotizing enterocolitis and volvulus in the premature neonate. *J. Pediatr. Surg.* **24**: 901–905.

Caniano D. A., Ormsbee H. S. *et al.* (1985) Total intestinal aganglionosis. *J. Pediatr. Surg.* **20**: 456–460.

Carcassonne M. & Delarue A. (1984) Management of Hirschsprung's disease: which, when, why and how. *Aust. NZ J. Surg.* **54**: 435–438.

Foster P., Cowan G. & Wrenn E. L. Jr (1990) Twenty-five years' experience with Hirschsprung's disease. *J. Pediatr. Surg.* **25**: 531–534.

Hocking M. & Young D. G. (1981) Duplications of the alimentary tract. *Brit. J. Surg.* **68**: 92-96.

Holschneider A. M. (1982) *Hirschsprung's Disease.* Hippokrates Verlag, Stuttgart.

Lloyd D. (1986) Meconium ileus. In: Welch K. J., Randolph J. G.,

Ravitch M. M., O'Neill J. A. & Rowe M. I. (eds), *Pediatric Surgery*, 4th edn, Vol. 2, pp. 849–858. Year Book Medical, Chicago.

Martin L. W. & Torres A. M. (1985) Hirschsprung's disease. *Surg. Clin. Nth Am.* **65**: 1171–1180.

Puri P., Guiney E. J. & Carroll R. (1985) Multiple gastrointestinal atresias in three consecutive siblings: observations and pathogenesis. *J. Pediatr. Surg.* **20**: 22–24.

Schiller M., Abu-Dalu K., Gorenstein A., Levy P. & Katz S. (1990) Endorectal pull-through for Hirschsprung's disease. Report of 78 cases. *Pediatr. Surg. Int.* **5**: 185–187.

Spigland N., Yazbeck S. & Desjardins J. G. (1990) Surgical outcome of necrotizing enterocolitis. *Pediatr. Surg. Int.* **5**: 355–358.

Stevenson R. J. (1985) Non-neonatal intestinal obstruction in children. *Surg. Clin. North Am.* **65**: 1217–1234.

8

Anorectal Anomalies

A perineum without an anal opening is described as 'imperforate', a term which embraces a number of anomalies. Most anorectal malformations communicate by a fistula with either the urinary or genital systems, or actually open to the skin of the perineum.

There is a wide range of anomalies which differ only in minute points of embryology. Rather than describe them in detail, the emphasis will be on the diagnostic points which identify two main groups, the associated anomalies and the factors which affect surgical correction, so that some idea of the prognosis can be conveyed to the parents at the time of diagnosis.

CLASSIFICATION

Development of the distal bowel is arrested at one of two levels, each with its own subtypes and clinical implications.

The principal distinction is in the relationship of the end of bowel to the chief muscle of continence, the puborectalis component of levator ani. Arrested development at or above levator ani (the supralevator lesions) produces rectal deformities; arrested development below levator ani (the translevator lesions) produces anal deformities. In each group the bowel may end blindly but usually communicates by a fistula with a neighbouring viscus or the perineal skin (Fig. 8.1).

Rectal deformities (high and intermediate lesions)

The classification (Table 8.1) distinguishes two main groups: supralevator (high and intermediate) and translevator (low).

Table 8.1 'Wingspread' classification of anorectal malformations (1984)

Male	Female
High	High
(1) Anorectal agenesis:	(1) Anorectal agenesis:
—with rectoprostatic/ urethral fistula	—with rectovaginal fistula
—without fistula	—without fistula
(2) Rectal atresia	(2) Rectal atresia
Intermediate	Intermediate
(1) Rectovestibular fistula	(1) Rectobulbar urethral fistula
(2) Rectovaginal fistula	(2) Anal agenesis without fistula
(3) Anal agenesis without fistula	
Low	Low
(1) Anovestibular fistula	(1) Anocutaneous fistula
(2) Anocutaneous fistula	(2) Anal stenosis
(3) Anal stenosis	
Cloacal malformations	
Rare malformations	Rare malformations

The bowel in the 'high' group stops above the levator sling, and is represented radiologically by gas shadows at or above the pubococcygeal line (see below); the 'intermediate' lesions lie on the sling but not through it, and the gas shadows lie at the radiological 'I point'. The subdivision of the supralevator lesions is necessary because of differences in the operative approach, but otherwise both sublevels have the prognostic implications common to the rectal deformities.

In rectal deformities the fistulous communications are more complex than in anal lesions and involve the

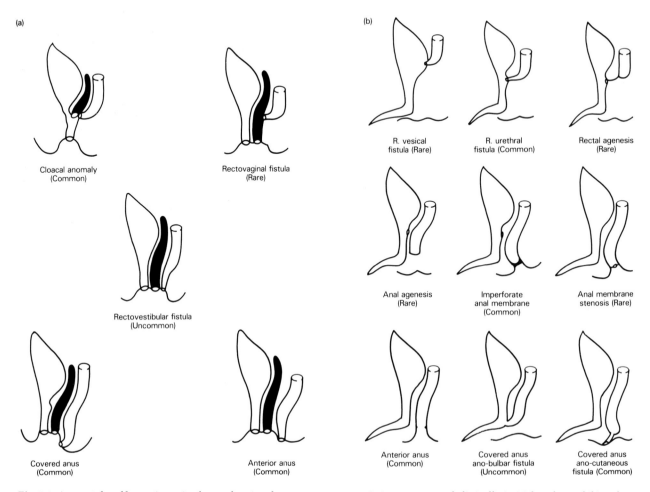

(a)

Cloacal anomaly
(Common)

Rectovaginal fistula
(Rare)

Rectovestibular fistula
(Uncommon)

Covered anus
(Common)

Anterior anus
(Common)

(b)

R. vesical
fistula (Rare)

R. urethral
fistula (Common)

Rectal agenesis
(Rare)

Anal agenesis
(Rare)

Imperforate
anal membrane
(Common)

Anal membrane
stenosis (Rare)

Anterior anus
(Common)

Covered anus
ano-bulbar fistula
(Uncommon)

Covered anus
ano-cutaneous
fistula (Common)

Fig. 8.1 Anorectal malformations. A schema showing the most common varieties encountered clinically in (a) females and (b) males.

urinary tract in boys and the genital tract in girls. Associated anomalies, which are more common in the rectal group, involve the urinary tract, the vertebral column, the alimentary canal and the heart; they are generally serious and may be lethal in themselves.

As well as the visceral connections shown in Fig. 8.1 there are defects in the muscular sphincters. The puborectalis is, as a rule, fully formed although it may be displaced. Occasionally part or all of the sacrum fails to develop, in which case the puborectalis may be deficient and lack a nerve supply. Incontinence then is inevitable.

The internal anal sphincter is absent in all these deformities, but the external sphincter varies from normal to rudimentary. Lack of these two sphincters does not produce faecal incontinence provided that the puborectalis is intact, but when the internal and external sphincters are deficient, there is often a partially open anal segment below puborectalis after reconstruction. This may lead to a slight staining of the underwear with mucus or faeces, because the external sphincter normally closes the anal verge.

The results of surgical reconstruction to bring the bowel through the puborectalis may be compromised because the muscle may be poorly formed and any operative damage reduces the effectiveness of faecal control. Because of these difficulties reconstruction may be delayed for some months and a colostomy is required in the interim to relieve the bowel obstruction.

Anal deformities (low lesions)

The bowel passes through the puborectalis, making surgical reconstruction much simpler and reasonable continence is assured. A colostomy in the neonatal period is not required and definitive correction can be completed within a day or two of birth by local perineal surgery (e.g. anal cutback). The fistulas usually do not involve other viscera and the coexistent anomalies are less common and less severe.

INCIDENCE

Anal or rectal malformations occur in 1 : 5000 live births with a slight preponderance in males, in whom there is a higher incidence of the more difficult rectal types, whereas in females most are of the anal type. The aetiology is unknown. No exogenous factors in pregnancy have been identified; evidence of a genetic determinant is meagre and only rarely is a subsequent sibling affected.

CLINICAL FEATURES

The newborn baby with a supralevator lesion presents with no visible anus and has intestinal obstruction (Fig. 8.2). However, in females the fistula to the genital tract is usually wide enough to decompress the bowel adequately. In males, a fistula to the urinary tract may lead to the appearance of meconium in the urine, an important diagnostic observation.

A fistula opening on the perineal skin is easily visible when it is filled with meconium, but can be very minute and requires a careful search with good illumination. The discovery of a fistula to the skin with even a tiny orifice is proof that it is an anal type of anomaly, whereas a completely 'blind' perineum may be due to either a rectal or anal anomaly, but usually the former.

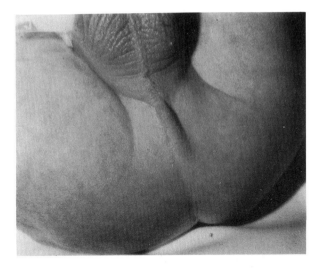

Fig. 8.2 The featureless perineum of a male baby with a recto-urethral fistula.

In females, a detailed search of each perineal orifice is essential, and the internal anatomy can be predicted when the site of the external opening has been located. For example, faeces may be described as coming from the vagina, yet rectovaginal fistulas are uncommon, and more careful examination will reveal a small orifice tucked into the vestibule just outside the vaginal orifice, that is the more common anovestibular fistula, which is quite simple to treat.

The exact nature of a non-communicating anomaly cannot be determined by clinical examination alone. X-rays are essential and their interpretation depends upon the presence of gas in the bowel or the distribution of radio-opaque dye introduced into the urinary tract.

Radiographic information is obtained by:

(1) X-rays of the spine for vertebral anomalies, especially sacral agenesis, which affects the neural pathways

(2) An X-ray of the pelvis at 12–24 h of age while the baby is held upside down, taken in an exact lateral projection, that is an invertograph. Gas rises to the apex of the blind bowel and its level is compared with various skeletal landmarks, which in turn correspond with the level of the puborectalis levator sling. A line drawn through the upper margin of the symphysis pubis and the sacrococcygeal junction in the lateral film constitutes the pubococcygeal (PC) line, and indicates the

uppermost and most lateral fibres of the puborectalis; a gas shadow at or cranial to the 'PC line' indicates a high rectal anomaly (Fig. 8.3a). The puborectalis then cones down like a funnel and its lowest and most medial fibres lie at the level shown by the skeletal landmark, the 'I point': the forward, lowermost tip of the comma-shaped ischial bone. A gas shadow between the 'PC line' and 'I point' is an intermediate rectal anomaly, although still supralevator. When the gas shadow is well caudal to the 'I point', the bowel has traversed the puborectalis sling and an anal anomaly is present (Fig. 8.3b)

(3) A micturating cysto-urethrogram (MCU) will

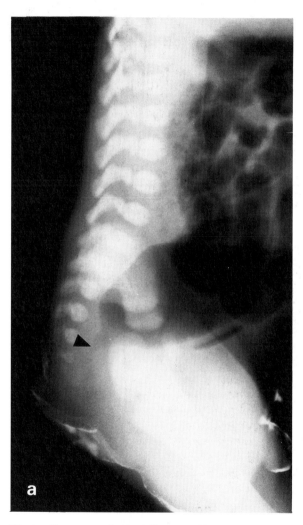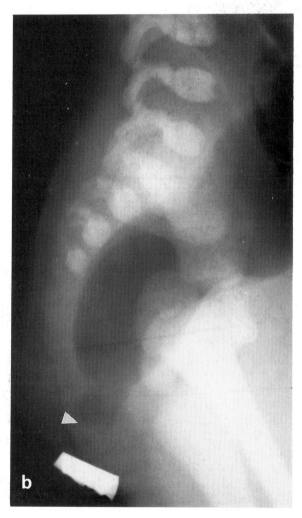

Fig. 8.3 'Invertogram'. Carefully centred lateral X-rays of the pelvis with the infant inverted (reversed to the upright position for clarity), showing (a) a 'high' lesion, for example anorectal agenesis. The gas-filled bowel extends just below the line between the crest of the pubis and the coccyx (PC line), which is the landmark for the cranial edge of the levator ani and the puborectalis muscles. The lowest point of the normal puborectalis corresponds to the lower edge of the ischial ossification centre (the 'I point'). (b) a 'low' lesion, for example imperforate anal membrane. The gas-filled bowel extends well below both the PC line and the 'I point'.

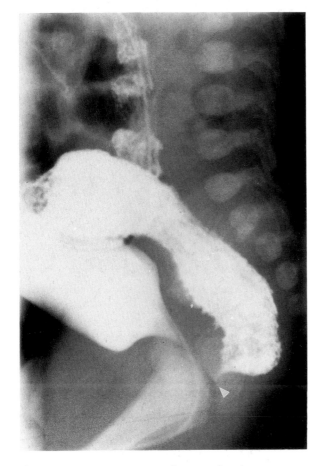

Fig. 8.4 A micturating cysto-urethrogram showing contrast in a recto-urethral fistula.

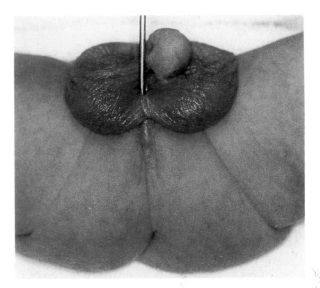

Fig. 8.5 Low imperforate anus: a male with an anocutaneous fistula opening in the midline of the scrotum as shown by the probe which has been inserted into it.

demonstrate a communication with the rectum, for example recto-urethral fistula, and other urinary tract abnormalities, for example vesico-ureteric reflux (Fig. 8.4)

(4) Computerized tomography, magnetic resonance imaging and pelvic ultrasound are used to obtain extra information in selected cases.

EXAMINATION AND DIAGNOSIS

The following plan of examination has been established by experience:

In males

(1) The perineum is examined to find an orifice, which may be:

(a) a normal anus in an anterior position—anterior perineal anus;

(b) a fistula opening onto the perineal skin anterior to the anus—anocutaneous fistula (Fig. 8.5);

(c) a small tight orifice at the normal site—stenosis of the anal membrane or anal stenosis due to covered anus or anorectal stenosis

(2) If no orifice is found, the urine is examined for the presence of meconium

(a) If there is no meconium, an invertograph is obtained and the terminal gas shadow will indicate one of three levels:

• high: anorectal agenesis (no fistula)—commonest

• intermediate: anal agenesis (no fistula)

• low: imperforate anal membrane or covered anus (complete)

(b) When meconium is present, this indicates that there is recto-urinary communication, and an inverto-

graph and MCU will then distinguish between:
- a high recto-urethral fistula or rectovesical fistula
- an intermediate rectobulbar fistula.

In females

(1) When some meconium is passed, the perineum and its orifices (the urethra and vagina) are examined for additional fistulous orifices:

(a) 'one hole'—cloacal anomaly
(b) 'two holes'—rectovaginal fistula
(c) 'three holes'
- anovestibular fistula, or rectovestibular fistula (Fig. 8.6)
- an anterior anus (perineal or vulvar); or
- a variety of covered anus (anocutaneous or anovulvar fistula).

These can be identified by their exact site, the size of the orifice and the direction taken by a probe introduced into the fistula

(2) When no meconium is passed there may be anal or rectal agenesis without fistula, a rarity in females, and

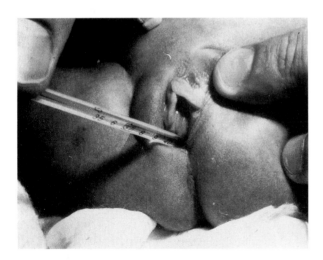

Fig. 8.6 Rectovestibular fistula: the fistula runs directly upwards parallel to the vagina as is shown by the thermometer. In the more common anovestibular fistula, the thermometer will be directed posteriorly towards the coccyx.

an invertograph is obtained; the same levels apply as in male deformities (above)

(3) Finally, the nerve supply to the bladder, the bowel, and the perineal muscles is examined, especially when X-rays show that the sacrum is abnormal.

Neurogenic bladder

A neurogenic bladder is usually expressible, and the sacral dermatomes are tested for response to pinprick. The sacral roots which supply the levator ani (S2, 3, 4) also supply the vesical sphincters, such that the perineal dermatomes provide a guide to the integrity of the levator ani and puborectalis.

When perineal sensation is absent and the bladder is expressible, faecal incontinence is certain, even if a rectoplasty is performed, for the levator ani is paralysed. Colostomy in the neonatal period is required for rectal deformities and further information concerning the anatomy of the fistula can be obtained by 'colograms'. The urinary tract is investigated by ultrasound and endoscopy.

TREATMENT AND PROGNOSIS

Certain generalizations can be made:

(1) The identification of a fistulous opening in the perineum indicates that there is an anal anomaly and the prognosis is good

(2) Meconium in the urine indicates the need for a preliminary colostomy, for all recto-urinary communications are supralevator

(3) In females a fistula should be expected and a thorough search made for it. Those with one or two orifices have a cloacal or rectal anomaly and a colostomy is required. In almost all those with three orifices, immediate local surgery is simple and the prognosis is good

(4) An anterior anus is by definition normal except for its ectopic situation and requires no treatment

(5) An expressible bladder, with perineal anaesthesia and malformation of the sacrum indicates a paretic levator ani and a permanent colostomy might be required

Anal deformities

The long term outlook for continence is good, apart from occasional slight smearing and staining of underwear, which usually is of little inconvenience.

An anocutaneous fistula in either sex, and anovestibular and anovulvar fistulas in females, require a cut-back along the fistula to display the covered anus. In females this may result in an anus contiguous with the posterior fourchette, but this nearly always functions normally. However, if there is a cosmetic problem or if faeces enter the vagina during defaecation, the anus can be transplanted to the normal site by a sacroperineal approach later in infancy or childhood.

Imperforate anal membrane and anal stenosis require simple incision and dilatation.

Rectal deformities

The outlook may be poor because of the associated neurological deficiency and other anomalies and the additional technical difficulties involved in correction. Provided there is no neural deficit, continence should be possible, but in practice, at least 20–30% lack good control. These children can be managed by supervision of their diet and the result is much better than with an abdominal colostomy alone; but some faecal soiling is common.

Infants with a rectal anomaly usually require a colostomy in the neonatal period and for the occasional surgeon an initial colostomy may be safer in both anal or rectal anomalies, even if it proves subsequently to have been unnecessary.

Rectoplasty is performed at 3–12 months, after a colostomy at birth. Various techniques are utilized, most depending on a sacroperineal approach to mobilize the rectum and bring it down to the perineum. It is difficult to locate the plane of the puborectalis from the abdominal approach alone, whereas it can be safely defined by the sacrococcygeal route or by careful dissection in the perineum. The preferred technique is sacroperineal rectoplasty, that is sacroperineal exposure of the puborectalis, division of fistula and mobilization of the bowel through the puborectalis sling to the perineum. For some high lesions sacro-abdominoperineal rectoplasty is required: this involves sacroperineal exposure of the puborectalis initially and the delineation of the puborectalis sling; then, through the abdominal route the rectum is mobilized, the fistula is divided and the bowel brought down within the previously defined puborectalis sling to the perineum.

COMPLICATIONS

(1) Anal strictures readily develop after anoplasty or rectoplasty, and the new anus must be dilated regularly for 3 months. A stricture is a serious matter, because it is followed by constipation and colonic inertia, the development of a large hypertrophied and dilated rectum and spurious incontinence (Chapter 22)

(2) Sloughing of the rectum due to ischaemia is most often the result of inadequate mobilization and excessive tension. Redundant and prolapsing rectal mucosa may require trimming later

(3) A perianal or pararectal abscess may develop and require drainage

(4) Recurrent fistulas occur when their initial closure has been inadequate

(5) Complications of the colostomy include prolapse of the colon, stenosis and intestinal obstruction

(6) Urinary complications are not uncommon (see below).

ASSOCIATED ANOMALIES

The mortality is influenced by the presence of other congenital abnormalities more than by any other factor. About 60% of those with a rectal deformity have a second anomaly.

The commonest associated abnormalities are genitourinary (30%), vertebral (30%), alimentary (10%), cardiac (10%), and a variety of other lesions, especially of the central nervous system (20%). Almost any anomaly may be present, but in the alimentary system, oesophageal atresia is not uncommon whereas Hirschsprung's disease is exceptionally rare.

Anomalies in the renal tract are especially important and may be:

(1) Urinary incontinence due to a spinal anomaly (e.g. sacral agenesis) or damage to the pelvic parasympathetics during operation.

(2) Urinary infection due to stasis in the upper urinary tract, for example megaureters, with or without vesico-ureteric reflux, duplex systems or from infection entering via a recto-urethral fistula.

The morbidity is further aggravated by the high incidence of hypoplasia, dysplasia or agenesis of the kidney.

FURTHER READING

De Vries P. A. & Cox K. L. (1985) Surgery of anorectal anomalies. *Surg. Clin. North Amer.* 1139–1170.

De Vries P. A. & Pena A. (1982) Posterior sagittal anorectoplasty. *J. Ped. Surg.* **17**: 638–643.

Goon H. K. (1990) Repair of anorectal anomalies in the neonatal period. *Pediatr. Surg. Int.* **5**: 246–249.

Matley P. J., Cywes S., Berg A. & Ferreira M. (1990) A 20-year follow-up study of children born with vestibular anus. *Pediatr. Surg. Int.* **5**: 37–40.

Ong N-T. & Beasley S. W. (1990) Comparison of clinical methods for the assessment of continence after repair of high anorectal anomalies. *Pediatr. Surg. Int.* **5**: 233–237.

Ong N-T. & Beasley S. W. (1990) Long-term functional results after perineal surgery for low anorectal anomalies. *Pediatr. Surg. Int.* **5**: 233–237.

Ong N-T., de Campo M. & Fowler R. Jr (1990) Computerised tomography in the management of imperforate anus patients following rectoplasty. *Pediatr. Surg. Int.* **5**: 241–245.

Pena A. (1988) Surgical management of anorectal malformations: a unified concept. *Pediatr. Surg. Int.* **3**: 82–93.

Rich M. A., Brock W. A. & Pena A. (1988) Spectrum of genitourinary malformations in patients with imperforate anus. *Pediatr. Surg. Int.* **3**: 110–113.

Rintala R., Lindahl H. & Louhimo I. (1991) Anorectal malformations—results of treatment and long term follow-up in 208 patients. *Pediatr. Surg. Int.* **6**: 36–41.

Stephens F. D. & Smith E. D. (1971) *Anorectal Malformations in Children.* Year Book Medical, Chicago.

Stephens F. D. & Smith E. D. (1986) Classification, identification, and assessment of surgical treatment of anorectal anomalies. *Pediatr. Surg. Int.* **1**: 200–205.

— 9 —

Abdominal Wall Defects

EXOMPHALOS AND GASTROSCHISIS

These two uncommon developmental abnormalities in the region of the umbilicus present at birth as neonatal emergencies that require urgent treatment.

The prevalence of exomphalos (omphalocele) and gastroschisis is relatively similar. Now that maternal ultrasonography is becoming routine in many developed countries, both conditions are recognized often in the first trimester. The high incidence of coexisting abnormalities in a fetus with exomphalos (35%) is often accepted as grounds for termination: if this becomes standard practice, exomphalos should be a rare clinical entity in the future.

In gastroschisis the defect can be identified by ultrasound early in the pregnancy, even before evisceration, which may not occur until much later, and is not usually an indication to terminate the pregnancy.

EXOMPHALOS

This congenital hernia into the base of the umbilical cord probably is caused by incomplete folding of the embryonic disc into three dimensions, with failure of the umbilical ring to form normally. The hernia is covered by fused amniotic membrane and peritoneum, which may rupture during or after birth.

Very occasionally, the membrane ruptures before birth and the eviscerated bowel becomes matted and indurated with dense adhesions, so that the bowel appears to be shorter than normal. The inflammation is believed to be caused by chemical irritation from the urine in the amniotic fluid. Rupture may occur during delivery, in which case the bowel is unaffected.

The size of the defect in the abdominal wall and the size (capacity) of the sac are variable. An intact sac is shiny and translucent but lacks a blood supply and begins to deteriorate at birth. Within 12 h it becomes opaque, yellowish, moist and malodorous; later it becomes black, inelastic, and desiccated.

The diagnosis is obvious (Fig. 9.1); the only difficulty may be in distinguishing a ruptured exomphalos from a gastroschisis. In the latter there are no sac remnants and the defect is small and separate from the umbilical cord (see below).

Coexisting abnormalities are common in exomphalos, particularly cardiac and renal malformations. Malrotation occurs in 12–20% of cases, but seldom

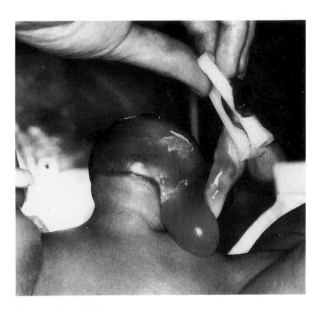

Fig. 9.1 Exomphalos.

causes volvulus, probably because of adhesions be-tween loops and 'secondary' fixation to the parietes. Beckwith-Wiedemann syndrome must be recognized early, because of the severe hypoglycaemia which requires immediate correction. These babies produce excess insulin during gestation, which leads to organo-megaly, exomphalos and excess bodyweight. The exomphalos appears to be secondary to the enlarged viscera, which cannot be accommodated inside the abdomen. Postnatal hypoglycaemia is transient but dangerous because of the risk of brain damage which it may cause.

Investigations

Chest X-ray and echocardiogram are required to exclude a cardiac lesion and intercurrent pulmonary conditions, for example atelectasis or meconium inhalation. The kidneys can be examined by ultrasonography. Careful physical examination may identify other serious ano-malies, which may modify or even preclude treatment.

Treatment

First aid and the method of transport to the tertiary centre are crucial for optimal treatment, and are dis-cussed at the end of this chapter. The aim of treatment is to provide skin coverage as soon as possible includ-ing repair of the muscle defect, if feasible. The method of treatment depends on: (i) the general condition of the infant (size, birthweight, maturity, suitability for anaesthesia); (ii) presence of other anomalies; (iii) whether the sac is intact or ruptured; (iv) the size of the defect; (v) whether part of the liver has herniated into the sac.

Immediate operation and complete repair is the best course when the defect is less than 5 cm in diameter, the infant is fit for surgery, and closure can be obtained.

Excision of the sac (or remnants if ruptured), and construction of a cylindrical tube (a 'silo') can be used for larger defects. A sheet of silastic and teflon is sewn to the edge of the defect. The volume of the silo is reduced in steps over 7–10 days by imbrication, so that the viscera are returned progressively to the abdomen. The prosthesis then is removed and the defect repaired. This method is often used when the sac has ruptured with massive evisceration, but it is not without problems, such as infection around the sutures that anchor the prosthesis to the edge of the defect.

Non-operative management is best when anaes-thesia is contra-indicated because of the poor condition of the infant (prematurity, cardiac anomaly, meconium inhalation) or when the defect is extremely large (> 5 cm in diameter) and contains herniated liver. The sac is painted with an astringent solution to make it a tough, dry eschar which separates when new skin has covered the area beneath it, after 8–12 weeks.

Mercurochrome has been used, but there is a risk of mercury poisoning (hepatic and/or renotubular dam-age) if applied excessively. A 1% aqueous solution applied once (2–3 mL total), with monitoring of the serum and urinary mercury is safe. Other 'tanning' solutions, such as gentian violet and alcohol may be effective, as well as being non-toxic. One advantage of mercurochrome is that it induces a thick layer of granulation tissue over which the skin grows. Subse-quent subcutaneous scarring reduces the hernia pro-gressively over 4–8 months and makes the definitive repair easier.

Once the eschar has formed, and normal feeding and stools are established, the infant can be managed safely at home, avoiding prolonged, costly and risky (because of cross-infection) hospitalization. The appear-ance of the hernia and eschar may be intimidating to the parents who need support and encouragement to achieve satisfactory bonding.

In the occasional infant with skin coverage (obtained by any method) the hernia enlarges more rapidly than the peritoneal cavity. Once the eschar has separated, careful measurements of the circumference and the diameter of the sac ('over the top') vertically and horizontally, should be taken at intervals of 1 month. If the dimensions are decreasing, repair can be deferred until the hernia is nearly flat. If the hernia is increasing, repair should be performed early, and on occasions may be assisted by external pneumatic compression.

GASTROSCHISIS

Recent antenatal ultrasound observations suggest gastroschisis results from rupture of a physiological hernia in the cord (6–10 weeks) or of a minor exomphalos. The fetus usually is normal genetically but has had an 'accident' affecting the umbilical cord. The abdominal wall defect is small (1–3 cm in diameter) and usually a little below and to the right of the umbilicus.

The evisceration may involve almost all the small and large bowel, which become densely matted and adherent with amniotic (chemical) peritonitis and fibrin (Fig. 9.2). The chemical peritonitis is believed to be secondary to urine in the amniotic fluid, particularly during the last trimester.

It differs from a ruptured exomphalos in that there is:

(1) A greater risk of hypothermia

(2) A smaller defect and no sac

(3) Lower incidence of serious coexisting malformations

(4) A greater (but still small) incidence of a small bowel atresia, sometimes 'occult', hidden by matted fibrin.

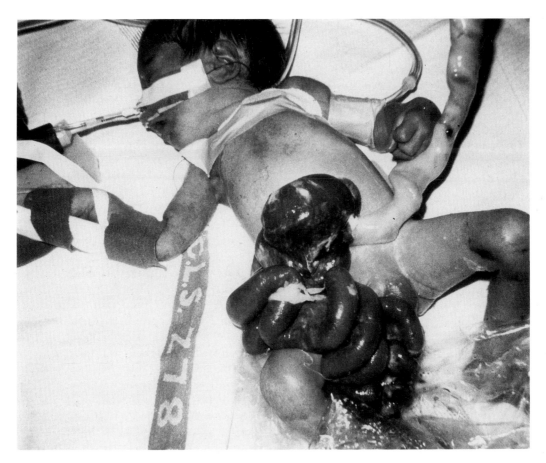

Fig. 9.2 Gastroschisis.

Treatment

Only two methods are available: (i) A prosthetic 'silo' as described above, reducing the viscera over 7–10 days, followed by definitive ('secondary') repair. (ii) Immediate operative reduction of the viscera and primary repair. This has become the method of choice, but success depends on a series of complementary adjuvant steps and requires expert intensive care and nursing. The method involves:

(1) Correction of any physiological disturbances (temperature, hydration, etc)

(2) Anorectal digital dilatation under anaesthesia to decompress the colon

(3) Nasogastric suction to minimize bowel gas

(4) Enlargement of the defect and intraperitoneal 'milking' of the bowel to evacuate as much meconium as possible through the anus

(5) Stretching of the scaphoid anterior abdominal wall to enlarge the capacity of the abdomen

(6) Postoperative mechanical ventilation to counteract splinting of the diaphragm caused by high intra-abdominal pressure when the viscera are 'reduced'

(7) Total parenteral alimentation until effective peristalsis has been restored, sometimes after many weeks

(8) Careful examination of the bowel at laparotomy to detect an 'occult' atresia

When all these are applied effectively, closure should be achieved and almost all infants should survive.

BLADDER EXSTROPHY (ECTOPIA VESICAE)

Failure of fusion of the lower abdominal wall during embryonic development leaves the bladder exposed as a flat plaque on the lower abdomen (Fig. 9.3). There is no covering muscle or skin. The pubic rami do not fuse in the midline. The ureters protrude from the exposed bladder and weep urine. The urethra is a flat strip and the bladder outlet sphincters are not functional. Bladder exstrophy, also known as 'ectopia vesicae', is rare, with an incidence of 1 : 40 000 births. Reconstructive surgery to close the bladder and abdominal wall with

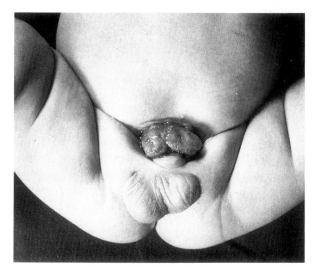

Fig. 9.3 Bladder exstrophy.

restoration of the bladder sphincters is one of the most difficult problems in paediatric surgery.

An even rarer variant of bladder exstrophy is known as cloacal exstrophy. In this condition, the right colon is fused onto the bladder exstrophy and there is an imperforate anus.

FIRST AID AT BIRTH

A baby with an anterior abdominal wall defect is at a greatly increased risk of heat and water loss (because of exposed viscera). Therefore, place the baby in a humidicrib, having wrapped the entire torso, including exposed viscera, in fresh plastic 'kitchen wrap' or aluminium foil, being careful not to twist exposed bowel at the level of the opening in the abdominal wall (Fig. 9.4). Do not use hot wet packs as these cool too quickly and chill the infant. The main objective is to prevent fluid and heat loss during transit to the neonatal surgical unit.

Insert a nasogastric tube to keep the bowel empty and do not feed the baby.

Give intravenous fluids of 10% dextrose + N/5 saline to prevent hypoglycaemia during transport, particularly if the baby has Beckwith's syndrome

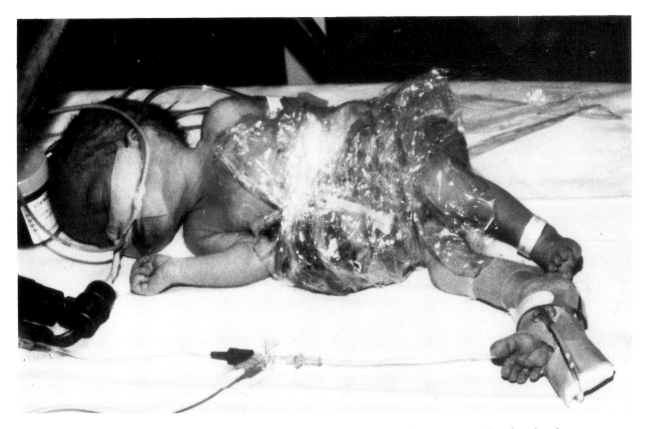

Fig. 9.4 First aid management of gastroschisis. The torso is wrapped in plastic 'kitchen wrap' to reduce heat loss from evaporation. A nasogastric tube keeps the bowel decompressed which facilitates operative reduction of the eviscerated bowel. An intravenous line has been inserted.

(organomegaly, exomphalos and hypoglycaemia secondary to excess fetal insulin production). Arrange transport via a specialized neonatal transport service, if available.

Transport

The infant with an abdominal wall defect should be referred to a fully equipped paediatric surgical centre without delay; if antenatal diagnosis has occurred, the delivery should be in a centre with paediatric surgeons standing by.

FURTHER READING

Beasley S. W. & Jones P. G. (1986) Use of mercurochrome in the management of the large exomphalos. *Aust. Paediatr. J.* **22**: 61–63.

Caniano D. A., Brokaw B. & Ginn-Pearse M. E. (1990) An individualized approach to the management of gastroschisis. *J. Pediatr. Surg.* **25**: 297–300.

Kirk E. P. & Wah R. M. (1983) Obstetric management of the fetus with omphalocele or gastroschisis: a review and report of 112 cases. *Am. J. Obstet. Gynecol.* **146**: 512–518.

Koff S. A. (1990) Technique for bladder neck reconstruction in exstrophy: Cinch. *J. Urol.* **144**: 546–549.

Lester W. M. & Torres A. M. (1985) Omphalocele and gastroschisis. *Surg. Clin. North Am.* **9**: 1235–1244.

Mabogunje O. A. & Mahour G. H. (1984) Omphalocele and gastroschisis. *Am. J. Surg.* **148**: 679–686.

Mitchell M. E., Brito C. G. & Rink R. C. (1990) Cloacal exstrophy reconstruction for urinary continence. *J. Urol.* **144**: 554–558.

Nakayama D. K., Harrison M. R., Gross B. H. *et al.* (1984) Management of the fetus with an abdominal wall defect. *J. Pediatr. Surg.* **19**: 408–413.

Taylor R. G. & Jones P. G. (1989) External pneumatic compression in the late repair of exomphalos major. *Pediatr. Surg. Int.* **4**: 107–109.

Torfs C., Curry C. & Roeper P. (1990) Gastroschisis. *J. Pediatr.* **116**: 1–6.

— 10 —

Spina Bifida

Spina bifida is one of the most crippling congenital anomalies. The primary abnormality is incomplete fusion of the neural tube and overlying ectoderm leading to a defect between the vertebral arches. There is protrusion and dysplasia of the spinal cord and its membranes. The resulting nerve deficit may cause paraplegia, incontinence and multiple orthopaedic deformities. Hydrocephalus is a frequent associated anomaly.

EMBRYOLOGY

Spina bifida and anencephaly are both neural tube defects. The fusion of the neural folds is completed by the fourth week of embryonic development. The mesoderm around the neural tube forms the meninges, vertebral column and muscles. The less severe anomalies involve failure of vertebral arch fusion and protrusion of the meninges to form a meningocele. More severe anomalies involve the neuro-ectoderm with protrusion of the neural tube itself to form a myelomeningocele. Failure of fusion of the brain causes an encephalocele (see Chapter 12) or anencephaly.

AETIOLOGY

The aetiology of spina bifida is unknown, but in 6–8% of cases there is a previous history of hydrocephalus, anencephaly or spina bifida. In these cases the risk of spina bifida in subsequent pregnancies is 1 : 20. With two affected children the risk is 1 : 8. Prenatal diagnosis in spina bifida is well established. Ultrasound may detect the sac and the vertebral defect. The open sac weeps fetal CSF into the liquor and this can be detected by α-fetoprotein estimation in maternal blood or amniotic fluid obtained by amniocentesis.

MYELOMENINGOCELE

This consists of a bifid spine with protrusion and dysplasia of the meninges and spinal cord. The dysplastic spinal cord is splayed over a meningeal sac filled with CSF and is associated with severe nerve deficits below the level of the lesion. This is the most common type and accounts for 94% of neonates with spina bifida. The malformation occurs in both sexes, with a slight predominance in females. The incidence varies widely from country to country and from one region to another within countries. There are also significant annual variations in incidence. The incidence in Australia is fairly high at 1 : 1000 live births.

Clinical features

The sac is in the midline, most commonly in the lumbosacral region (Figs 10.1, 10.2). The size of the sac is variable; there is an area of well-developed skin at the periphery but this is thin at the apex, which is covered

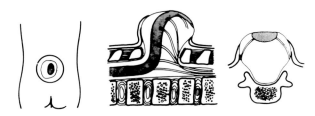

Fig. 10.1 Myelomeningocele. Tissue of the spinal cord forms part of the wall of the sac as well as its contents.

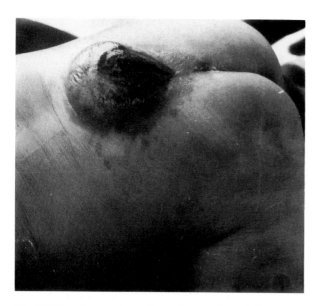

Fig. 10.2 Lumbar myelomeningocele: a moderately large sac with well-developed skin at its periphery. The glistening arachnoid membrane and nervous tissue is exposed on the apex of the sac.

by delicate glistening arachnoid membrane with nervous tissue visible on the surface.

If untreated the central area becomes ulcerated and infected, with a consequent risk of meningitis. Epithelialization occurs slowly, leaving a puckered cicatricial mass covered with poor quality skin liable to ulceration. The coverings may rupture before or during birth, or soon after, with escape of CSF. In rachischisis, the most severe form, the neural tube lies open, no sac is present, and the spinal cord is a flattened, red, velvet-like ribbon down the centre of the back (Fig. 10.3).

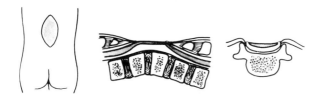

Fig. 10.3 Rachischisis. There is no sac and the central canal of the spinal cord lies wide open on the broad deficiency in the posterior laminae of the vertebrae.

Motor loss

There is a flaccid paralysis of the lower motor neurone type, the extent depending on the level of the neurological lesion. In some patients, upper motor neurone spastic paralysis is present also and is due to either isolated normal sections of the cord below the lesion, or to cerebral or spinal-cord damage from hydrocephalus or meningitis.

Children can be grouped according to the level of the lesion. The motor loss can be assessed by observing the infant's voluntary (not reflex) movements, and the determination of the level is helpful in assessing the probable extent of the ultimate disability (Table 10.1).

Table 10.1 Assessment of level of paralysis

Level of lesion	Incidence (%)	Motor function
Cervical/upper thoracic	1	Paralysis of legs and trunk
Lower thoracic	27	Complete paraplegia including psoas
Upper lumbar	23	Hip flexion and adduction present
Low lumbar/ upper sacral	45	Hip movements, knee extension, foot dorsiflexion
Lower sacral	4	All normal movements

Sensory loss

Sensory loss corresponds closely to the level of motor loss, although the lower level of normal sensation is usually about one segment higher than the lower level of normal motor power. Loss of sensation is most important in the feet, the buttocks and the perineum, because of the risk of pressure sores in these areas.

MENINGOCELE

This is a simple meningeal sac lined by arachnoid membrane and dura, containing CSF and only occasionally

Fig. 10.4 Meningocele. The sac contains CSF only and the cord is normal.

nervous tissue (Fig. 10.4). It is relatively uncommon (6% of cases of spina bifida cystica) and it may be associated with cutaneous lesions.

The sac may be of any size from a small bulge to an enormous protrusion. It may be tense, but more often is soft and fluctuant; some become tense when the baby cries or when pressure is applied to the fontanelle. The skin over the sac is generally intact but is occasionally ulcerated, although this is more typical of myelomeningocele.

Hydrocephalus has been reported but is rare. The mental state of the child is normal and there are no neurological abnormalities. Deaths are rare and are usually due to meningitis developing before or after operative repair.

Treatment consists of repair of the sac, and when the skin is sound there is no urgency; the repair can be done at any convenient time during infancy. If the sac is ulcerated it should be repaired immediately after birth, but if this opportunity is missed, epithelium should be allowed to cover the sac, which is then excised at a convenient time later in infancy.

VARIANTS OF SPINA BIFIDA

The vertebrae may be bifid without a meningocele or myelomeningocele sac. This may be a normal variant of spinal arch fusion; 'spina bifida occulta' is seen with incomplete fusion of the fifth lumbar or first sacral vertebral arches. In fact this minor fusion anomaly is not associated with any nerve defect and does not deserve to be considered in the same context as myelomeningocele.

There are, however, some spina bifida variants of more serious note. Dysplasia of the skin over the spine is a sign of a potentially serious spina bifida: a hairy patch, pigmented naevus, haemangioma, lipoma or a sinus may be present. A dermal sinus over the spine may link with an intraspinal dermoid cyst. If this becomes infected an intraspinal abscess may form with destruction of the adjacent spinal cord.

A spinal lipoma may be indicated by a pigmented, hairy patch over the lumbosacral region or a bulge under the skin. The lower lumbar and sacral nerves run through the fibrolipomatous tissue and progressive nerve damage may occur through spinal cord tethering. These lesions will be demonstrated on computerized tomography or magnetic resonance imaging.

ASSOCIATED ANOMALIES AND SEQUELAE OF SPINA BIFIDA

Hydrocephalus

Hydrocephalus is the most important associated anomaly, for it is present to some degree in almost all cases of myelomeningocele in early infancy. In about 70% it needs investigation and treatment. Hydrocephalus is relatively more common when the myelomeningocele is in the lower thoracic and upper lumbar areas, but it may occur with a myelomeningocele at any level.

The three most common causes of hydrocephalus are the Arnold-Chiari malformation, stricture of the aqueduct of Sylvius and failure of the subarachnoid space to open up at the level of the tentorium.

Hydrocephalus is an important factor which influences the basic decisions in the neonatal period, the child's survival and subsequent mental state.

Orthopaedic deformities

Orthopaedic deformities are very common and greatly complicate management of the paraplegia. They include: kyphosis, lordosis, scoliosis, paralytic dislocation of the hips, flexion contractures of the hips and knees, and deformities of the foot. They are caused by inequality of muscular action and bony immobility leading to inadequate growth stimulus to the skeleton.

Urinary tract abnormalities

Ninety-five per cent of children with myelomeningocele have a neuropathic bladder. The kidneys are usually normal at birth, but there is a high incidence of progressive renal damage during the first few years of life if the problems of high pressure vesicoureteric reflux and chronic pyelonephritis are not treated effectively.

Other anomalies

Other anomalies may be associated with spina bifida, many of them lethal, for example cardiac defects and visceral malformations.

Complications

Meningitis

Meningitis accounts for approximately one-third of all deaths from spina bifida cystica; it arises either from infection of the ulcerated sac (especially if ruptured) or after surgical repair.

Mental retardation

Mental retardation is related to hydrocephalus although separate cerebral deficiencies may occur also. Less than 10% of children without clinical hydrocephalus are retarded, but in children with hydrocephalus who survive without treatment, 38% have normal intelligence, 35% are retarded, and 27% are grossly retarded. With treatment, for example ventriculoperitoneal shunts, these figures are 66, 30 and 4 respectively. Overall, in all children with myelomeningocele who survive to school age intelligence is normal in approximately 77%; retarded but educable in special schools in 21% and grossly retarded in 2%.

Pressure sores

These may develop on the feet, sacrum and perineum; in the latter two sites the problem is accentuated by urinary and faecal soiling. Prevention and treatment of pressure sores is of great importance. For deep, extensive sores in the buttock and sacral area, full-thickness skin grafts may prevent recurrent breakdown.

Special senses

Paralytic squint (i.e. sixth nerve palsy) is a common complication of hydrocephalus, and optic atrophy with blindness occasionally occurs from raised intracranial pressure, usually in older children. Deafness also occurs occasionally, apparently unrelated to the hydrocephalus.

Urinary infection

Stasis in the neurogenic bladder contributes to urinary tract infection and leads to chronic pyelonephritis, which if untreated causes progressive renal scarring. Long term low dose antibiotics and regular drainage of the bladder by intermittent catheterization may prevent or limit these problems.

At 2–3 years of age intermittent catheterization is commenced. The parents pass a 'clean' catheter four to five times a day. In 80% of cases the child wets a little between catheterization, but parents regard this as satisfactory; 10% of children are completely dry between catheterization. In 10% there is marked wetting and the bladder storage capacity may be increased by using α-adrenergic or anticholinergic drugs.

In spina bifida the neurogenic bladder pattern is usually that of retention leading to overflow incontinence; the rationale of 'clean intermittent catheterization' is to empty the bladder frequently, before overflow incontinence occurs.

Paradoxically, catheterization usually lowers the incidence of urinary tract infections by removing stagnant residual urine. However, many children on this regimen will also need low dose antibiotics, for example nitrofurantoin or Co-trimoxazole, daily in one-eighth of the therapeutic dose.

As children grow older the wetting becomes less acceptable. The main two causes of failure of intermittent catheterization are: (i) poor urine storage due to deficient bladder outlet sphincters; (ii) a small bladder capacity with a thick-walled, low compliance bladder. When these children reach school age the bladder storage can be improved by the implantation of an artificial bladder sphincter or by augmentation cystoplasty. Even after these operations intermittent catheterization is still required to empty the bladder.

Faecal incontinence

During early childhood, 'accidents' are common; normal training should be offered and the child taught to evacuate the stool by contraction of the abdominal muscles. Most children are constipated and the aim is to produce a firm stool that is not soft enough to dribble out and not so hard as to impact. This is achieved by diet, laxatives and bulking agents. After adolescence, most patients are clean and regular and evacuate a firm and hard stool. A few patients require a daily suppository or enema. Gross impaction with overflow is cleared by bowel washouts. Biofeedback techniques are useful for some children.

PSYCHOLOGICAL AND SOCIAL MANAGEMENT

Many children show some psychological disturbances as a result of their disabilities, especially in adolescence, though only a few are seriously disturbed. The disturbances are not directly proportional to the degree of disability or to the level of intellectual functioning; nor are they specific to children with spina bifida. Counselling is generally sufficient but some children require additional psychiatric treatment.

Many parents need help to enable them to accept their child's disability realistically. This aspect presents few problems if they have been given a full picture of the condition soon after birth and have been directly involved in treatment, but it can be difficult with parents with previous psychiatric or marital problems.

ASSESSMENT IN THE NEWBORN

Careful assessment by a team of specialists is essential in the neonatal period. A treatment plan should be formulated as early as possible and the following points should be noted:

(1) The presence of other congenital abnormalities, especially those likely to lead to death in infancy or childhood

(2) The type of spina bifida, that is myelomeningocele or meningocele

(3) The level, size and state of the sac

(4) The presence of hydrocephalus and, in the older child, mental retardation

(5) The presence of meningitis

(6) The severity of the orthopaedic disability, recorded by charting muscle activity, especially that of the psoas major, quadriceps and the dorsiflexors and plantar flexors of the ankle

(7) The presence of a neurogenic bladder and bowel, as shown by dribbling urine, a patulous anus, perineal anaesthesia and an expressible bladder

(8) The presence of other urinary tract abnormalities, especially in the upper urinary tract, and of urinary infections

(9) The adequacy of the family. Special problems exist with families who are unable to cope with the considerable strains imposed.

Most of the above points can be evaluated in the neonatal period, and the predicted disabilities should be fully discussed with the parents as soon as possible.

TREATMENT

The aim is to produce an ambulant patient, dry and free of the smell of urine and faeces, functioning to the best of his intellectual and physical potential, educable and capable of employment and independent living. The severity of the disease in some children precludes the attainment of all these objectives. The adverse factors, carrying a high mortality and less satisfactory quality of life in the survivors are: high level lesions associated with complete paraplegia (especially if associated with spinal kyphosis); hydrocephalus clinically present at birth; rapidly developing and progressive hydro-cephalus; meningitis or ventriculitis; other severe con-genital abnormalities; other life-threatening diseases; gross renal pathology.

Initial examination and regular supervision in a special co-ordinated clinic are required for accurate assessment and optimum results.

The sac

The primary decision in the neonatal period concerns operation on the sac. Early operation reduces the inci-dence of meningitis, shortens the stay in hospital, re-lieves the parents of the necessity for constant dressings of the back at home and encourages acceptance of the child by the parents. Early repair of the sac has no significant influence on the development of hydro-cephalus. However, in some children the prognosis is very poor and repair of the sac in these children should be deferred.

The guidelines for treatment are as follows:

Treatment at birth

Caesarean section and immediate postnatal repair may preserve neurological function in some babies where antenatal ultrasound demonstrates good leg movement. There is mounting evidence that trauma during delivery accentuates the degree of neurological deficit. Immedi-ate repair of the sac is indicated in all low lesions in the absence of the adverse factors listed above.

Deferment of sac repair is appropriate in the pres-ence of any of the adverse factors. If the sac is covered with sound skin there is no urgency for repair. If there is a small flat sac repair may never be required.

Subsequent treatment

After the sac is repaired at birth active treatment is given for all subsequent problems, for example shunting for hydrocephalus.

Many children where active treatment was ini-tially deferred will die in the first few months of life, or, because of the severity and progression of the disease, can be expected to die in infancy; active treatment in these children is deferred further unless it is clear that they will survive.

The parents will require sympathetic understand-ing and continuing support during this difficult period and in many cases the child will require terminal care in hospital.

Hydrocephalus

The ventriculoperitoneal shunt is the main technique for the correction of hydrocephalus (Chapter 12).

Orthopaedic treatment

This is aimed at motor development, which should be as near normal as the degree of paralysis will allow. The child with extensive paralysis is given a supportive chair at the age of 3 or 4 months; physiotherapists and occupational therapists encourage activities appropriate to the child's age but which otherwise would be delayed by the paralysis. Standing and walking are encouraged as soon as the child is mature enough to cooperate with these activities; for the severely paralysed child this will be at a later age than normal. Few children fail to achieve walking, but many of those with high lesions will later cease walking because their mobility is greater in a wheelchair than with extensive orthoses and crutches. One-third of affected children walk well with-out orthoses. Children with high lesions (above L3) generally walk in long orthoses with extensions to the lower trunk and with elbow crutches. They tend to develop fixed flexion deformity of the hips and knees which may require surgical release.

The presence of an active quadriceps muscle enables the child to stand by extending the knee joint, so long calipers are not required. When the muscles acting on the feet are weak or inactive, plastic ankle–foot orthoses (AFO) are used to stabilize the feet.

In the common situation in which the dorsiflexors of the ankle are strong but the calf is paralysed, transfer of the tendon of the tibialis anterior posteriorly to the tendo Achilles and calcaneum will prevent progressive deformity.

No orthopaedic treatment is required for children with low sacral lesions.

Other deformities which require treatment are kyphosis and scoliosis. Correction and fusion of paralytic spinal deformities in spina bifida require an operation on the vertebral bodies from in front and on the intact vertebral arches from behind. Internal fixation devices are inserted through both approaches.

Schooling and employment

Most children with spina bifida have a need for assistance at school. Difficulties with access, mobility and continence need to be overcome. Some children with shunted hydrocephalus have specific learning problems. Varying degrees of difficulty with concentration span, attention control and fine motor and perceptual functioning have been noted.

Almost all children with spina bifida cystica attend normal school, 5–10% require special schools for the physically handicapped and a few attend special schools for the mentally handicapped.

Because of the extensive assistance required, those children with the highest lesions may need to attend special school.

During the early years in secondary school, vocational guidance is required to orientate education and training towards suitable employment. Many professional, commercial, clerical and bench-type jobs are suitable for paraplegic patients.

PROGNOSIS

Recently, the mortality of myelomeningocele has been 35–40%. The causes of death have been hydrocephalus (35%), meningitis (51%), with other congenital abnormalities and intercurrent infections contributing in 30%. Most deaths (83%) occur before the age of 1 year, 37% between birth and 28 days, 46% between 29 and 364 days, and 17% at 12 months of age and over.

Deaths after 1 year of age are usually due to excessive intracranial pressure after failure of a shunt for hydrocephalus, or to urinary complications. Many children, even with severe disabilities, reach adult life.

The outlook for children with spina bifida has been transformed in the last two decades and changes in approach and treatment are having a marked effect on the number now expected to survive, and on the facilities that will have to be provided for them.

With the elimination of skeletal tuberculosis and of poliomyelitis, spina bifida is, in Australia now, second only to cerebral palsy as the commonest serious crippling disorder in children.

FURTHER READING

Cass A. S. et. al. (1984) Clean intermittent catheterization in the management of neurogenic bladder in children. J. Urol. **132**: 1526.

Foster L. S., Kogan B. A., Cogen P. H. & Edwards M. S. B. (1990) Bladder function in patients with lipomyelomeningocele. J. Urol. **143**: 984–986.

Hendren W. H. & Hendren R. B. (1990) Bladder augmentation: experience with 129 children and young adults. J. Urol. **144**: 445–453.

Hensle T. W., Connor J. P. & Burbige K. A. (1990) Continent urinary diversion in childhood. J. Urol. **143**: 981–983.

Hutson J. M. & Beasley S. W. (1988) Spina bifida. The Surgical Examination of Children. Heinemann Medical, Oxford.

McLawrin R. L., Oppenheimer S., Dias L. & Kaplan W. E. (eds) (1986) Spina Bifida. A Multidisciplinary Approach. Praeger, New York.

Menelaus M. B. (1980) The Orthopaedic Management of Spina Bifida Cystica, 2nd edn. Churchill Livingstone, Edinburgh.

Minns R. (1986) The management of children with spina bifida and associated hydrocephalus. In: Gordon N. & MacKinlay I. (eds) Neurologically Handicapped Children: Treatment and Management, pp. 109–147. Blackwell Scientific Publications, Oxford.

Raimondi A. J. (1987) Pediatric Neurosurgery. Springer-Verlag, New York.

Shurtleff D. B. (1986) Myelodysplasias and Extrophies: Significance, Prevention and Treatment. Grune and Stratton, Orlando, FL.

11

Ambiguous Sexual Development

No part of a newborn infant's anatomy arouses as much interest initially as the external genitalia. Throughout the pregnancy the parents have contemplated whether their child will be a boy or a girl. The announcement of the gender of the child triggers a set of socially pre-determined and gender-related responses in other members of the family and in friends. These responses traditionally are expressed in gifts, congratulations and celebrations, giving the parents pride and pleasure.

It is therefore an extremely serious matter, a crisis, if the infant's genitalia are abnormal so that the gender is in doubt (Fig. 11.1). The urgency of the situation is heightened by the fact that a genital malformation in the newborn may be the outward sign of a life-threatening internal disorder.

The responsibilities of the attending doctor are: to minimize the distress of the parents and family and to arrange for the immediate diagnosis and treatment of the medical disorder of which the ambiguity is but a part.

DEFINITION

Genitalia are described as ambiguous when: the phallus is too large for a clitoris and too small for a penis; the urethral opening is proximal, near the labioscrotal (genital) folds; the genital folds remain unfused, giving the appearance of labia or a cleft scrotum; testes are either not descended or impalpable (Fig. 11.1).

THE CLINICAL PROBLEMS

When confronted with a newborn baby with ambiguous genitalia, the parents should be told as soon as possible that sexual development is incomplete, that the gender

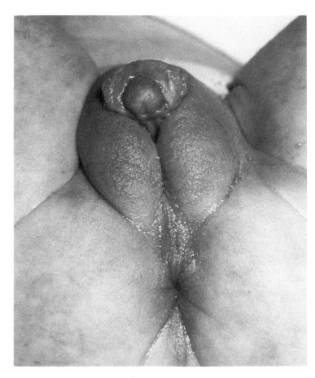

Fig. 11.1 Completely ambiguous appearance of the external genitalia. Is it a boy or is it a girl?

cannot be assigned, and that the necessary information will be sought with the utmost urgency. A consultation with the appropriate specialist will be arranged immediately, and it will be the specialist's role to outline the steps required to obtain the necessary information to determine the sex of rearing. The investigations of this complex problem are outlined below, but two specific entities are the principal sources of ambiguity in the newborn: severe hypospadias with undescended testes, and congenital adrenal hyperplasia.

Severe hypospadias with undescended testes

This condition comes within the definition of ambiguity, although the phallus may be large enough to indicate that the infant is essentially male. In fact, the chromosomal karyotype usually is normal and male (46 XY), and a contrast urethrogram demonstrates a normal male urethra without a vagina or uterus. The testes may be impalpable (in the canal or abdomen) or palpable near the pubic tubercle, on one or both sides.

Treatment consists of urethroplasty and orchidopexy at the appropriate times.

Congenital adrenal hyperplasia

This life-threatening condition occurs in 1 : 8000 live births, and should be identified with urgency by investigations which take priority over all other considerations in the management of ambiguous genitalia.

When congenital adrenal hyperplasia (CAH) occurs in females, the appearance of the external genitalia may be such that the sex is difficult to determine (Fig. 11.2). The ambiguous appearance results from a genetic abnormality, with autosomal recessive inheritance, involving a deficiency of the adrenocortical enzyme, 21-hydroxylase. This enzyme is necessary for the biosynthesis of both cortisol and aldosterone. Cortisol levels therefore are low, and this causes the secretion of pituitary adrenocorticotrophic hormone to increase markedly, resulting in adrenal hyperplasia; because of the enzyme block only androgens are produced, and in a female, these cause virilization.

It is more usual for the degree of virilization to be less severe (Fig. 11.3). If the degree of clitoral enlargement is minor the diagnosis may be overlooked—a potentially dangerous situation because of the associated biochemical defect.

Investigations

(1) The serum electrolytes and blood glucose should be obtained with utmost urgency—within the hour.

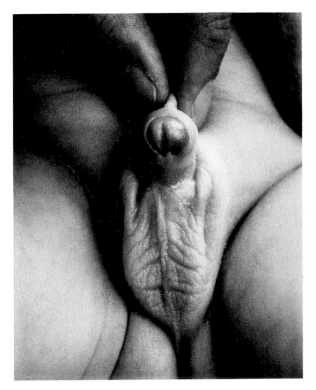

Fig. 11.2 Apparent hypospadias and impalpable testes (actually a female with CAH). (Reproduced with permission from Scheffer I. E., Hutson J. M., Warne G. L. & Ennis G. (1988) *Pediatr. Surg. Int.* **3**: 165–168.)

They reveal low sodium and high potassium, and also hypoglycaemia

(2) Serum 17 hydroxy-progesterone is estimated and the result obtained in 12–24 h. This metabolite is high in all except rare forms of CAH

(3) Chromosomal analysis is arranged (result obtainable in 3 days to 3 weeks)

(4) A 24 h urine specimen is collected for estimation of pregnanetriol and to obtain a gas–liquid chromatography steroid profile. The result is obtainable in 5 days

(5) A urogenital sinugram shows a masculinized urethra but the presence of a vagina and cervix

(6) A pelvic ultrasound confirms the presence of a uterus and fallopian tubes.

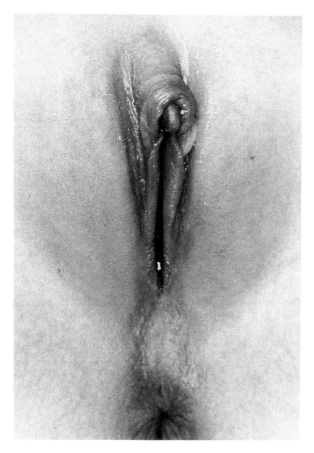

Fig. 11.3 An enlarged clitoris in a girl with CAH.

Treatment

(1) Intravenous rehydration, initially with 0.9% saline

(2) Hypoglycaemia is monitored and corrected with intravenous glucose–saline solution

(3) Cortisone acetate or hydrocortisone are given as soon as blood and urine have been collected for examination.

The anatomy should be established as soon as the biochemical status is stabilized, but with less urgency. For the information, while confirming the diagnosis, is required to enable planning of subsequent surgical correction: that is clitoroplasty and vaginoplasty. It is important to realize, and to inform the parents, that females with CAH have normal reproductive potential.

Other types of ambiguity

This complex subject is beyond the scope of this chapter, but the background is summarized in the following sections.

Internal genitalia

Gonadal differentiation is determined by the karyotype, the Y chromosome being essential for testicular development. Other internal organs develop as persistent parts of the paired embryonic ducts, the Wolffian and Müllerian ducts which are present initially in both males and females.

The testes *in utero* secrete two hormones: testosterone and Müllerian inhibitory substance (MIS), the latter a protein which acts in promoting regression of the Müllerian ducts. Absence of the Müllerian structures (uterus, fallopian tubes and upper vagina) is evidence that MIS must have been secreted and that a testis must be present.

Development of Wolffian ducts requires local stimulation by testosterone, in the absence of which the Wolffian ducts atrophy, with failure of development of their derivates (the epididymis vas deferens and seminal vesicles).

Chromosomal regulation of sexual differentiation

X, Y, and autosomal chromosomes are responsible for sexual differentiation; the Y chromosome directs development of the testis.

Normal development of the ovaries requires two X chromosomes, and the gene encoding for androgen receptors is also located on the X chromosome. The enzymes required for the synthesis of testosterone are regulated by autosomal genes, as is the enzyme 5 α-reductase.

PRACTICAL DECISIONS IN MANAGEMENT

Three aspects are important in the management of infants with ambiguous genitalia:

(1) The specific diagnosis

(2) The sex of rearing

(3) The explanation and counselling given to the parents.

Diagnosis

To reach a specific diagnosis, the advice of a paediatric endocrinologist, and detailed biochemical and anatomical investigations, are required because:

(1) There may be genetic implications affecting counselling

(2) The potential fertility of the infant should be established

(3) Urgent medical treatment may be required, for example in CAH

(4) A plan for surgical management is necessary.

However, in many children no specific diagnosis is possible.

Sex of rearing

The appropriate sex of rearing maximizes the patient's prospects of fertility and minimizes the risk of psychological damage.

Fertility in the male depends upon testes capable of spermatogenesis, a patent pathway and a penis with sufficient erectile tissue for erection and insemination. A good-sized phallus is rarely present in male infants with ambiguous genitalia, and fertility is usually impossible.

In the female, ovulation and a pathway to the uterus are required, but future developments in *in vitro* fertilization, using donor gametes and transplantation of an embryo, may permit pregnancy in a female with a uterus and vagina but no ovaries or fallopian tubes. There are greater opportunities, therefore, for active participation in the reproductive process in those raised as females where a uterus is present.

Psychological damage is much more likely when a patient is raised unsuccessfully as a male than in those reared electively as a female. Embarrassment due to a micro-phallus, inability to void standing and a phallus inadequate for intercourse, all create major or insuperable problems.

There is, therefore, an onus to demonstrate the appropriateness and practicality of rearing as a male before irrevocably deciding on this course for a particular patient.

Counselling parents

Parents should never be allowed to think of their child as somewhere 'in between' male and female. They should be frankly told when the gender is unclear, that tests will be carried out urgently and how long this will take, and promises must be kept.

The gender is the sex of rearing, and once decided, should be reinforced at every opportunity by referring to the infant as 'he' or 'she', never 'it'. It is important to reassure parents that genital ambiguity and malformations do not lead to homosexuality, a fear many parents experience but rarely express. It is helpful to explain to parents that in both sexes, the genitalia go through an undifferentiated stage; and that differentiation is extremely complex and not always complete.

FURTHER READING

Donahoe P. K. & Crawford J. D. (1986) Ambiguous genitalia in the newborn. In: Welch K. J., Randolph J. G., Ravitch M. M. O'Neill J. A. & Rowe M. I. (eds), *Pediatric Surgery*, 4th edn, Vol. 1, p. 589. Year Book, Chicago.

Grumbach M. M. & Conte F. A. (1985) Disorders of sexual differentiation, In: Wilson J. D. & Foster D. W. (eds), *Williams Textbook of Endocrinology*, 7th edn, p. 313 Saunders, Philadelphia.

Hutson J. M. & Beasley S. W. (1988) Ambiguous genitalia: is it a boy or a girl? In: *The Surgical Examination of Children* pp. 257–266. Heinemann Medical, Oxford.

New M. I., Pang S. & Levine L. S. (1985) An update in congenital adrenal hyperplasia, In: Lifshitz F. (ed.), *Pediatric Endocrinology—A Clinical Guide*, p. 203. Marcel Dekker, New York.

Saenger P. (1984) Abnormal sexual differentiation. *J. Pediatr.* **104**: 1–17.

12

The Skull and Brain

THE INFANT WITH A LARGE HEAD

When suspicion arises that an infant's head is enlarging too rapidly, measurements must be repeated over a period of weeks or months, and compared with the normal curve for this dimension. Deviations from normal (Fig. 12.1) are grouped as follows:

(1)   A steadily increasing divergence above the normal curve, commencing at birth

(2)   A normal curve interrupted by some event, for example a subdural haemorrhage or an infection, with subsequent increase greater than normal

(3)   An accelerated rate of growth initially, followed

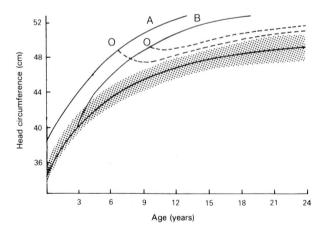

Fig. 12.1 Variations in the growth curve of the infant head, showing the average and the 90th and 10th percentiles. The two additional curves represent: (a) hydrocephalus present from birth; (b) acquired hydrocephalus following meningitis, indicated by a deviation above normal limits at 3 months of age. In each case operation (○) is followed by a return towards normal.

by less rapid growth which continues at a high level but parallel to the normal curve.

The first two groups need treatment, but in the third, unless the accelerated growth in the initial period is very great, operation may be deferred until stabilization occurs.

An enlarging head may be the result of factors other than the accumulation of CSF, although these are uncommon. The infant's head may enlarge because of thickening of the skull bones, as in diffuse osteofibromatosis, and be readily recognizable in X-rays. The brain itself may be large, without any increase in the size of the ventricles. This condition, macrocephaly, is diagnosed by finding ventricles of normal size. The intelligence is sometimes above normal, but the reverse is more common: the larger the head the more the patient is retarded.

Localized expanding lesions, for example subdural haematoma, simple intracerebral or arachnoid cysts or, very occasionally, a cystic neoplasm, may also cause enlargment of the head.

Hydrocephalus

Most infants with a large head suffer from excess CSF caused by: (i) excessive production; (ii) obstruction along the CSF pathway; or (iii) impaired absorption into the veins.

Increased production of CSF causing hydrocephalus is rare and is limited to two conditions: papilloma of the choroid plexus; and arteriovenous malformations involving the great vein of Galen.

Obstruction to the flow of CSF is the commonest cause of hydrocephalus, and is further subdivided as follows:

(1) Non-communicating or internal hydrocephalus in which there is no communication between the subarachnoid space and the ventricles. The latter are greatly enlarged without distension of the basal cisterns or cerebral sulci (Fig. 12.2)

(2) In communicating hydrocephalus the ventricles communicate with the basal cisterns, but there is an obstruction between these and the subarachnoid spaces in the region of the sagittal sinus.

The most frequent causes of obstruction are a primary developmental anomaly or obstruction secondary to haemorrhage or infection. Intracerebral haemorrhage in premature babies is now common. Tumours may obstruct the ventricular system in the older child, but only 5% of cases of hydrocephalus in infancy are caused by a neoplasm.

Failure of absorption of the CSF may occur temporarily, as a result of inflammatory exudate around the arachnoidal villi. Permanent and severe derangement

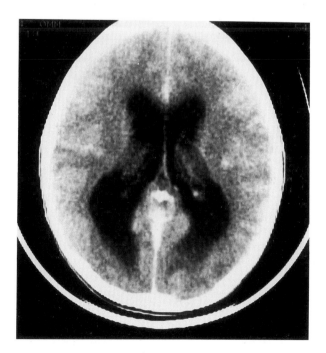

Fig. 12.2 Non-communicating hydrocephalus. CT scan showing massive dilatation of the ventricles.

follows thrombosis of the sagittal or lateral sinuses in the newborn as a result of dehydration; the result is a sudden enlargement of the head. Inadequate absorption of CSF also may occur when the intracranial venous pressure is raised, for example an arteriovenous malformation involving the venous sinuses, but this is extremely rare.

Summary of causes

Although there are many possible causes of hydrocephalus, only three are common:

(1) Subarachnoid obstruction at the level of the tentorium

(2) Stricture of the aqueduct

(3) Obstruction of the CSF at any level by tumours or cysts.

In planning the correct approach to the problem of hydrocephalus, in estimating the prognosis and in deciding which operative procedure is best, the cause and the rate of enlargement must be determined. Sometimes this is possible after a consideration of the history, the physical signs, and a chart of the rate of growth (Fig. 12.1), but more often special investigations are needed.

Clinical signs

A skull circumference which is increasing faster than the normal increments for the age of the infant is the main clinical feature and the indication for investigation and treatment. The deviation is depicted by plotting the measurements of the circumference obtained at regular intervals on a graph of the normal curve (Fig. 12.1).

The shape of the head becomes abnormal (Fig. 12.3). The frontal region is prominent in all types, but in stricture of the aqueduct, expansion of the lateral ventricles produces an 'occipital overhang' above the small posterior fossa as well. The opposite occurs when the fourth ventricle is expanded as a result of occlusion of its foramina; the external occipital protuberance is pushed upwards.

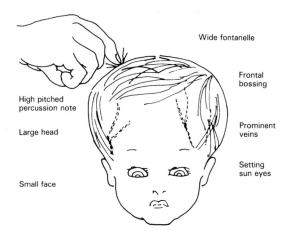

Wide fontanelle

Frontal bossing

High pitched percussion note

Prominent veins

Large head

Setting sun eyes

Small face

Fig. 12.3 Hydrocephalus. Seven clinical signs are illustrated in a diagram of a typical case.

Raised intracranial pressure produces a wide anterior fontanelle, separation of the cranial sutures, and a raised or drum-like note on percussion of the skull.

Abnormal neurological signs from hydrocephalus alone are unusual. The sixth cranial nerve is vulnerable because of its long course and, a lateral rectus palsy causing internal strabismus may occur. Persistent downward deviation of the eyes ('setting sun') is present with certain types of hydrocephalus. There may be brain-stem signs when the obstruction is acute and hydrocephalus develops rapidly, that is increased extensor tone with rigidly extended lower limbs and clenched hands with the fingers over the infolded thumb. Retraction of the head and opisthotonus also may be present.

Transillumination of the head by a beam of bright light in a darkened room often will show characteristic patterns. General transillumination indicates a gross and uniform dilatation of the ventricles. Unilateral translucency may indicate a subdural collection of fluid, and other localized bright areas may indicate large cysts or a large dilated fourth ventricle.

Investigations

Ultrasound imaging is a non-invasive means of diagnosing hydrocephalus in infancy. Once closure of the fontanelle occurs, the technique is no longer applicable. Little or no special preparation is required; the procedure is risk free and can be repeated as often as necessary.

Computerized tomography (CT) is used in the older child, and in infants, if more detail is required. A CT scan gives a clear image of the intracranial anatomy and provides a precise means of detecting the presence of hydrocephalus, determining its extent and frequently demonstrates the site and cause of obstruction.

Magnetic resonance imaging (MRI) is required rarely, but may be of assistance in defining the aetiology. The CSF dynamic scan involves the use of a solution containing a radionuclide tracer injected into the CSF pathway, and its passage through the ventricles and subarachnoid space is followed. Obstructions and abnormalities in the passage of CSF, from production to final absorption, can be recorded.

Angiography is employed infrequently. In certain cases intracranial pressure monitoring may help to determine the need, or otherwise, for treatment. Plain X-rays are generally of no great value but may be of use in confirming a diagnosis of raised intracranial pressure.

Treatment

Not all infants with enlargement of the head require operation, but if there is evidence of a continued deviation from the normal curve and/or signs of raised intracranial pressure the child should be investigated in the manner described above. Operation is indicated when there is sustained deviation from the normal curve in infants without obvious evidence of hopeless brain damage.

There are various methods of controlling an expanding head, but all depend on one of three principles:
(1) Reduction of CSF production
(2) Reconstitution of CSF pathways within the cranium
(3) Diversion of CSF to a site outside the cranium.

Production of CSF can be reduced by a drug which acts directly on the choroid plexus to reduce production (carbonic anhydrase inhibitor) or by an osmotic agent.

Control is frequently incomplete and of short-term benefit only.

Removal of a mass may allow CSF to return to a normal flow pattern. Tumours in the posterior fossa frequently cause hydrocephalus and excision of the tumour leads to a rapid resolution in most cases. Internal shunt operations are rarely performed now, but ventriculocisternostomy occasionally has a place in the treatment of hydrocephalus due to stricture of the aqueduct in older patients.

External removal of CSF is the usual method of treating this disorder. In some types of hydrocephalus, particularly in premature infants, removal may be undertaken intermittently, via lumbar puncture (communicating hydrocephalus), or via a ventricular reservoir; this controls the hydrocephalus until normal pathways are re-established.

A ventriculoperitoneal shunt, a more definitive procedure, is usually the operation of choice in children of all ages. This shunt comprises a ventricular catheter, a valve or flushing device beneath the scalp, and a long kink-resistant tube passing along the chest wall to enter the peritoneal cavity. A long length of tube is placed within the peritoneal cavity to allow for subsequent growth of the patient. Less frequently a ventriculo-atrial shunt to divert the CSF into the right atrium is performed.

Complications

(1) Obstruction. Most frequently the ventricular tube becomes clogged with choroid plexus or cerebral tissue. The lower end may be obstructed by the growth of the child which displaces the lower end into an unsuitable position, by adherence to the greater omentum and by fracture of the tube. Rarely, the valve may malfunction.

(2) Infection. The shunt system becomes colonized by pathogenic organisms.

These complications are often difficult to diagnose, and catastrophic in their results. They must be assessed and corrected urgently.

A child with a shunt must be reviewed at regular intervals during the growing years, and parents must be informed of the nature of the procedure and the possible complications. In general, if the diagnosis is established before hydrocephalus is advanced, if there are no other significant brain anomalies, and if the treatment is appropriate and maintained, then the patient has every chance of developing normally. Such children should be encouraged to lead a completely normal life.

CONGENITAL ABNORMALITIES OF THE CRANIUM

Errors in the development of the scalp, skull and brain are not as common as those of the spinal cord, but they present the same bewildering variety of abnormalities. Only the more common or important ones are shown here.

Dermoid sinus

This is found most frequently in the occipital region and may communicate with a more deeply situated dermoid cyst containing sebaceous material and hairs. The sinus may have some fine hairs protruding from it and usually discharges sebaceous material. The deeper component can cause all the signs of an intracranial tumour with cerebellar signs predominating; it may also become infected.

An intracranial dermoid can occur without an external sinus. Infection is uncommon and the cyst presents by causing obstruction of the CSF. Rarely, the cyst ruptures, leading to aseptic meningitis.

Dermoid cysts are common near the orbital margin and are described in Chapter 16.

Craniosynostosis

Premature closure of the sutures between the bones of the vault, which act as lines of growth, restricts development of the region, although compensatory growth occurs at other suture lines. The subsequent distortion in the shape of the skull is a severe cosmetic defect, but only occasionally does it cause sufficient diminution of the intracranial capacity to limit the growth of the brain and cause mental retardation.

The shape of the deformity depends on which suture or sutures are involved. There are three common forms and three others less easily recognized, and all produce characteristic deformities.

Scaphocephaly

The sagittal suture is fused and growth continues at the coronal and lambdoid sutures. The head is long and narrow—like an upturned boat—and often has a prominent frontal region (Fig. 12.4).

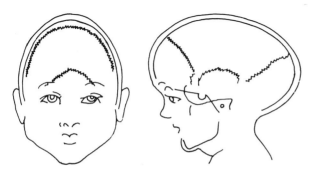

Fig. 12.4 Scaphocephaly, caused by fusion of the sagittal suture, is the commonest form of craniosynostosis.

Brachycephaly

The coronal sutures are closed and the head has a short anteroposterior and wide biparietal diameter; the eyes are widely separated and 'bulging' (Fig. 12.5).

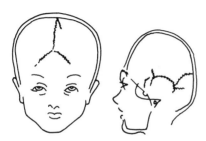

Fig. 12.5 Brachycephaly. The head is short and wide and the eyes are prominent, following fusion of the coronal sutures.

Turricephaly

The coronal and sagittal sutures are obliterated; the skull enlarges vertically with a high vault, a 'tower skull' (Fig. 12.6).

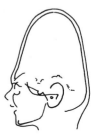

Fig. 12.6 Turricephaly. The head is narrow, short and high, after fusion of all sutures except the lambdoid.

Unilateral closure of one coronal suture produces a severe disturbance of growth of the forehead and the orbit with flattening of the forehead on the affected side, bulging on the other, and a deformed orbit which interferes with binocular vision.

Premature closure of the metopic suture leads to a narrow, pointed forehead with the eyes closely set together. The lambdoid suture is affected less frequently and produces asymmetry of the back of the head.

The diagnosis can be made by observation of the shape of the head and is confirmed by radiography.

Treatment

The appearance and the risk of mental retardation are the two indications for treatment by the craniofacial surgical team. The cosmetic defect can be severe if nothing is done. Early operation, before 3 months of age, results in a head of almost normal size and shape.

Mental retardation probably occurs in only 10% of these children, and its likelihood is to be suspected when radiographs show signs of increased intracranial pressure, that is digital impressions and separation of the unfused sutures. Headache, vomiting and papilloedema are rare, but exophthalmos and ophthalmoplegia are not infrequent.

Operation consists of either simple linear craniectomy (excision of a strip of bone along the fused suture) or radical removal and repositioning of the vault bones. In the former, the bone edges are covered to delay refusion while expanding brain moulds the head into a normal shape.

In recent years major advances have been made in the surgical reconstruction of the face and cranium when severely deformed by malformations such as the Crouzon's syndrome and Apert's syndrome. Very considerable cosmetic improvement can now be obtained.

Cranium bifidum (including encephalocele)

Defects in the neural folds at the cephalic end of the embryo are much less common than in the lumbar region. The same basic types occur, mostly in the occipital region, but in some countries, for example Thailand, they are more common in the frontal area.

The herniations are in the midline (Fig. 12.7), well covered with skin and lined by meninges, and may contain CSF alone or, more frequently, brain (encephalocele). Occasionally, the herniation occurs into the nasal cavity, and the sac is then covered by mucosa, not skin.

Other intracranial abnormalities also may be present, so an ultrasound or a CT scan is necessary to detect these before surgical repair.

Simple excision of the sac and its contents, and sound closure of the dura and the bone defect usually can be effected. Encephaloceles cause severe brain dysfunction (mental retardation, blindness, hydrocephalus), which may preclude treatment.

Plagiocephaly

This is a common deformity which affects the entire skull. One frontal region and the opposite occipital region are flat and the contralateral areas are full and rounded; for example right frontal and left occipital flat, left frontal and right occipital rounded (Fig. 12.8). On the side with the flat frontal area, the ear and the parietal eminence are placed more posteriorly and the face is wider. The effect is that the longest diameter is displaced from the sagittal axis towards the side with the prominent frontal contour.

Plagiocephaly is either congenital or acquired, and when present at birth it may have been caused by

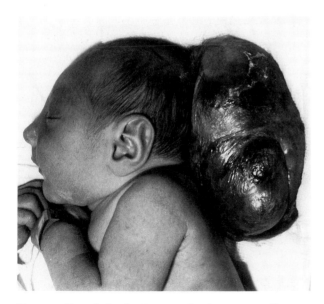

Fig. 12.7 Encephalocele. An example of a severe midline herniation with cranium bifidum, which is a neural tube defect.

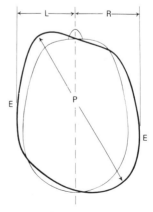

Fig. 12.8 Plagiocephaly. The long axis (P) is deflected from the sagittal plane. The right ear (E) is more posterior and the right half of the face appears wider.

contact of the fetal head with the maternal pelvis or with some irregularity of the uterine wall, for example fibroids. In some patients, there may be inadequate growth in the lambdoid suture on one side.

Plagiocephaly can be acquired in the first 3–4 months after birth in torticollis causing one occipital area to bear the weight of the cranium and the brain, which determines the shape of the thin and largely membranous calvarium. The deformity can be minimized by placing babies with postural or sternomastoid torticollis in such a way that they sleep on each side alternately and never supine.

The deformity tends to return towards normal after the age of 6 months and usually in the first 2 years. A minor degree probably persists indefinitely, though this is not readily detected when hair obscures the contours of the skull. Surgery generally is not indicated except in infants with a significant deformation due to abnormal function of the lambdoid suture.

INTRACRANIAL TUMOURS

Tumours of the central nervous system are the largest group of malignancies, excluding leukaemia, in childhood. Even the benign tumours, because of their inaccessible sites, the inexpandable nature of the surrounding tissue and their tendency to infiltrate and recur locally, must be considered as malignant in the broadest sense. Unless operation is carried out at an early stage, there is little hope of extirpation or reasonable prospect of survival.

Mode of presentation

The mode of presentation in children differs in many ways from that seen in adults:

(1) The common types of tumour and their sites of origin are different; for example the preponderance of tumours in the posterior fossa in childhood (Fig. 12.9)

(2) Children adapt better to an expanding intracranial lesion; accommodation for weeks or even months is possible, but once this fails, the final decline is often catastrophic

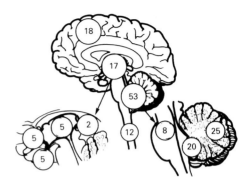

Fig. 12.9 Cerebral tumours. The percentage distribution of 300 consecutive tumours treated at the Royal Children's Hospital, Melbourne.

(3) Many tumours arise close to the CSF pathways in relatively 'silent' areas, so neurological signs are few or absent until the flow of CSF is obstructed, when signs of raised intracranial pressure; for example headache, vomiting and papilloedema, develop with alarming suddenness

(4) Early signs often affect the vision, but loss of acuity or diplopia are not appreciated in early childhood and never arise as symptoms in infants

(5) Neurological signs may present clearly, while evidence of raised intracranial pressure appears much later. In infants and younger children, the dramatic development of raised intracranial pressure may initiate a search for localizing signs which only then are recognized.

Intracranial tumours can be divided into three main groups, each of which produces a more or less typical clinical pattern.

Group I: Glial tumours of the cerebral hemispheres

These are five times less common than those in the posterior fossa and tend to be highly malignant. In the few relatively benign tumours, the fibrillary astrocytoma and the haemangioblastoma, cysts form and grow slowly, and the survival rate is good.

The clinical picture is similar to that of adults, and diagnosis and management follow the same lines.

Group II: Tumours in the region of the third ventricle

These form a very important group in childhood. Their progress is often insidious until there are signs of ventricular obstruction. Those situated anteriorly produce defects in vision, and those at the back of the third ventricle cause disturbances in ocular movements. The four types in this group tend to cause diagnostic localizing signs early: optic glioma; craniopharyngioma; pineal tumours; posterior gliomas.

Gliomas of the optic chiasm

Gliomas of the optic chiasm and optic nerves cause bizarre field defects and loss of visual acuity before obstructing the third ventricle. The optic discs show no papilloedema, but rather the white disc of optic atrophy. Frequently, they are associated with generalized neurofibromatosis. Impaired vision, squint and proptosis are common.

Infants may present with hydrocephalus or with involvement of the hypothalamus causing wasting and anorexia known as the 'diencephalic syndrome', and a similar lesion in older children may cause precocious puberty.

Specific treatment is difficult and shunts to relieve ventricular obstruction sometimes are necessary. Long term survivals are not uncommon.

Craniopharyngioma

The craniopharyngioma grows extremely insidiously. It arises in, above or behind the sella turcica from a remnant of the primitive Rathke's pouch and compresses the pituitary gland, slowing growth and development and gradually depressing vision. The tumour is usually not suspected until the child has had defective sight for years, growth and development have lagged behind or the child tires easily and is unable to keep up with his peers.

When the tumour is detected early, it can be removed totally without damage to the optic nerves or the pituitary gland. Later operations may be incomplete and followed by persistent pituitary deficiency. Steroid and other hormone replacement therapy has improved the outlook for these patients.

Tumours of the pineal gland

These occur in three forms:
    (1)   A small infiltrating tumour of the brain stem
    (2)   A more massive tumour containing much calcification; or
    (3)   A large teratoma with solid and cystic areas.

Often they obstruct the aqueduct before local signs develop so that headache, vomiting, papilloedema and impaired consciousness are the presenting features. Later, involvement of the oculomotor nuclei causes a loss of upward gaze, a distinctive localizing sign.

When there is extensive calcification diagnosis by CT scan is easy.

Management begins with relief of the obstruction by ventriculoperitoneal shunt, followed by removal of the pinealoma. This may be incomplete, but radiotherapy controls further growth effectively.

Glial tumours near the aqueduct

These present in the same fashion, but extend more widely. They are treated by a shunt and radiotherapy. The prognosis is variable, with some long term survivors.

Group III: Tumours of the posterior fossa

These form 50% of all intracranial tumours in childhood, and those in the cerebellum cause ventricular obstruction early, so that headache and vomiting—characteristically in the early morning—appear before neurological signs such as incoordination, ataxia, hypotonia and tremor. In brain-stem gliomas, gross incoordination, ataxia and cranial nerve palsies may precede signs of increased intracranial pressure. There are four common tumours in this region.

Medulloblastoma

This is a cellular tumour of the vermis forming a massive growth which blocks the fourth ventricle (Fig. 12.10). It spreads out into the basal cisterns and characteristically disseminates widely throughout the CSF pathways, particularly in the spinal canal.

The tumour occurs more often in males at about 2 years of age, with a typical history of morning headaches and vomiting, change in personality and clumsiness of gait. The patient is usually a good-looking, attractive child, with a wan facial expression as if forewarned of his fate. Papilloedema and truncal ataxia are the common neurological signs and there may be tilting of the head when the child sits up. The skull has a high-pitched note on percussion with the fingertip ('cracked pot' sign). At presentation, there is often a large tumour in the fourth ventricle with CSF seedlings. After excision, the tumour may recur locally and disseminate unless it responds to adjuvant new radiotherapeutic techniques and chemotherapy.

Astrocytoma of the cerebellum

This presents a brighter picture, but the prognosis still depends upon the histological pattern. Fast growing tumours recur early, while those with a fibrillary matrix and few mitotic figures can be cured if excised completely.

An astrocytoma may be solid and well-defined or a nodule of tumour in the wall of a cyst or even the lining of a simple cyst. Children are older (about 5 years) than those with a medulloblastoma; the length of the history

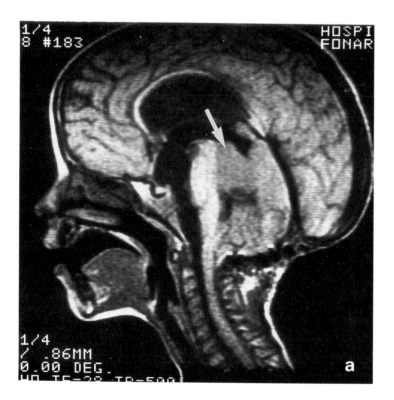 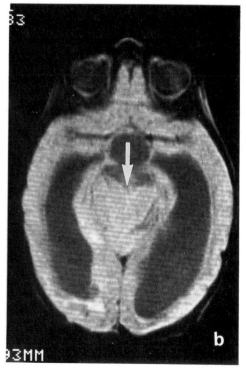

Fig. 12.10 Medulloblastoma. A MRI scan showing a massive posterior fossa tumour blocking the fourth ventricle in (a) sagittal section and (b) transverse section.

is 3–6 months rather than weeks, beginning with morning headaches and vomiting. Much later, usually in the 2–3 weeks before diagnosis, squint, incoordination and ataxia appear. The clinical signs are fairly constant: papilloedema, squint, mild ataxia and incoordination of hand movements.

There is usually a localized tumour, in one lateral lobe, which is removable completely. Radiotherapy is not advised for the benign fibrillary types; otherwise, its effectiveness is related to the histological picture.

Glioma of the brain-stem

This causes brain-stem enlargement without much evidence of a localized tumour. The age incidence is wide and the signs are caused by cranial nerve palsies and involvement of the long tracts passing through the brain-stem: gross strabismus, facial weakness, difficulty in swallowing, hemiparesis and ataxia occur. The child is miserable and pathetic, quite different from those with other types of posterior fossa tumours.

The diagnosis is confirmed by CT or MRI scanning, and it is rare that the tumour can be removed surgically. Radiotherapy is used, with variable results. In most patients, the signs resolve rapidly during treatment but recur within 3–6 months. A few seem to achieve a longer period of relief.

Ependymoma

The mode of presentation is similar to medulloblastoma. At operation, the tumour frequently is attached to the floor of the fourth ventricle and, like the medulloblastoma, the tumour has the same tendency to metas-tasize in the CSF pathways. The overall prognosis is worse.

TUMOURS IN THE SPINAL CANAL

In childhood these usually arise from paravertebral structures, and neuroblastoma is the commonest. Primary vertebral and intrathecal tumours are so rare that in the first 2–3 years of life the commonest lesion is a metastasis from a medulloblastoma.

In later childhood other intrathecal tumours appear, for example neurofibromas of the nerve roots and ependymomas of the spinal cord. Slowly progressive weakness of the lower limbs, with abnormal reflexes, is suggestive and the diagnosis is established by myelography, a spinal CT or MRI scan.

FURTHER READING

Albright A. L., Price R. A. & Guthkelch A. N. (1983) Brain stem gliomas of children. A clinicopathological study. *Cancer* **53**: 2313.

David J. O., Poswillo D. & Simpson D. (1982) *The Craniosynostoses*. Springer Verlag, Berlin.

Hooper R. S. (1976) Intracranial and spinal tumours: In: Jones P. G. & Campbell P. E. (eds), *Tumours of Infancy and Childhood*, pp. 231–294. Blackwell Scientific Publications, Oxford.

Milhorat T. H. (1978) *Pediatric Neurosurgery*. F. A. Davis, Philadelphia.

Raimondi A. J. & Tomita T. (1981) Hydrocephalus and infratentorial tumours. Incidence, clinical picture and treatment. *J. Neurosurg.* **55**: 174.

Szymonowicz W., Yu V. Y. H. & Lewis E. A. (1985) Posthaemorrhagic hydrocephalus in the preterm infant. *Aust. Paediatr. J.* **21**: 175–179.

Till K. (1975) *Paediatric Neurosurgery for Paediatricians and Neurosurgeons*. Blackwell Scientific Publications, Oxford.

13

The Eye

Ocular signs and symptoms (Table 13.1) in children can aid the diagnosis of both systemic and local diseases, and their early detection also may preserve sight. In infancy the only history is by a parent, so a careful examination is crucial. The points to be observed when examining the eyes are summarized in Table 13.2.

Suspected poor vision

When parents suspect that their infant is blind, the problems facing the clinician are complex, for the blindness may be irreversible, and objective assessment of vision is difficult.

The macula is not differentiated fully until about 4 months of age, when the fovea becomes visible. The macula contains a high density of cone cells responsible for acute vision and colour perception, whereas the fovea contains only cone cells. When the visual field is plotted, the macula is represented by its centre, and 'macular viewing' is referred to as 'central vision' or 'central fixation'. Macular damage in infants may cause nystagmus known as 'fixation nystagmus'.

Table 13.1 Common ocular symptoms and signs in children

Suspected poor vision
Strabismus (squint)
The white pupil (leukocorea)
Epiphora (watering eye)
The 'small' eye
The 'large' eye
Abnormal head posture
Conjunctival discharge
Headache

Table 13.2 What to look for during examination of the eye

Clarity of the optic media
A clear cornea
A black pupil
Normal pupillary reflexes
Absence of nystagmus
Ability to fix on a light by the age of 6 weeks
Ability to follow a moving object at 4 months (macular function established)
Ability to pick up coloured beads and small objects

Infants will fix on a face, especially the mother's, within the first few days of life. Regular eye contact should be obtained by 6–8 weeks of age. Consistent absence of these phenomena suggests delayed visual development which may be cortical in origin. In infants blind from birth, unsteady fixation and searching movements of the eyes mimicking nystagmus appear at about 4 months of age. The onset of nystagmus in a child less than 4 years of age strongly suggests interference with the visual pathway.

Nystagmus along with poor 'following' is strong evidence of blindness, whereas good 'following' despite nystagmus suggests disturbance of motor control of the eyes.

Visual acuity in older children, that is 3–3.5 years and older, can be determined fairly accurately by the 'E' test. Only the letter E is presented, but it can be pointed up, down or to either side. An 'E chart', similar to the ordinary Snellen's Test Chart, is used and the child points his finger (or an E on another card) in the same direction as in the one presented.

In the Sheridan Gardener test the child is given a card with seven different letters on it, and the examiner holds up letters asking the patient to point to the one on the card which is the same.

STRABISMUS (SQUINT)

This occurs when there is a failure of co-ordination of the eyes (Fig. 13.1). Normally, the macula of each eye is able to look at an object simultaneously from 2 to 3 months of age; strabismus after this age requires immediate investigation to prevent suppression of vision (amblyopia) in the deviated eye. Suppression may become permanent if left untreated. Surgery is often performed in the first year of life. Binocular vision can be obtained in about half, emphasizing the need for early diagnosis and treatment.

Causes

Co-ordinated use of the eyes requires a reflex arc: the afferent arc is the visual pathway, the efferent arc is the motor nerves supplying the ocular muscles, while the central connections lie in the occipital cortex and brain-stem.

Sensory or 'afferent' causes of strabismus include corneal scarring, cataracts or diseases of the central retina (e.g. toxoplasmosis), all of which may interfere with co-ordination and lead to strabismus. Every child with a squint should be regarded as having a potentially blind eye, because of a structural abnormality or because of suppression of the vision in the deviated eye.

Motor or 'efferent' causes include birth injuries of the oculomotor nerves, congenital abnormalities of the extraocular muscles or of their innervation, and congenital abnormalities of the orbit.

A refractive error also interferes with afferent impulses, for if there is a marked difference in the refractive properties of the two eyes, there is a tendency to suppress the vision in the eye with the greater error. Hypermetropia (long sight) causes a convergent strabismus, and myopia sometimes results in a divergent strabismus. When an object is observed at a short distance from the eye, three changes occur:

(1) Constriction of the pupil

(2) Convergence of the eyes

(3) Accommodation, that is focusing on the object.

These are all interrelated, so that any increase in the effort required to focus may cause disharmony and result in overconvergence, as seen in some children who are long-sighted. Glasses can correct the hypermetropia and restore harmony between convergence and focusing, with disappearance of the squint.

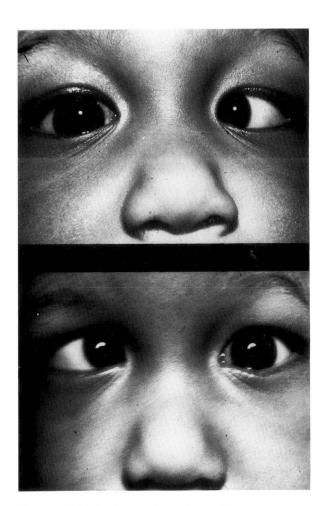

Fig. 13.1 Child showing an alternating strabismus.

Diagnosis

(1)   A light shone on the eyes should produce symmetrical corneal reflections in the two eyes

(2)   Covering the non-squinting eye leads to movement of the deviated eye so that it takes up macular fixation to obtain a clear image, and hence ceases to deviate. However, when structural ocular disease prevents a clear image or when a long-standing squint leads to severe functional suppression, vision may be so poor that macular vision is absent and no shift occurs

(3)   An abnormal head posture may be adopted to achieve binocular vision; this is most likely when a 'vertical' muscle is affected.

Epicanthic folds

Epicanthic folds give a false appearance of a squint, referred to as 'pseudostrabismus', and this is probably the basis of the incorrect belief that children tend to 'grow out' of childhood strabismus. Epicanthic folds require no treatment and usually disappear with growth of the base of nose, before the child is 10 years old. However, epicanthic folds and strabismus may coexist.

Treatment

The management of strabismus includes surgery, correction of any refractive error, especially hypermetropia, and prevention and treatment of amblyopia.

Early diagnosis of a squint may detect poor vision, which can be corrected by simply covering (occluding) the non-squinting eye. This can be achieved by an adhesive patch, by a patch placed in a pair of glasses or by atropine drops to blur the vision in the good eye. The disadvantage of atropine drops is that pupillary dilatation causes discomfort in bright light. Simple occlusion is less successful for the chronic squint, particularly if the child is more than 6 years of age.

Operative treatment of strabismus in one or both eyes results in little discomfort and the eyes are not padded. Most children are operated on as day cases.

THE WHITE PUPIL (LEUKOCOREA)

A white 'reflex' is an extremely important sign in the examination of an infant with strabismus (Fig. 13.2). The white pupil is the commonest presentation of a retinoblastoma in infancy. The differential diagnosis

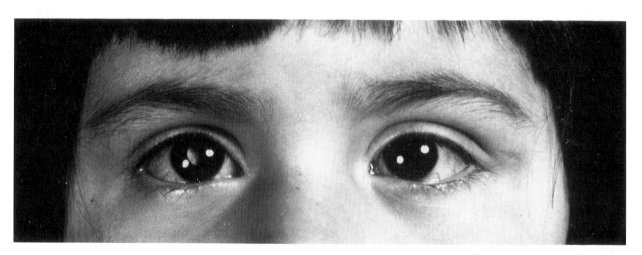

Fig. 13.2 The 'white' reflex: photograph of a tumour behind the lens, reflecting incident light to produce a 'white' pupillary reflex.

includes retinoblastoma, cataract, retinopathy of prematurity, persistent primary hyperplastic vitreous, and granulomatous uveitis, due to toxoplasmosis, or toxocara (a parasite in the gut of kittens and puppies).

Congenital (developmental) cataracts

Congenital cataracts are present at birth, although the term often includes cataracts which develop later but have been congenitally determined. Half the babies have a second ocular anomaly, for example microphthalmos, nystagmus, amblyopia, strabismus or aniridia.

Common types of congenital cataract are:

(1) Hereditary cataract with autosomal dominant inheritance or less commonly autosomal recessive and rarely sex-linked inheritance

(2) 'Persistent hyperplastic primary vitreous' describes failure of regression of a vascular membrane which normally encloses the embryonic lens. There may be associated microphthalmos which distinguishes it from retinoblastoma. The lesion usually occurs in normal full-term infants and is unilateral

(3) Post-rubella cataract. Maternal rubella during the first trimester usually leads to bilateral cataracts. When unilateral, the contralateral retina shows pigmentary changes of rubella retinitis. The cataract may continue to develop postnatally and almost invariably is associated with microphthalmos and hypoplasia of the iris, and frequently with deafness, mental retardation and cardiac anomalies such as pulmonary stenosis and patent ductus arteriosus.

(4) Cataracts also occur in galactosaemia, diabetes, trisomy 21 and in association with a variety of syndromes, including oxycephaly and stippled epiphyses.

Surgical treatment of cataracts is determined by the severity of visual loss, since successful early surgery diminishes the incidence of subsequent amblyopia. However, early surgery is more difficult despite new microsurgical methods and the final result may be frustrated by other ocular abnormalities. Contact lenses can be used in unilateral cases to prevent amblyopia. Intra-ocular lenses are not used in children. Unilateral cataracts lead to significant amblyopia.

Retinopathy of prematurity

This used to be known as 'retrolental fibroplasia' and occurs after exposure to excessive oxygen, particularly in infants of less than 32 weeks gestation, weighing less than 1500 g and those with intermittent apnoea. It is still one of the commonest causes of blindness in infancy.

Exposure to excessive oxygen causes irreversible obliteration of immature retinal vessels. New vessels grow into the vitreous humour, accompanied by glial deposits behind the lens. This leads to a contracture which causes retinal detachment and a secondary cataract. In less severe forms there is high myopia, and retinal detachment may occur in the second or third decade.

Granulomatous uveitis

Toxoplasmosis or infestation with *Toxocara canis* can cause a mass lesion at the macula which may mimic a retinoblastoma. The morphology of the mass, the presence of eosinophilia and specific skin tests help to confirm the diagnosis of *Toxocara* infestation.

EPIPHORA (THE WATERING EYE)

Development of the lacrimal gland and the nasolacrimal duct is incomplete at birth, but the moisture produced is sufficient to maintain the corneal epithelium and to lubricate the conjunctiva.

Nasolacrimal duct obstruction at birth is due commonly to epithelial debris in the duct or, in 10% of cases, to an occluding membrane. Rarely, epiphora is caused by agenesis or atresia of the lacrimal duct.

There is little need to probe or syringe the duct in the first 6 months. Spontaneous resolution is common and active treatment is indicated only when there is recurrent infection or epiphora persisting after the age of 6 months. Conservative treatment includes frequent massage of the tear sac and the instillation of antibiotic drops.

Epiphora associated with photophobia is serious because it indicates corneal irritation. The cause may be: congenital glaucoma, corneal foreign body, keratitis or defects of ocular pigmentation, for example albinism.

Congenital glaucoma

Fluid secreted by the ciliary body circulates in, and drains from, the eye at the iridocorneal angle. In congenital glaucoma the outflow of aqueous humour is obstructed, causing increased intraocular pressure and enlargement of the cornea. Photophobia and epiphora are the earliest signs. The rising intra-ocular pressure stretches the cornea and ruptures its lining. This causes haziness and irritation, reflex secretion of tears and photophobia.

Emergency surgical division of the obstructing membrane results in normal eye pressure in about 90% of children. Long term regular review is required.

Corneal foreign bodies

These can be removed with a sterile disposable hypodermic needle, and in young children a general anaesthetic usually is necessary. The cornea is only 0.5 mm thick, and deep foreign bodies should be removed with an operating microscope. After removal the cornea is often rough leading to irritation and delay in healing. A foreign body should be removed as soon as possible, and antibiotic ointment placed in the conjunctival sac.

Corneal ulceration

Herpes simplex causing a characteristic dendritic ('branching') ulcer is the commonest infective corneal ulcer in childhood. The diagnosis is made by staining the cornea with fluorescein strips. Fluorescein drops should be avoided because of the risk of contamination with *Pseudomonas pyocyaneus*, which can destroy the eye in 24 h.

Initial treatment is with guttae Idoxuridine (1%) hourly or oculentum Idoxuridine (0.5%) six times daily. Newer antiviral medications are oculentum Vidarabine and oculentum Acyclovir. Guttae atropine (1%) daily and an occlusive pad over the eye may be required.

Keratitis

Allergic conjunctivitis with keratitis is common in children with asthma or eczema. It may be difficult to distinguish allergic keratitis from herpes simplex keratitis, particularly when bilateral, and the treatment of the two conditions is different. The initial treatment of allergic (vernal) keratitis is guttae Antistine Privine, four times daily. Cortisone should be used with caution, for if herpes simplex is present, it can result in rapid exacerbation and even perforation of the cornea.

THE 'SMALL' EYE

One eye looks small when the globe itself is small or the palpebral fissure is narrow. Unilateral microphthalmos is a developmental anomaly associated with persistent hyperplastic primary vitreous or rubella. A narrowed palpebral aperture due to true ptosis may be muscular (e.g. congenital hypoplasia of the levator palpebrae superioris or a muscular dystrophy) or neural, (e.g. a congenital Horner's syndrome or congenital third nerve palsy). The commonest cause of ptosis is congenital familial levator hypoplasia. An evaluation for coexistent ocular abnormalities should be made.

In severe unilateral ptosis vision may be obstructed, leading to amblyopia. However, in most cases binocular vision is maintained in the lower half of the visual field by inclining the head backwards. Shortening of the levator is the best treatment unless levator function is poor or absent, when a fascial sling from the eyebrow is preferred.

THE 'LARGE' EYE

The appearance of a large eye may be caused by actual enlargement of the eyeball, (e.g. megalocornea); high myopia or congenital glaucoma; retraction of the lid (e.g. with a facial nerve palsy or thyrotoxicosis); or proptosis from trauma or a tumour.

ABNORMAL HEAD POSTURE

Ocular causes are postural compensations for: (i) a 'vertical' squint; (ii) nystagmus, where the eyes point in the direction in which the excursion of the nystagmus is least; (iii) partial visual field loss, for example blindness in one eye, where the child tilts the head while reading to bring the words into the centre of the visual field of the remaining eye.

CONJUNCTIVAL DISCHARGE

Inflammation of the conjunctivae causes a characteristic 'sticky' discharge which may be caused by infection, allergy or chemical irritants. Acute neonatal conjunctivitis may be due to maternal infection with gonorrhoea or chlamydia.

Neisseria gonorrhoea needs urgent treatment with penicillin drops and crystalline penicillin, because ulceration and perforation of the cornea may occur rapidly. Trachoma inclusion conjunctivitis (TRIC) is due to vaginal chlamydial infection. Swabs should always be taken for culture and antibiotic sensitivity.

Conjunctivitis later in the first year of life nearly always is related to obstruction of the nasolacrimal duct. Recurrent conjunctivitis at any age is suggestive of obstruction, with the tear sac forming a reservoir of infected fluid.

Suitable antibiotic eye drops or ointment are sulfacetamide (10%), neomycin (0.5%), chloramphenicol (1%), polymyxin, bacitracin and oxytetracycline, or combinations of these agents, for example Terramycin and Chloromyxin. Oxytetracycline is used to treat viral infections, especially those of the larger viruses, for example TRIC. Antibiotic drops should be administered frequently, for example every hour or every 2 h, and supported by the use of ointment at night. With this regimen, infections can usually be overcome within a few days.

Steroids are indicated for serious intra-ocular inflammation, allergic conjunctivitis and blepharitis. They are contraindicated in herpetic keratitis and therefore should not be used unless the diagnosis is certain and the cornea is not involved.

HEADACHE

Headache is difficult to evaluate in infancy because the child cannot describe it. Headache in school age children is a frequent complaint. The common ocular causes of headache are refractive error, for example hypermetropia, astigmatism and, less commonly, raised intracranial pressure, for example caused by a cerebral tumour.

A careful history is essential to determine the basis of the headache. In the early stages the headache of raised intracranial pressure is vague, and careful evaluation of the patient and the optic discs is essential. This is not easy because some normal children have apparently swollen optic discs.

OCULAR INJURIES

Every suspected eye injury should be treated as a penetrating injury until proven otherwise.

The eye should be examined under general anaesthesia if there is any doubt about the diagnosis.

Eye injuries associated with head injuries

In children there may be facial abrasions and lacerations and severe trauma of the middle third of the face. The important symptoms and signs are loss of sight; epiphora; diplopia; proptosis or enophthalmos.

Loss of vision

An estimate of sight should be made as soon as feasible, because failing vision suggests compression of the optic nerve which may be relieved by surgical intervention. In unilateral loss of vision, the retention of the consensual light reflex (producing constriction of the pupil) in the absence of direct light reflex suggests sensory damage to the vision in that eye, that is an afferent pupil defect.

Epiphora

Overflow of tears results from irritation of the cornea. Intra-orbital trauma and fractures of the middle third of the face may damage the lacrimal drainage apparatus, which should be repaired early.

Damage to the canaliculus should be suspected if there is injury to the medial half of the eyelid or the canthal region; primary repair of this injury offers the best result.

Diplopia

Double vision is secondary to interference with ocular movements and may be due to:

(1)   Muscle entrapment, that is catching of an extra-ocular muscle in an orbital fracture. Circumduction of the globe under anaesthesia confirms the diagnosis, which should be recognized early to avoid fibrosis in the muscle

(2)   Damage to the nerves supplying the extra-ocular muscles, for example in orbital fractures or secondary to severe intracranial injury

(3)   Displacement of the eye, for example following an intra-orbital haemorrhage which is usually accompanied by detectable proptosis.

Diplopia is rarely a long term problem in children, because: (i) binocular vision can often be restored by placing the head in an abnormal posture (and subsequently by strabismus surgery); (ii) the ability of children to suppress the confusing second image usually ensures that troublesome double vision is ultimately eliminated, sometimes at the cost of amblyopia.

Proptosis

Proptosis may be the result of:

(1)   Intra-orbital swelling (commonest)

(2)   Compression of the orbit following displacement of its walls

(3)   Orbital haemorrhage; the direction of the proptosis depends on the site of the haemorrhage, for example a fracture of the orbital roof with a subperiosteal haematoma causes displacement forwards and downwards

(4)   Caroticocavernous fistula; this should be suspected when proptosis develops a day or so after a severe head injury. It causes pulsating exophthalmos, oedema of the conjunctivae and oculomotor paralysis. Neurosurgical treatment is required.

Enophthalmos

Enophthalmos is caused by a fracture of the orbital margin, for example a depressed zygomatic bone. There is an irregularity of the orbital margin, a flattened cheek, possible infra-orbital anaesthesia and difficulty in closing the jaw. Perforation of the eyeball with extrusion of some of its contents is less common.

Blow-out fracture of the orbit

A 'blow-out' fracture of the orbit usually occurs through the orbital floor following a sudden increase in the intra-orbital pressure, for example by blunt injury to the eyeball and eyelids, caused by a first or large ball.

The signs of a 'blow-out' injury are: enophthalmos, infra-orbital anaesthesia or double vision due to entrapment of the inferior rectus or inferior oblique muscle in the fracture. X-rays of the maxillary sinus may reveal the prolapsed orbital tissue as a 'polyp'. Early recognition and repair of the orbital floor from above give the best results.

Delayed ecchymosis in the upper lid or conjunctiva usually indicates a fracture of the roof of the orbit, which may involve the optic canal. The level of visual acuity is determined as a baseline for subsequent observations.

Isolated direct injuries of the eye

Abrasions and superficial foreign bodies

The symptoms are pain, photophobia and spasm of the eyelids. When inspecting the eye and opening the lids, do not press on the globe itself. A drop of local anaesthetic from a freshly opened bottle may encourage spontaneous opening of the eyelids. The simplest method is to pull the lower lid down, push the soft tissues against the orbital rim and then to ask the child to look straight ahead before gently lifting the skin of the brow, lid and soft tissues against the orbital rim.

A foreign body is seen best by shining a light obliquely on the cornea and observing the irregularity of the reflection. Fluorescein strips may be used to stain the corneal epithelium and demonstrate the irregularity once a penetrating injury has been excluded. An irregular pupil, with prolapse of the iris through a hole in the cornea, may mimic the appearance of a corneal foreign body.

When no cause for the symptoms can be found, a careful search for a foreign body in the conjunctival fornices should be made, including eversion of the upper lid to exclude a foreign body on the back of the tarsal plate.

Recurrent abrasion may occur months after the initial injury when the corneal epithelium has not healed correctly. At night the epithelium becomes stuck to the under surface of the eyelid; opening the lids tears the corneal epithelium. Herpes simplex keratitis affects about 10% of corneal abrasions. A mycotic keratitis should be considered when an abrasion has been caused by agricultural material.

After instillation of local anaesthetic and removal of the foreign body, the conjunctiva should be irrigated with normal saline. An antibiotic ointment and an eye pad should be supplied.

Rupture of the eyeball

A 'black eye' from a severe periorbital haematoma may hide a 'blow out' fracture of orbit (see above) or rupture of the eyeball. Rupture of intra-ocular structures may cause dislocation of the lens or intra-ocular haemorrhage and mask underlying retinal detachment or lead to secondary glaucoma. The commonest site of rupture of the globe is at the limbus, that is, the junction of the cornea and the sclera.

A ruptured globe leads to decreased vision, absence of the 'red reflex' (seen by using an ophthalmoscope set at 0 and viewed from 25 cm) or a 'soft' eye. A subconjunctival haemorrhage may be caused by rupture of the sclera.

If a rupture or a penetrating injury of the eyeball is suspected, the eye should be protected with a large dressing and the patient referred to an ophthalmologist as an emergency, for examination and repair under anaesthesia. If uveal tissue (i.e. iris, ciliary body or choroid) is extruded, there is a serious risk of sympathetic ophthalmia developing (see below).

Retinal detachment

A grey 'mound' disturbs the normal red reflex. When the retinal detachment is associated with prolapse of the retina or other structures through a penetrating injury, blindness usually follows. However, retinal detachment most commonly is delayed after a blunt injury and should be suspected whenever there is late failure of vision after ocular trauma.

Hyphema

Moderately severe blunt injuries to the globe often cause hyphema, that is a haemorrhage into the anterior chamber between the cornea in front and the lens and iris diaphragm behind. The most important treatment is immediate rest in bed and immobilization of the child. No drops are instilled initially and the hyphema usually absorbs spontaneously in 6–7 days. Secondary haemorrhage or glaucoma are complications of hyphema. If either develops, the pressure should be controlled with acetazolamide and/or osmotic agents such as mannitol. Evacuation of the blood clot sometimes may save the sight and is deferred just long enough to allow the intra-ocular pressure to stop the bleeding.

Lacerations and penetrating injuries

When an eyelid is lacerated the eye itself is at risk. When the globe also has been lacerated, it should be repaired before the eyelid.

The signs of corneal perforation are obvious collapse of the eye; a distorted pupil (due to prolapse of iris); hyphema; prolapse of the lens, vitreous, retina or choroid. The prolapsed tissues are mixed with blood, so attempts to wipe away 'clots' are dangerous and may precipitate further prolapse of the contents. The eye should be kept covered until the child is anaesthetized; the lids then can be separated without danger of squeezing the globe or rotating the eye, either of which can result in extrusion of further intra-ocular contents.

The prognosis for sight is determined by the extent of the injury, but meticulous microsurgical repair can salvage the eye. Early repair in the first 24 h often will produce a good result.

Sympathetic ophthalmitis

The management of a perforating injury causing prolapse of uveal tissue is fraught with the risk of sympathetic ophthalmia, which is currently regarded as an autoimmune disease based on sensitivity to uveal pigment. This results in an inflammatory phenomenon in the uninjured eye, causing blindness which may be total.

The risks of sympathetic ophthalmia must be weighed against the possibility of useful vision following careful repair of the injured eye. Sympathetic ophthalmia occurs in 4% of children with neglected prolapse of uveal tissues. It may occur at any time up to 2 years after the injury. Removal of an eye with prolapsed uveal tissue within 10 days of the injury appears to afford the most complete protection from sympathetic ophthalmia.

Burns

Radiation burns

Sunburn of the eyelids rarely is serious, but permanent damage from solar retinitis may follow gazing at the sun for as little as 10 s. The danger is greatest during an eclipse of the sun, which arouses the interest and attention of children who are unaware of the risks of staring at the sun.

Thermal burns

Flame burns rarely affect the eye directly, because of reflex spasm of the eyelids. Delayed secondary effects arise from exposure of the eyeball caused by scar contraction in the eyelids, and these should be anticipated when the eyelids are burnt.

Chemical burns

Alkalis and acids can devastate the eyes. Emergency treatment is immediate, copious irrigation with innocuous fluid. One way is to partially submerge the child's head in a bucket or a basin of water, and encourage him to open his eyes under water. Irrigation should never be delayed until special fluids have been obtained, because alkalis continue to coagulate tissue for as long as they are present undiluted. Acid burns, on the other hand, tend to coagulate a superficial layer of tissue only. The cornea may appear to be clear when in reality it is becoming thinner and there is a danger of rupture; an urgent corneal graft may be required.

OCULAR TUMOURS IN CHILDREN

Ocular tumours in infants lead to progressive failure of vision but this may be difficult to detect clinically. Structural loss of vision prevents the transmission of a clear image from the eye, resulting in nystagmus or strabismus. Functional loss of vision may be due to failure to receive a clear image on the retina, for example a bulky lesion of the eyelid. Space-occupying lesions arising in the orbit may distort the globe and deform it so that errors in refraction occur.

Proptosis is the commonest sign of an expanding lesion in the orbit and is best seen from above the patient's forehead. Proptosis which is pulsating, intermittent or reducible by gentle pressure on the closed eyelids, is likely to be caused by a benign condition, for example a bony or vascular abnormality; inflammatory or neoplastic masses are firm and non-compressible.

Strabismus may be caused by unilateral blindness or paralysed ocular muscles, either by compression or invasion of the muscles or their motor nerves. Impairment of eye movements leads to secondary loss of vision (i.e. amblyopia).

Buphthalmos (i.e. ox's eye) is enlargement of the globe, for example as in infantile glaucoma. Buphthalmos may be secondary to a tumour involving the outflow of aqueous humour.

Diagnosis

The age of the patient indicates the likelihood of a benign or malignant tumour being present. Evidence of systemic disease, for example cafe-au-lait spots, may clinch the diagnosis of optic nerve glioma in a patient with neurofibromatosis, as may an abdominal mass of neuroblastoma because of its tendency to produce orbital metastases.

Radiology includes computerized tomography of the skull, orbit and optic canals. Fluorescein angiography may help define vascular abnormalities, and ultrasound is useful for both orbital and intra-ocular tumours.

Malignant tumours of the orbit

Rapidly growing tumours

These produce signs suggestive of an acute inflammatory condition. Rhabdomyosarcoma is the most important primary malignant tumour arising in the orbit in the first decade. Its rapid growth may be mistaken for orbital cellulitis. The differential diagnosis includes orbital cellulitis, maxillary osteomyelitis, chronic inflammatory conditions, lymphomas and haematoma. Orbital rhabdomyosarcomas are treated by a combination of chemotherapy and radiotherapy.

Metastatic orbital tumours include: metastatic neuroblastoma, by far the commonest cause of malignant proptosis in childhood (Fig. 13.3); orbital deposits in leukaemia or malignant lymphoma; extension from nasopharyngeal tumours; radiation-induced sarcomas, extension of a retinoblastoma.

Slowly growing lesions

These often present late. An optic nerve glioma affecting the chiasm presents with nystagmus, raised intracranial pressure or failure to thrive, while those involving the optic nerve in the orbit present with proptosis, strabismus or both. Nystagmus due to a chiasmal glioma must be distinguished from 'congenital' nystagmus. The optic disc, appears abnormal, for example pallor and/or papilloedema.

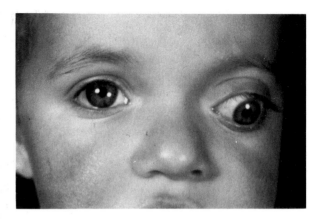

Fig. 13.3 Metastatic neuroblastoma is the commonest cause of malignant proptosis in childhood.

Retinoblastoma

Retinoblastoma is a rare malignant intra-ocular tumour of infancy and childhood. Its early recognition is life-saving. Death is usually due to direct spread to the central nervous system along the optic nerve, by haematogenous spread or by invasion of the orbital tissues.

Hereditary retinoblastoma is an autosomal dominant with the penetrance of the gene related to the clinical presentation. Sporadic bilateral retinoblastoma is almost certainly a germinal mutation with 100% penetrance, so that in the offspring of a survivor there is a 50% chance of developing the tumour. Unilateral retinoblastoma (which accounts for two-thirds of cases) carries only a 10% incidence in the progeny. When a child develops a retinoblastoma and the parents are normal with no family history, there is a 4% chance that a subsequent sibling will be affected. Regular re-examination of children born to a parent who has retinoblastoma enables early detection of a tumour.

Signs and symptoms

The two commonest signs are: a 'white' reflex in the pupil (Fig. 13.2), a finding that demands urgent referral to an ophthalmologist, and a convergent strabismus.

Poor vision is only obvious in very young children when there is massive involvement of the eye(s).

Treatment

This depends on the extent of the tumour and on whether one or both eyes are involved. Local measures include: external sclerally-applied radiation using ^{60}Co; light coagulation; cryotherapy. General treatment of the retina as a whole can be achieved by enucleation or radiation. Chemotherapy is used if there is evidence of systemic metastasis.

FURTHER READING

Gardiner P. A. (1979) *ABC of Ophthalmology*, 2nd edn. BMA London.

Isenberg S. J. (ed.) (1989) *The Eye in Infancy*. Year Book Medical, Chicago.

Kerrigan P. (1989) Ocular problems in practice (symposium) *Practitioner* **233** (entire issue).

Lubeck D. & Coster D. (1989) *Eye Infections. Modern Med.* **32**: 24–36.

Reich J. (1986) Examining the eye. *Aust. Fam. Phys.* **15**: 1329.

Vaughan D. & Ashbury T. (1989) *General Ophthalmology*, 12th edn. Lange Medical, Norwalk, Conn. USA.

14

The Ear, Nose and Throat

SINUSITIS AND RHINITIS

The complaints of continuous and recurring headcold are difficult to manage for three main reasons. The essential pathology is infection of respiratory mucosa with swelling and production of purulent secretions, so there is no clearly defined difference between normal children and those with problems. The second difficulty is that no laboratory test can show why the upper respiratory mucosa in some children is excessively susceptible to infection. The third frustration is that surgical, drug or other treatment rarely produces worthwhile improvement.

The natural history, however, is encouraging as few older children or adults have these complaints or show any residual damage or disability resulting from rhinitis or sinusitis in early childhood.

Investigations

No specific bacteria are implicated. White blood cell and blood antibody tests seldom find any abnormality. The osseous and cartilaginous anatomy of the nose, sinuses and ostea is normal in these children. Plain X-rays of maxillary sinuses are equivocal or misleading in more than 30%, and unerupted teeth can make their interpretation even more uncertain. Thin section computerized tomography (CT) scans in the coronal plane provide precise and accurate imaging where needed, but when imaging is done for unrelated reasons, for example neurosurgery, mucosal thickening in the sinuses is often shown in asymptomatic patients. Thus investigations, including X-rays, rarely contribute to management when the complaint is chronic or recurrent purulent nasal discharge.

Reassurance

Treatment of the nose and sinuses does not influence lower respiratory problems, such as cough and bronchospasm. Post-nasal secretions are swallowed and do not cause cough by entering the larynx and trachea. Bronchitis and asthma are often related, rather than secondary, problems. Parents also need to realize that most children with purulent noses have normal energy and overall good health. There is no irreversible damage to any upper respiratory structure or tissue.

Treatment options

The surgical treatment considered most often is the creation of extra naso-antral windows (intranasal antrostomies) with the idea of improving aeration and drainage of the maxillary sinuses. Unfortunately, results are consistently disappointing. Precise endoscopic surgical enlargement of the natural osteum with ablation of some adjacent ethmoid cells is a new surgical option which is being evaluated. Large obstructing adenoids are not a common finding and their removal often causes little reduction in purulent discharge.

Desensitization to aeroallergens does not produce improvement in purulent rhinosinusitis. Similarly, there is no evidence that food allergy is important. Antibiotics produce short-term improvement, but do not influence the long term course. It is reasonable to use them to treat acute exacerbations. Topical and oral decongestants and topical steroids are not effective when the discharge is purulent. Regular γ-globulin infusions seem to benefit a few severe sufferers, even when γ-globulin levels are in the normal range.

Most children are best left untreated because most treatment is ineffective and the medium to long term prognosis is favourable.

UPPER AIRWAYS OBSTRUCTION

Restricted intranasal airway

In nearly all neonates and in some infants, nose-breathing is obligatory. In older children, constantly poor nasal airways result in mouth-breathing without any difficulty. Choanal atresia presents immediately after birth as cyanosis or respiratory distress relieved by crying. If any air flow can be demonstrated (e.g. by condensation on a cold surface) choanal atresia is not present. Hypoplasia of the nasal bones is a more common cause of inadequate nasal airways in a neonate and, if severe, may require nasopharyngeal intubation. Another cause in infants is non-specific or infective swelling of the nasal mucosa. Most patients can be managed by the occasional application of a topical steroid antibiotic preparation, alternating with a decongestant.

In older children, poor nasal airways are most often due to mucosal swelling, either intrinsic or related to asthma or allergy. If the child complains, it will be because of being unable to nose-breathe when in bed. Treatment includes anti-allergy measures and surgical reduction of mucosa by cautery or trimming. A good initial surgical result may fail months later from recurrence of mucosal hypertrophy. Oral decongestants are useful when used infrequently but unhelpful when used regularly. Topical vasoconstrictors and decongestants cause mucosal irritation, so long term use increases mucosal swelling and inflammation. Topical steroids (e.g. Beclamethazone) often help when allergic symptoms such as wetness and sneezing are pronounced. However, most children soon reject this regular preventative medication. Steam inhalations can give some relief. Many children with chronic hypertrophic rhinitis are best left untreated.

Treatment of choanal atresia

Surgery involves the accurate removal of the thickened posterior end of the nasal septum and complete removal of bone occluding the posterior nares. Keeping mucosal damage to a minimum reduces the likelihood of re-stenosis and the need for months of intranasal stenting. This surgery can be performed effectively transnasally, using telescopes for visualization via the nose and mouth. Only rarely is a transpalatal approach preferable.

Large adenoids obstructing the nasopharynx

The usual age group is 4–7 years, and adenoidal obstruction is uncommon under the age of 2 years. Most children mouth-breathe without complaining. If mouth-breathing is laboured and obstructed during sleep, there is also likely to be oropharyngeal obstruction caused by large tonsils. The severity of airways obstruction during sleep is a guide to the need for treatment. In atypical or doubtful cases sleep studies may be indicated. In children under 5 years, obstruction is a more common indication for tonsillectomy and adenoidectomy than is recurring infection. In a few young children with poor nasal airways, breathing during sleep is obstructed because the child is still an obligatory nose-breather. If asleep mouth-breathing is not laboured and there is no middle ear disease secondary to poor eustachian tube function, adenoidectomy is optional and tonsillectomy is not indicated. Orthodontic problems can be an indication for adenoidectomy. Removal of obstructing adenoids and possibly tonsils in mid or early childhood may prevent adult snoring.

The hypopharynx, larynx and upper trachea

Upper tracheal problems are uncommon but include tracheomalacia and congenital cysts. Symptoms begin soon after birth and stridor is both inspiratory and expiratory. Idiopathic bilateral vocal cord paralysis presents soon after birth with marked inspiratory stridor and obstruction requiring airways assistance. Tracheostomy is usually needed, but occasionally the airways are tolerable despite the lack of vocal cord movement. If there is no spontaneous recovery after several years, arytenoidectomy is an alternative to permanent tracheostomy. Congenital malformations (e.g. sub-glottic stenosis, cysts and vocal cord webs) also cause obstructed breathing and stridor. Laryngeal papillomatosis is uncommon but has characteristic progressive voice change and airways restriction. Papillomas are treated by microlaryngoscopy and laser vaporization. The natural history is variable and recurrence is common. Laryngomalacia (soft and prolapsing supraglottic structures) is the most common cause of mild stridor and obstruction developing soon after birth. Stridor increases during times of increased respiratory effort producing a characteristic inspiratory noise. If the clinical picture is typical, endoscopy is often unnecessary.

In doubtful cases, fibreoptic transnasal laryngoscopy has the advantage of not needing a general anaesthesia and is performed as an outpatient procedure. Structures at vocal cord level and above can be seen adequately, and the technique is especially useful when the suspected pathology is dynamic, as with vocal cord paralysis and laryngomalacia. Direct and rigid telescope endoscopy has the disadvantage of requiring general anaesthesia but the view is superior.

TONSILLITIS

Typical features of acute tonsillitis are rapid onset, fever, lethargy and malaise, vomiting, throat pain (which may be absent in young children) and decreased oral intake.

Recovery occurs after 2–5 days of treatment with penicillin. If the history is not clear-cut, examination during an attack should document fever, redness and swelling of tonsils, exudate and tenderness and swelling of neck lymph nodes. Where the pre-operative diagnosis has been correct, these illnesses will cease after removal of tonsils. Pharyngitis can still occur after tonsillectomy, but episodes are less frequent and throat pain less severe. Serious complications of tonsillectomy are rare but include death from either excessive blood loss or upper airways obstruction. In Australia, the overall mortality rate is less than 1 : 10 000 operations. Other ill-effects are rare. Removal of the tonsillar lymphoid tissue has no ill-effects. Tonsillectomy is indicated when the morbidity of recurring tonsillitis is greater than the morbidity of removal. In healthy, older children this usually means more than four attacks of severe tonsillitis per year for several successive years. Toddlers and children just beginning school often have poor defences against infections. In this age group, surgery is avoided, except in severe cases, because spontaneous improvement is likely.

QUINSY

In quinsy, peritonsillar cellulitis progresses to single or multiple abscesses between the tonsillar capsule and the pharyngeal muscle. There is swelling of the soft palate and tonsil, trismus, marked systemic upset and a raised neutrophil count and fever. Peritonsillar cellulitis and abscess are often indistinguishable. In these children, intravenous fluids and high dose penicillin are given for 48 h. In peritonsillar cellulitis, there will be improvement by 36 h. Antibiotic therapy will not resolve a peritonsillar abscess and drainage by incision or tonsillectomy is needed.

The differential diagnosis is infectious mononucleosis and this diagnosis should be considered if the clinical course is protracted, swelling is confined to the tonsils without involvement of peritonsillar tissues and there is no trismus. The typical peripheral blood film is usually found but it may often take 1–2 weeks for antibody tests for infectious mononucleosis to become positive. Often there is no enlargement of the liver or spleen.

EAR, NOSE AND THROAT INJURIES

Small nasal bones are difficult to palpate accurately, so considerable skill is required. Nevertheless, palpation remains the mainstay of diagnosis. Facial bone fractures heal rapidly and complications, such as infection, are rare. Undisplaced or minimally displaced nasal bone fractures need no treatment. If a fracture with displacement is left untreated, the deformity will increase as the child grows. X-rays rarely contribute because they fail to detect many minor fractures and are a poor indication of the degree of displacement.

Fracture reduction is monitored by palpation, so treatment has to be delayed until most swelling has subsided. However, it should not be delayed for more than a few days because by 1 week bone union will be substantial. Fracture reduction can be performed very satisfactorily under local anaesthesia in older children.

Nasal septal haematoma

This is an uncommon complication of nasal injury, but it is important because without treatment, it will progress to abscess formation, cartilage necrosis and eventually saddle-nose deformity. The diagnosis is made by inspection of the septum and assessment of the nasal airways. If there is doubt about the diagnosis, a topical anaesthetic and decongestant should be applied and the septum palpated. Irreversible damage will occur within 24–48 h, which makes this a surgical emergency. Adequate surgery will often involve a general anaesthetic and surgery similar to a septoplasty.

External neck injuries

Injuries from sharp edges (e.g. fence wire) tend to be more severe than those produced by blunt objects (e.g. elbow). Fracture of tracheal rings or laryngeal cartilages may cause airways obstruction and voice change, and air may escape into the neck or produce pneumomediastinum and pneumothorax. The recurrent laryngeal nerves can be damaged, but the oesophagus and neurovascular structures are damaged rarely.

Children who have sustained minor injuries with no subcutaneous emphysema, minimal breathing difficulty or voice change, need only observation. In more severe injuries, tracheostomy or open exploration may be required. Full evaluation includes soft tissue X-rays and examination under anaesthesia, with direct laryngoscopy, microlaryngoscopy and use of direct and angleviewing telescopes. Vocal cord movement needs to be assessed with the patient awake, using a rod telescope through the mouth or a fibreoptic endoscope through the nose.

Tympanic membrane rupture

This can occur with a pressure wave such as an openhanded slap across the ear or a fall into water with the side of the head taking the impact. Direct trauma (e.g. stick or cotton bud) is also a common cause. The majority will heal spontaneously but it is a slow process, taking from several weeks to 6 months. The ear must be kept dry to prevent infection. In a small percentage, the rupture produces a triangular flap with the edge rolled inwards which prevents healing. This is the only indication for early surgical intervention. Damage to the ossicular chain or inner ear is very rare.

Temporal bone fracture

Considerable force is required to produce this injury; in most cases there is loss of consciousness and blood or CSF issues from the ear. The bone is elastic, so disruption can occur even when there is no residual bone displacement. A CT scan will often demonstrate a fracture. The injury may include: tearing of deep ear canal skin or tympanic membrane; ossicular chain fracture or dislocation; facial nerve paralysis; disruption of the inner ear and labyrinth; CSF leak; and perilymph fistula.

Examination may be prevented by blood clot in the ear canal and attempts at removing the clot cause more bleeding. Inspection is delayed for several weeks until lacerations have healed. If there is no deafness on audiometry, no vertigo or nystagmus, no facial weakness and no CSF leak, the prognosis is excellent.

A CSF or perilymph leak can be present behind an intact tympanic membrane. The diagnosis is suspected if meningitis develops weeks or months after a skull injury. Where there is total loss of hearing in the damaged ear, a perilymph fistula is likely. The leak occurs through or near the oval or round window in the medial wall of the inner ear. The ear surgery necessary to plug a perilymph leak is less complex than intracranial exploration. If there is no major sensorineural deafness, meningitis is most likely secondary to CSF leak through the roof of the middle ear. This is repaired by a middle cranial fossa approach. Facial nerve repair will improve the outcome of facial paralysis only if the nerve is completely transected and the ends separated. This is never the situation in delayed-onset paralysis or if paralysis is incomplete. Spontaneous recovery can take more than 12 months.

OTITIS MEDIA

Serous otitis media includes a spectrum of middle ear pathology ranging from a symptomless air–fluid mixture in the middle ear, to severe glue ear and finally, to its complications (Table 14.1).

Table 14.1 Enlarged tonsils

? Symmetrical—No—Consider lymphoma/tumour
Yes
? Airways obstruction—No—Reassure
Yes
? Recurrent infections (> 4–6/year)—No—Consider sleep studies
Yes
? Preschool age—Yes—Avoid operation and await improvement
No
T's and A's

The normal state

The middle ear is filled with air because the eustachian tube opens with yawning and swallowing. If the eustachian tube is partly blocked, the air pressure in the middle ear will be low and some tympanic membrane retraction will occur.

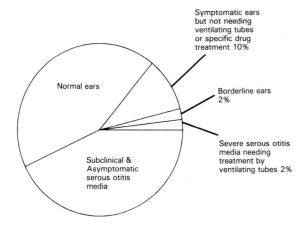

Fig. 14.1 Spectrum of middle ear disease in children.

Mild serous otitis media

Only a small amount of air passes up the eustachian tube, resulting in a mixture of air and seromucous fluid in the middle ear. This is found in 30% of kindergarten and early school age children. Conductive deafness is usually minimal, unilateral and of short duration. The medium and long term prognosis is excellent. It is important to distinguish mild glue ear not requiring treatment, from severe glue ear.

Severe glue ear

The severity of deafness and the damage to the ear dictate the need for insertion of ventilating tubes. Where the middle ear is completely fluid-filled there will be moderate conductive deafness with thresholds at 30–40 db. When this is bilateral and chronic, the child needs treatment. The severity of ear damage also needs to be considered. In most, there is no tissue necrosis and a perfect recovery is expected. When damage does occur, the tympanic membrane is the first structure affected. Unimportant damage includes slight generalized retraction, small areas of thin scar and small areas of white fibrosis or calcification. Localized areas of deep retraction in the attic or postero-superiorly in areas of thin scar, progress to ossicular erosion or cholesteatoma formation. Recurring ear abscesses may lead to chronic perforation. Progressive damage is not common but can occur, even when deafness is minimal and there is no earache. Ear-drum examination is the only way to assess progressive damage.

Recurring acute otitis media

This is superimposed often on a background of serous otitis media. If there is sufficient nuisance value from nights of severe earache, insertion of ventilating tubes may be warranted even if there is no hearing handicap, no developing ear damage and if the prognosis is excellent.

Treatment of serous otitis media

Ideal treatment would be to improve eustachian tube function. However, antibiotics, oral decongestants and topical decongestants are ineffective. Direct eustachian tube surgery has been abandoned. A few children develop serous otitis media, despite adequate eustachian tubes, by excessive sniffing. Fortunately, eustachian tube function spontaneously improves in more than 95% of children before mid-primary school age and continues to improve until growth ceases. In less than 2% of children, eustachian tube and middle ear problems persist throughout life. Children with mild serous otitis media should be left untreated. Most parents accept this management plan when they realize that there is no damage occurring and the long term prognosis is excellent. Children with severe glue ear have an unacceptable hearing handicap and may suffer progressive damage and excessive earache: these children benefit from insertion of ventilating tubes.

Treatment of acute otitis media

Drug treatment has no effect on the natural history of acute otitis media. Most parents are happy to find the minor episodes of acute otitis media can be treated symptomatically. Antibiotics are reserved for: severe bouts with pain persisting more than 6 h; associated systemic upset and fever; complications.

Treatment with ventilating tubes

Tube insertion requires day surgery and 5–10 min of general anaesthesia. The child resumes normal activities the next day. Small-sized tubes are most often used and these extrude spontaneously after 6–9 months. The recurrence rate of severe glue ear requiring re-insertion of ventilating tubes is about 20%. This occurs because there has not been sufficient spontaneous improvement in eustachian tube function. Larger ventilating tubes that take 12–18 months to extrude can be used. However, the larger tubes lead to slightly more residual tympanic membrane scarring and the residual perforation rate rises from 1 to 5%. Infection with discharge will complicate 20% of ears with ventilating tubes, particularly if they get wet.

CHRONIC TYMPANIC MEMBRANE PERFORATION

This is usually the result of recurrent episodes of acute suppurative otitis media. More than 70% of acute perforations caused by trauma or infection heal spontaneously. Most small chronic tympanic membrane perforations cause little deafness and can be symptomless, requiring no treatment. The main objective of drum grafting is often to produce an ear that will not develop discharge and infection after swimming. The success rate for tympanic membrane grafting is 90%. Complications apart from recurrent perforation are rare. If eustachian tube function is inadequate and grafting is successful, glue ear or middle ear infection will recur. For this reason, tympanic membrane grafting is usually delayed until at least 9 years of age. A variety of non-epithelial tissues can be used for grafting, for example temporalis muscle fascia.

ACUTE MASTOIDITIS

The features of acute mastoiditis include ear pain, postauricular swelling (displacing the pinna), tenderness, systemic upset and conductive deafness. Very young children diagnosed early respond to intensive antibiotics and suction myringotomy. Frequently, bone necrosis in the mastoid causes a subperiostial abscess requiring drainage. Diseased bone is removed and a communication established with the middle ear space to allow adequate drainage. Often there is full recovery with no residual ear symptoms or deafness.

CHOLESTEATOMA

In this condition, a thin part of the ear-drum becomes deeply retracted into the middle ear space because of poor eustachian tube function. Retraction pockets are most often seen in the attic region or in the postero-superior part of the pars tensor after it has ruptured during bouts of acute suppurative otitis media. If retraction pockets have wide mouths and limited depth, they can be self-cleaning and symptomless. In other cases, wax and epithelial debris collect and expand the sac which eventually engulfs the ossicles, and then fills the attic region and the mastoid cell system. The usual presenting symptom is ear discharge refractory to treatment. Less often, it is conductive deafness. Infection may spread intracranially or to the inner ear. Treatment aims to prevent these complications, stop ear discharge, improve hearing and provide an intact tympanic membrane (i.e. a wettable ear). Effective surgery requires complete removal of all the epithelial wall of the cholesteatoma.

PROCEDURES AND TECHNIQUES

Otoscopy

Wax may obscure the tympanic membrane, but its removal by syringing is time-consuming, and for young children is upsetting. The alternative is to use a small wax ring or tiny cotton wool swab on a dental broach. Instrumentation cannot be done through a hand-held otoscope but a binocular spectacle-frame-mounted otoscope makes these procedures relatively easy. Once the ear canal is clear, the tympanic membrane can be inspected by a hand-held otoscope, a head-worn binocular otoscope or even an operating microscope. The static appearance of an ear-drum is often not diagnostic. Acute otitis media should be diagnosed only if there is an accompanying history of pain and malaise. In serous otitis media, the drum may be brown or purple. Sometimes air/fluid interfaces can be seen, for example bubbles or menisci. The most important role of static otoscopy is to look for evidence of tympanic membrane damage that is likely to be progressive and serious, such as localized areas of deep retraction.

Pneumatoscopy

A sealed viewing system is required and the tympanic membrane is forced in and out by changing air pressure in the ear canal generated by the doctor or child squeezing a rubber bulb. In experienced hands this examination will diagnose the presence and severity of serous otitis media in more than 90% of cases. In a normal air-filled middle ear tympanic membrane movement is extensive and rapid. If the middle ear is completely fluid-filled then drum movement will be slow and minimal. No movement suggests an inadequate seal between the speculum and the ear canal or a tympanic membrane perforation. An air/fluid mixture in the middle ear produces variable drum movement. Air/fluid interfaces may be revealed by the motion of the drum.

Removal of foreign bodies

Forceps are not the best instrument for removal of most foreign bodies, which they tend instead to push further in. Some, such as insects, tend to break up. Most are best removed with a fine probe with the terminal 2–4 mm bent to a right angle. This hook is passed beyond the foreign body and then rotated to withdraw and remove it. A head light and viewing system is essential. If these techniques are used, few objects need to be removed under general anaesthesia. Before removal of a nasal foreign body is attempted, topical anaesthesia and vasoconstriction is induced. Five centimetre lengths of 8 mm ($\frac{1}{2}$") ribbon gauze are dampened with cocaine and adrenaline. These are introduced 1 or 2 cm into the nose in a non-frightening way with fingers, rather than instruments.

Nasal cautery for epistaxis

The application of a local anaesthetic and vasoconstrictor is an essential preliminary. The object of cautery is to produce thrombosis and necrosis of the appropriate blood vessels. Hot wire cautery is used where possible because it will be effective even in the presence of blood and mucus and it can be very accurately controlled. If heat cautery is not available, or is inappropriate because the patient is very young and apprehensive, chemical cautery is used. However, it must be very accurately applied to dry mucosa to be effective. A convenient way to achieve good access and vision is to use a large-sized ear speculum directed medially against the involved part of the nasal septum.

Audiometry

Pure-tone testing with headphones is feasible for children aged four years and older. For most even younger children, hearing can be tested adequately in a free field situation using behavioural response. For a conventional audiogram where thresholds are at 10 dB or better, hearing is within the normal range. With severe glue ear causing obvious deafness, thresholds are often at 35–45 dB for all frequencies. An air/fluid mixture in the middle ear produces thresholds of about 30 dB for lower frequencies, but close to normal for the higher frequencies. This is usually barely noticeable and not a hearing handicap. The maximum degree of deafness that can be caused by middle ear problems is about 50 dB. If thresholds are at 50 dB or worse, then at least some of the deafness must be sensorineural.

Tympanometry (impedence audiometry)

A continuous sound is introduced into the ear canal by a fine tube, and another fine tube measures how much of the sound is reflected back from the tympanic membrane. Thus the degree of sound absorbed by the tympanic membrane, and the middle ear can be assessed. The ear canal is sealed so that air pressure can be changed to move the tympanic membrane in and out. The result is a 'tympanogram' which is a graph of sound absorption against the pressure of air in the ear canal (Fig. 14.2). In a normal result (type 'A' tympanogram), there is a peak of sound absorption when the canal pressure is atmospheric, but as the ear-drum is stretched either inwards or outwards, sound absorption is less. If the middle ear is air-filled but air pressure is low because of intermittent eustachian tube obstruction, a similar peak of sound absorption can be obtained only when the air pressure in the ear canal is lowered to match that in the middle ear. This is called a type 'C'

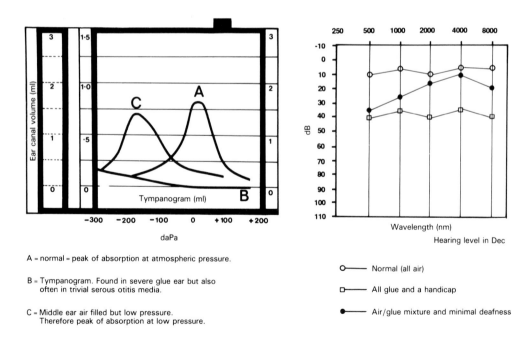

A = normal = peak of absorption at atmospheric pressure.

B = Tympanogram. Found in severe glue ear but also often in trivial serous otitis media.

C = Middle ear air filled but low pressure. Therefore peak of absorption at low pressure.

Fig. 14.2 Tympanogram, showing the 'A', 'B' and 'C' types. The 'A' type is normal. The 'B' type occurs with fluid-filled ears as well as some other conditions. The 'C' type indicates eustachian tube obstruction and a low pressure in the air-filled middle ear. The righthand graph is an audiogram showing the effect of glue ears on hearing.

tympanogram. If the middle ear is fluid-filled, sound absorption will be poor and will not change as ear canal pressure is varied. This is called a flat or type 'B' tympanogram. Unfortunately, this result is seen also with a variety of conditions, many of which are trivial and do not need treatment. Type 'B' tympanograms will be seen with middle ear air/fluid mixtures; tympanic membrane perforations; patent ventilating tubes; and even with air-filled middle ears if the tympanic membrane is stiff and air pressure is low. Thus type 'A' and type 'C' tympanograms are helpful and specific, whereas type 'B' tympanograms can mean severe glue ear, but also can reflect trivial problems which do not require treatment.

COMMON CONDITIONS OF THE MOUTH

Mucous retention cysts

Goblet cells in the buccal mucosa may become blocked and form a pale pedunculated retention cyst up to 1 cm in diameter on the inner aspect of the lip, the gingivolabial sulcus, or the lining of the cheek. They sometimes evacuate spontaneously, but usually annoy the patient, worry the parents, and occasionally interfere with feeding. They are best removed.

Ranula

A ranula is a larger sessile cyst 2–3 cm in diameter in the floor of the mouth under the tongue. It is lax, bluish grey or translucent, and may become large enough to interfere with speech and swallowing. It should be deroofed (marsupialized).

Tongue-tie

In tongue-tie, the lingual frenulum is short and may be attached to the very tip of the tongue. It never interferes with the infant's sucking or swallowing, and only rarely interferes with speech. When tongue protrusion is not possible in a child over 2 years of age, the tight frenulum can be divided under general anaesthesia.

FURTHER READING

Balkany T. J. & Pashley N. R. T. (eds) (1986) *Clinical Pediatric Otolaryngology*. C. V. Mosby, St Louis.

Benjamin B. (1990) *Diagnostic Laryngology. Adults and Children*. W. B. Saunders, Philadelphia.

Bluestone C. D. & Klein J. O. (1988) *Otitis Media in Infants and Children*. W. B. Saunders, Philadelphia.

Bluestone C. D. (1989) Modern Management of Otitis Media. *Pediatr. Clin. North Am.* **36**: 1388.

Grundfast K. M. (ed.) (1989) Recent Advances in Pediatric Otolaryngology. *Pediatr. Clin. North Am.* **36**.

Lusk R. P., Lazar R. H., Muntz H. R. (1989) The diagnosis and treatment of recurrent and chronic sinusitis in children. *Pediatr. Clin. North Am.* **36**: 1422.

McCormick B. (1988) *Screening for Hearing Impairment in Young Children*. Croom Helm, London

Myer C. M. & Cotton R. T. (1988) *A Practical Approach to Pediatric Otolaryngology*. Year Book Medical, Chicago.

Tweedie J. (1987) *Children's Hearing Problems: Their Significance, Detection and Management*. John Wright, Bristol.

— 15 —

Cleft Lip and Palate

A cleft lip is a cleft of the 'primary' palate and involves the lip, the alveolus between the lateral incisor and canine and the anterior portion of the hard palate to the incisive foramen. The cleft is caused by failure of the mesoderm to merge between the medial frontonasal process and the maxillary process of the first branchial arch, between 4 and 7 weeks of gestation.

A cleft palate involves the 'secondary' palate, which forms the hard and soft palate behind the incisive foramen. These clefts are caused by failure of fusion of the two hemi-palatal shelves between 7 and 12 weeks of gestation.

INCIDENCE, AETIOLOGY AND RISK

Congenital clefts of the lip and palate are common malformations. They occur in approximately 1 : 600 live births but with slight racial variation. Cleft lip with or without cleft palate makes up about 75% of patients and is seen more commonly in boys. Cleft palate alone accounts for 25% of cases and is more common in girls.

Cleft lip and palate are inherited in a multifactorial polygenic way. There may be a positive family history. The risk of having a second child with a cleft is 4% with one affected child and 16% if the parent is affected as well.

While most clefts are isolated anomalies they may be part of a multiple malformation syndrome. In all patients other congenital anomalies should be looked for as some may be life-threatening.

CLASSIFICATION

Clefts of the lip may be incomplete, complete, unilateral or bilateral (Fig. 15.1). Bilateral clefts need not be symmetrical. Two-thirds also have a cleft of the second-

ary palate, involving both the hard and soft palate posterior to the incisive foramen. In a minority, a small band of tissue (Simonartz band) bridges the lip just below the nose, masking the cleft in the nasal floor and

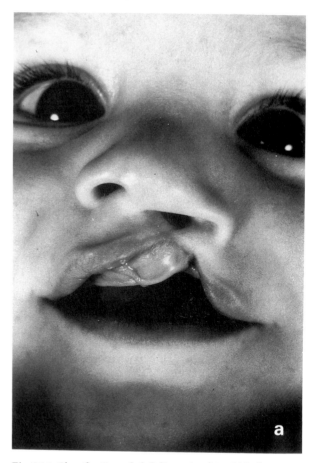

Fig. 15.1 Classification of cleft lip and palate: (a) Left unilateral complete cleft lip involving the nose, lip, alveolus and primary palate.

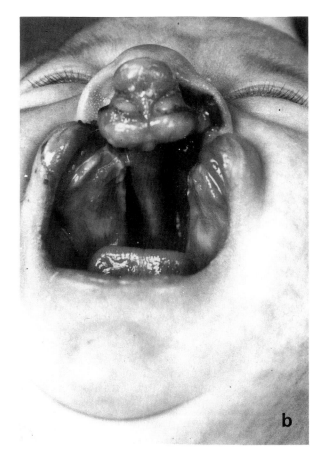
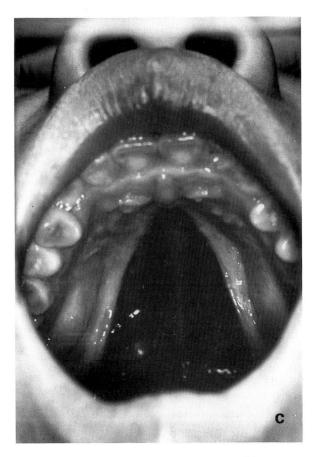

Fig. 15.1 Classification of cleft lip and palate: (b) Bilateral complete cleft lip and palate. (c) Isolated complete cleft of the secondary palate.

alveolus. Cleft palate may be complete, incomplete or submucous. Cleft lip with or without cleft palate is considered as a different clinical group from isolated cleft palate.

Pierre Robin anomalad

Many isolated cleft palates are associated with a small lower jaw. If this is severe there may be problems with swallowing and breathing as the tongue is too large for the oral cavity, and is retroposed. The tongue may become wedged in the wide cleft causing complete respiratory obstruction. These patients may have feed-

ing difficulties, failure to thrive and apnoeic episodes.

Careful nursing in a neonatal unit should allow these children to outgrow their anatomical problems. Occasionally, an oropharyngeal airway or operation to produce a tongue-lip adhesion may be required to prevent the tongue from falling back before the palate is repaired.

MANAGEMENT

Clefts of the lip and palate are managed by neonatal referral to the surgical team. The deformity affects not only the patient's appearance but also feeding, hearing, speech, and dental and maxillofacial development. The cleft lip and palate team includes specialists from many disciplines so that problems in all of these areas can be diagnosed, assessed and treated.

The proposed management is discussed with the parents as early as possible. The presence of a cleft can be a severe shock for parents, and considerable support and explanation of the likely outcome are necessary. This can be facilitated by referral to the plastic surgeon on day 1.

Feeding

Sucking presents no difficulty for the baby with a cleft of the lip alone. Breast feeding is normal. However, babies with clefts involving the secondary palate are unable to generate enough negative intra-oral pressure to make suction through the mouth possible. These babies swallow normally.

A bolus of feed is delivered to the back of the tongue, usually by means of a squeeze bottle (Fig. 15.2).

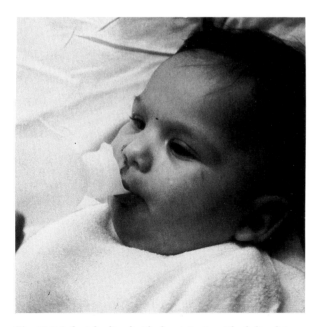

Fig. 15.2 Infant feeding bottle for patients with cleft palate. (The infant has also had lip repair.)

The baby will swallow normally. Nasogastric feeding is unnecessary in an otherwise normal infant with a cleft palate. However, premature infants or infants with other anomalies may require gavage feeding.

Lip repair

Repair of the lip is carried out at about 3 months of age. In patients with bilateral clefts or wide unilateral clefts, presurgical orthopaedics can be used to guide the palatal segments into a better position prior to surgery. Alternatively, a lip adhesion operation may be performed at 6 weeks of age.

The aim of lip repair is to obtain definitive closure of the skin, vermilion and the orbicularis oris muscle. In addition, the nasal deformity can be corrected. If the cleft includes the primary palate this and the nasal floor are also closed (Fig. 15.3). A bilateral cleft usually is repaired at one operation, although there are two-stage procedures.

Palate repair

Clefts of the secondary palate are repaired between 9 and 12 months of age, prior to the acquisition of speech. Unnecessary delay in palate repair may affect the prognosis for normal speech as the child develops compensatory speech patterns which are difficult to correct later with speech therapy. The aims of the procedure are to lengthen the palate and repair the soft palate musculature so that the oral and nasal cavities can be separated during speech by normal elevation of the soft palate to the posterior pharyngeal wall.

Submucous cleft palate

A submucous cleft palate often is overlooked. In these patients the uvula is bifid and the soft palate grooved in the midline where the muscle is cleft. There is also a palpable notch in the posterior margin of the hard palate. These patients require careful assessment and may need surgical repair in the same manner as an overt cleft palate.

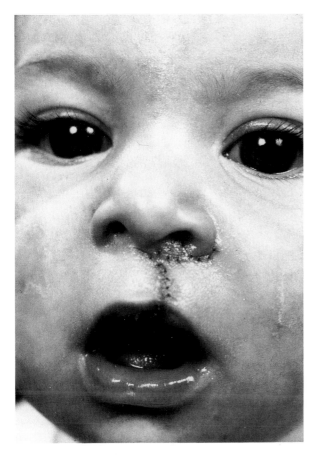

Fig. 15.3 Repair of the cleft lip.

Speech

Speech should be assessed at intervals following surgery. Speech therapy will benefit patients with articulation problems or those who use compensatory mechanisms to produce certain sounds. However, an operation is needed if the nasopharynx is incompetent and allows nasal escape of air during speech.

Between 80 and 85% of patients with cleft palate will achieve normal or acceptable, intelligible speech. Correction of nasopharyngeal incompetence is performed with a pharyngoplasty, where local pharyngeal tissue is mobilized and repositioned either into the upper surface of the soft palate or onto the posterior pharyngeal wall. This procedure is designed to help the soft palate close off the narrowed nasopharyngeal port during speech.

Pharyngoplasty is indicated also for patients with nasopharyngeal incompetence due to unoperated, late diagnosed, submucous cleft palates, as well as other less common lesions.

Problems in the ear and nose

Children with cleft palate have abnormal eustachian tubes leading to a very high incidence of middle ear disease (80%), and about 60% of these will require tubes for middle ear ventilation. Tubes often are inserted at the time of palate repair. Hearing may be impaired and these patients require frequent otoscopic and audiologic evaluation.

Tonsils and adenoids occupy a significant space in the pharynx. Their removal is contra-indicated in cleft palate patients unless recurrent infections cannot be controlled and then only after consultation with an otolaryngologist.

Dental and orthodontic treatment

Virtually all children with cleft lip and/or palate will require orthodontic treatment necessitating good dental hygiene. The cleft alveolus usually is bone-grafted to allow for proper eruption of the adult canine teeth. Supernumerary or abnormal teeth in the cleft may require removal.

A few patients require orthognathic surgery to reposition the hypoplastic maxillary arch to obtain functional occlusion. Rarely, surgery will be required on both jaws.

Secondary surgery

Secondary surgery may be required to correct residual cosmetic and functional deformities, particularly of the nose. Initial procedures are performed prior to school entry to minimize the obvious deformity in bilateral cleft lip where the columella is distinctly short. Definitive

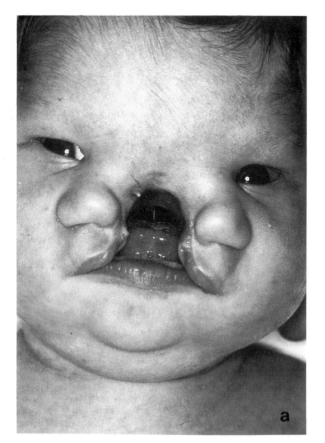

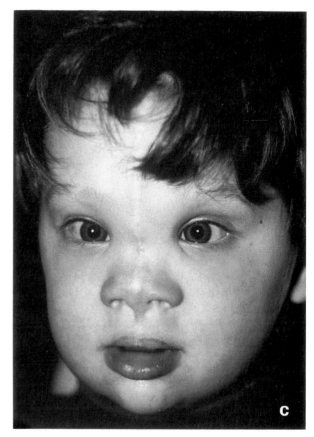

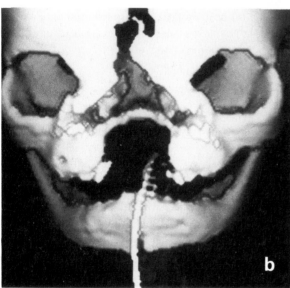

Fig. 15.4 An example of a rare craniofacial cleft and the result of its surgical correction. The bony deformity is well displayed on the three-dimensional CT scan: (a) clinical view pre-operatively; (b) three-dimensional CT with endotracheal tube *in situ*; (c) and postoperative appearance.

nasal and septal correction is usually reserved until the completion of nasal growth.

Minor procedures on the lip and vermilion can be performed at any time.

RARE FACIAL CLEFTS/CRANIOFACIAL SURGERY

There are other rare disorders in which there are clefts involving the lip and/or palate which are apparent on inspection of the baby. These types of cleft problems are managed best by a team approach and should be referred early to a craniofacial surgical unit. The same basic principles of management apply, although the technical details are greatly different (Fig. 15.4).

FURTHER READING

Dykes E. H., Raine P. A. M., Arthur D. S., Drainer I. K. & Young D. G. (1985) Pierre Robin syndrome and pulmonary hypertension. *J. Pediatr. Surg.* **20**, 49–52.

Kernahan D. A. & Rosenstein S. W. (eds) (1990) *Cleft Lip and Palate: A System of Management.* Williams & Wilkins, Baltimore.

Muir I. F. K., McLay K. A. & Wright G. (1987) Cleft lip and palate. In: Muir I. F. K. (ed.) *Plastic Surgery in Paediatrics*, pp. 11–67. Lloyd-Luke (Medical Books), London.

Stricker M. *et al.* (eds) (1990) *Craniofacial Malformations.* Churchill Livingstone, Melbourne.

— 16 —

Abnormalities of the Neck and Face

The neck is one of the commonest sites for cystic and solid swellings during childhood. Lesions are either 'developmental anomalies' arising from remnants of the branchial arches, the thyroglossal tract, the jugular lymphatics or the skin; or 'acquired', as in diseases in the lymph nodes, salivary glands or the thyroid gland (Table 16.1).

Table 16.1 Swellings in the neck

| **Developmental anomalies** |
| Branchial |
| cysts |
| sinuses |
| fistulae |
| cartilage |
| Thyroglossal cyst |
| Ectopic thyroid |
| Cystic hygroma |
| Epidermal cyst |
| **Acquired lesions** |
| Inflammation of cervical lymphatics |
| acute lymphadenitis |
| MAIS lymphadenitis |
| acute lymph node abscess |
| Lymph node tumours |
| primary neoplasia |
| secondary neoplasia |
| Submandibular gland |
| calculus |
| Parotid gland |
| sialectasis |

BRANCHIAL CYSTS, SINUSES, FISTULAE AND OTHER REMNANTS

These arise from the branchial arch system. Branchial clefts may give rise to an epithelial-lined lesion: for example branchial cyst, branchial sinus (blind-ending tract) or branchial fistula (communication between two epithelial-lined surfaces). The branchial arch itself may give rise to mesodermal remnants, usually cartilaginous, lying along the line of development of the arch.

Sinuses and fistulae most commonly arise from the second branchial cleft, occasionally from the first and rarely from the third branchial cleft. In the second branchial cleft defects, the tract commences in the tonsillar fossa and passes with the glossopharyngeal nerve between the internal and external carotid arteries to end on the skin at the anterior border of the lower third of the sternomastoid muscle. First cleft fistulae run from the external auditory canal to the skin below the lower border of the mandible. The rare third branchial cleft fistula opens internally into the piriform sinus and externally on the skin overlying the lower end of the sternomastoid muscle.

Branchial fistulae usually present in early childhood when a drop of mucus is observed leaking from the external orifice or when a persisting damp patch is noticed on the clothing. Sinuses may present at any time during childhood and sometimes may be complicated by infection. The treatment for both is surgical excision.

Branchial cysts are uncommon in childhood. They usually arise from the second cleft and emerge from beneath the anterior border of the sternomastoid in the upper third of the neck. They may extend upwards behind the angle of the jaw to the base of the skull or antero-inferiorly towards the midline, lying on the carotid sheath. The fluid contents are milky and contain cholesterol crystals. They may become infected and these cysts should be excised.

Branchial arch remnants usually arise from the second branchial arch and present as an unsightly protuberance at the anterior border of the lower third of the sternomastoid. These lesions are excised for cosmetic reasons.

THYROGLOSSAL CYST

The descent of the thyroid anlage from the floor of the fetal mouth leaves a track from the foramen caecum of the tongue to the thyroid isthmus. A cyst lined by respiratory epithelium may arise anywhere along the track, but is usually close to and adherent to the hyoid bone (75%). Typically, there is a tense rounded cyst in the mid-line or just to one side, which moves on swallowing and on protrusion of the tongue. The cysts also may be submental (15%), lingual (2%) and suprasternal (8%) in position. Infection may supervene and form an abscess (Fig. 16.1). An infected thyroglossal cyst may be mistaken for acute bacterial lymphadenitis in the submental lymph nodes. The thyroglossal cyst and the entire thyroglossal track should be excised,

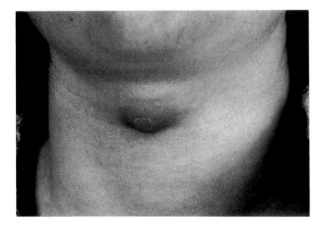

Fig. 16.1 Thyroglossal cyst which has become infected.

preferably before infection occurs; this excision should include the middle third of the hyoid bone to minimise the risk of recurrence (Sistrunk operation).

ECTOPIC THYROID

Ectopic thyroid is a rare cause of midline neck swelling. The swelling tends to be softer than that of a thyroglossal cyst but the diagnosis may not be apparent until at operation when the lesion is found to be solid and vascular. If this lesion is suspected pre-operatively, a thyroid isotope scan should be performed to determine the distribution of all functioning thyroid, because the ectopic thyroid may be the only functioning thyroid tissue present. In this situation, it is not excised: the mass is divided in the midline and rotated on its vascular pedicle laterally to lie behind the strap muscles. Other thyroid swellings in children are rare. Neonatal goitre may result from excessive maternal iodine ingestion. Thyrotoxicosis is rare in young children. Adenoma and papillary carcinoma are seen occasionally in older children.

CYSTIC HYGROMA

A cystic hygroma is a hamartoma of the jugular lymph sacs. It presents in infancy and is more common in boys than girls (Fig. 16.2). Cystic hygromas are of two types: first, a simple multicystic lesion without involvement of other structures; second, a complex lesion which involves other structures including the mouth, pharynx, larynx or mediastinum and may contain cavernous haemangiomatous elements. This type resembles lymphangiomas found elsewhere in the body.

Simple cystic hygromas are commoner and are usually found as unilateral fluctuant, transilluminable swellings centred on the carotid triangle. The cysts are of varying sizes and contain clear fluid. They may enlarge suddenly and rapidly due to viral or bacterial infection or haemorrhage. The effect of this will depend on the site and size of the cysts. A clinical emergency may arise if the increased swelling compromises the airways. In the absence of these complications surgical excision is undertaken for cosmetic reasons and the prognosis is good.

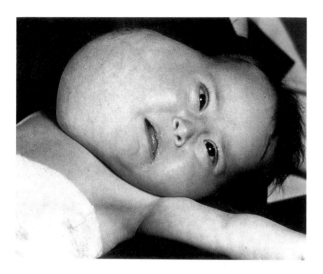

Fig. 16.2 Cystic hygroma in a baby with Down syndrome.

Complex cystic hygromas are less common and complications arise because of extensive soft-tissue involvement. These malformations may involve the oropharynx leading to difficulty with speech and swallowing, or the larynx and trachea leading to a life-threatening respiratory obstruction. Involvement of the mediastinum and pleural cavity likewise may lead to respiratory embarrassment. They present on the first day of life and emergency care may necessitate insertion of an endotracheal tube and sometimes a tracheostomy. Surgical excision is undertaken relatively early and involves debulking the extensive lesion.

EPIDERMOID CYSTS

Inclusion dermoids arise from ectodermal cells detached during fetal growth. They are often in the midline or along lines of fusion, for example the midline cervical dermoid which may be mistaken for a thyroglossal cyst. They contain sebaceous 'cheesy' material surrounded by squamous epithelium. They enlarge slowly and should be removed. The commonest inclusion dermoid is the external angular dermoid at the orbital margin (see below).

Less common varieties include the sublingual dermoid which lies between the mylohyoid and genioglossus muscles in the floor of the mouth. It may interfere with speech and swallowing and can be excised through a submental incision. It may be confused with a ranula or mucocele of the floor of the mouth, a lesion which contains mucus and is treated by marsupialization of its roof.

An unusual developmental anomaly found in this region is the midline cervical cleft, a vertical open groove which results from failure of fusion of the branchial arches. Surgical repair should be undertaken.

PERIORBITAL CELLULITIS

Infection in the soft tissues around the eye can cause periorbital cellulitis with rapid extension across the face (Fig. 16.3). The danger with this infection is that it may spread to the cavernous sinus, which is potentially lethal. Children with periorbital cellulitis should be admitted to hospital for treatment with intravenous antibiotics.

DISEASES OF THE LYMPH NODES

Infection is the commonest cause of lymph node enlargement in childhood. It may be caused by bacteria, viruses or non-tuberculous mycobacteria. In many cases the lymph nodes are reacting to an upper respiratory tract or ear infection; this is known as non-specific reactive hyperplasia. Lymph nodes also may become enlarged due to primary or secondary malignancy. When the diagnosis is in doubt or if persistently enlarged lymph nodes (>3 cm) are present for longer than 4–6 weeks a surgical biopsy is indicated. In 1 year at the Royal Children's Hospital, 102 children underwent a biopsy of lymph nodes.

Reactive hyperplasia

Persistently enlarged lymph nodes are seen in many children with frequent upper respiratory tract infections. These nodes are not painful and are a normal

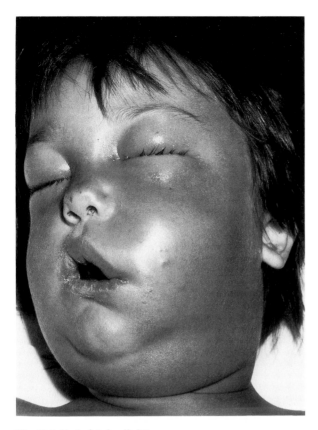

Fig. 16.3 Periorbital cellulitis.

response to infection. Occasionally a markedly enlarged hyperplastic node may come to excision biopsy to exclude tumour or other diagnoses.

Acute lymphadenitis

Acutely tender enlarged lymph glands are commonly seen during upper respiratory tract infections. Lymphadenitis usually settles with rest, analgesia and—if bacterial infection is suspected—antibiotics.

Acute lymph node abscess

Lymphadenitis may progress to an abscess, particularly in children aged 6 months to 3 years. The swelling enlarges over 3 or 4 days and may become fluctuant. An abscess in deeper nodes may not exhibit fluctuation. The overlying skin is red and, if untreated, the abscess will eventually point and discharge. The management of an abscess in a child is incision and drainage under general anaesthesia. Damage to the mandibular branch of the facial nerve must be avoided when submandibular abscesses are incised.

'MAIS' lymphadenitis

Mycobacteria avium, intracellulare and scrofulaceum (MAIS) cause chronic cervical lymphadenitis and 'collar stud' abscesses in children. In most Western countries, Human TB and Bovine TB strains almost have been eradicated. However, MAIS lymphadenitis is still a problem in the preschool child. The MAIS mycobacteria are found in the soil and infection is from the child's dirty hand to the mouth and then to the tonsillar lymph node. Initially the node is enlarged and firm, but nontender. Over a period of 4–6 weeks the node produces a collar stud abscess in the subcutaneous tissue causing the overlying skin to become a characteristic blue-purple colour. Untreated, the collarstud 'cold' abscess will ulcerate through the skin and lead to multiple discharging sinuses. MAIS mycobacteria do not respond to antibiotics and require surgical excision to remove the infected lymph nodes. The mandibular branch of the facial nerve may be at risk during excision of an affected jugulodigastric lymph node. The diagnosis of MAIS lymphadenitis is confirmed by histological examination of the lymph node and culture of the pus and lymph node tissue. Skin tests based on the reaction of intradermal purified protein derivative of Mycobacterium avium may provide further evidence of infection.

Lymph node tumours

Primary neoplasia

Hodgkin's and non-Hodgkin's lymphomas may occur in cervical lymph nodes in older children.

Secondary neoplasia

Nasopharyngeal and thyroid tumours and neuro-blastoma may present with cervical node enlargement. In most cases the marked enlargement and rocky hardness of the lymph nodes makes the diagnosis of neoplasia obvious. In other circumstances the differential diagnosis between a large hyperplastic lymph node and a neoplastic node is difficult and necessitates excision biopsy.

THE SUBMANDIBULAR GLAND

The commonest cause of enlargement is a small calculus in the submandibular duct. It produces rapid and painful enlargement of the gland during eating. The gland becomes hard and tender and fluctuates in size. The submucous part of the duct in the floor of the mouth should be inspected for a tiny calculus impacted near the orifice under the tongue. An X-ray of the floor of the mouth may show an opaque calculus which is too small or too proximal to be seen with the naked eye. The submandibular duct calculus can be removed by simple incision of the duct.

THE PAROTID GLAND

Recurrent enlargement is more common in the parotid than in the submandibular gland and is due to recurrent parotitis associated with sialectasis, a condition analogous to bronchiectasis, which affects the lesser ducts and their tributaries. Parotid calculi are extremely rare.

Symptoms of sialectasis usually commence at 2–4 years of age, and the first attack may be misdiagnosed as mumps, although both sides are seldom swollen at the same time. One or both parotids are affected and the attacks are unilateral or alternate from side to side. The gland becomes generally enlarged and mildly tender; fever and malaise are mild or absent.

Purulent fluid issues from the orifice when the duct is compressed, and *Streptococcus viridans* or other weakly pathogenic organisms may be found on culture. The attacks are self-limiting and last 3–4 days, but the symptoms may persist intermittently for several years.

The diagnosis is clinical. However, if a sialogram is performed it will show a snowstorm of sacculations 2–4 mm in diameter along the radicles of the gland (Fig. 16.4) but no duct obstruction. The changes are often present in both glands, even when the symptoms have been confined to one side.

The condition is troublesome but not serious and the attacks can be shortened or made less frequent by massage of the parotid, tart drinks to promote the flow of saliva, and occasionally by antibiotics if infection supervenes. In most children there is a marked decrease in the number of attacks at about 10 years of age, and sialograms during adolescence often show that the sialectasis has disappeared. Parotidectomy is not necessary.

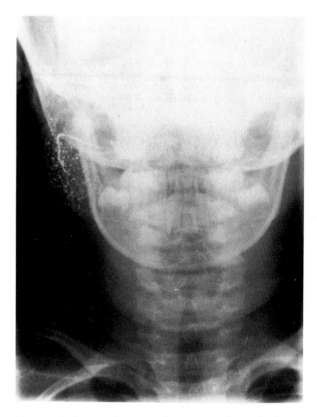

Fig. 16.4 Sialogram showing sialectasis. A radiograph of radio-opaque material in the parotid duct showing a 'snowstorm' of saccular dilatations of the lesser ducts in the enlarged parotid.

DEVELOPMENTAL ANOMALIES OF THE FACE

External angular dermoid

This is a common anomaly of fusion between the frontonasal and maxillary processes during formation of the head and face (Chapter 12). The cyst is noticed in infancy as it enlarges gradually and progressively (Fig. 16.5). Often it is beneath the pericranium, which gives it a firmer consistency than may be expected. Occasionally, it is misdiagnosed as a bony lump. Excision through a small eyebrow incision is curative.

Many varieties of facial clefts have been described and classified, but most of them are rare. Cleft lip and palate, by contrast, are very common, and hence are described in a separate section (Chapter 15).

Hemifacial microsomia

Malformations of the structures derived from the first pharyngeal arch may cause microstomia, a misshapen ear, absence of the external auditory canal, a rudimentary middle ear, hypoplasia of the mandible and its teeth, hypoplasia of the malar–maxillary complex and, sometimes, facial paralysis. The condition may be bilateral.

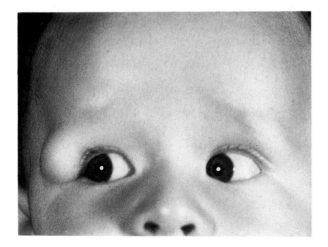

Fig. 16.5 External angular dermoid.

Mandibular dysostosis (Treacher Collins syndrome)

Children with Treacher Collins syndrome have bilateral absence of the malar bone, microtia, colobomata of the eyelids and hypoplasia of the masseter and temporalis muscles. Complex defects of the facial skeleton such as this are managed by sophisticated craniofacial surgery.

DEFORMITIES OF THE EAR

Accessory auricles

Any number of small tags of skin and cartilage may be present, usually close to the tragus, but sometimes along a line extending to the angle of the mouth. They are removed for cosmetic reasons.

Pre-auricular sinus

This is a common condition, often bilateral and asymptomatic. There is a tiny hole just in front of the upper crus of the helix, from which an epithelial track extends deeply forwards. The track is often short, but sometimes extends deeply towards the pharynx and is extremely difficult to trace among the important structures in this area.

Where there are no symptoms or only an occasional bead of watery discharge, it is best left alone. If it becomes infected with purulent discharge and the opening becomes sealed, a large abscess may develop. In such cases the abscess should be deroofed and the sinus excised, which is curative.

Microtia

A rudimentary ear, of irregular skin and cartilage, is associated with absence of the external auditory canal, a rudimentary middle ear and a small mandible on the same side (Fig. 16.6). When the site of the ear is acceptable, it can be used as the basis for a reconstruction, which is preferable to an artificial prosthetic ear.

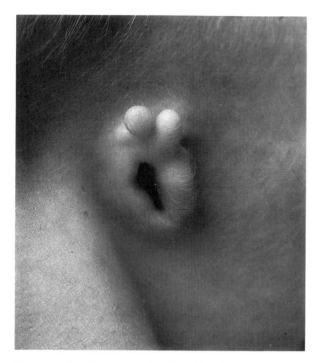

Fig. 16.6 Microtia, associated with maldevelopment of the dorsal ends of the first and second branchial arches. The external auditory canal is a shallow pit.

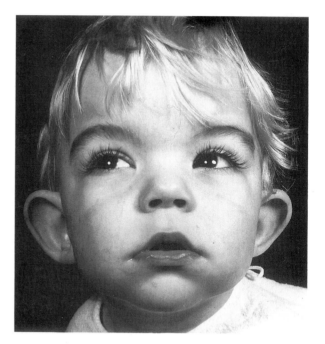

Fig. 16.7 Bat ears.

Only when the condition is bilateral is it necessary to create an external auditory canal and it is important to provide a hearing aid within the first few months of life to enable the infant to hear and develop speech. Further operations are required in later years.

Bat ears

Bat ears, both unilateral and bilateral, are common and often familial (Fig. 16.7). The concavity of the concha extends to the rim which stands out farther than normal. The ear is often bigger than normal as well as more protuberant.

Corrective surgery is advisable when there is gross protrusion, particularly when there are adverse comments from other children. Strapping in the neonatal period achieves nothing, and removal of skin from the post-auricular groove is inadequate. The fold of the antihelix must be fashioned, shaping and fixing the cartilages in a new relationship, and holding them in position for the approximately 3 weeks required for union of the cartilages.

'Shell' ears

Shell ears are similar to bat ears in protruding from the scalp, but they are small, and the rim of the helix is so short that the ear cannot be readily folded back into the normal position. Surgical repair usually has to be done in stages and is much more difficult than in bat ears.

FURTHER READING

Doi O., Hutson J. M., Myers N. A. & McKelvie P. A. (1988) Branchial remnants: a review of 58 cases. *J. Pediatr. Surg.* **23**: 798–792.

Friedberg J. (1988) Clinical diagnosis of neck lumps: a practical guide. *Pediatr. Ann.* **17**: 620–628.

Joshi W., Davidson P. M., Jones P. G., Campbell P. E. & Roberton D. M. (1989) Non-tuberculous mycobacterial lymphadenitis in children. *Eur. J. Pediatr.* **148**: 751–754.

Kennedy T. L. (1989) Cystic hygroma–lymphangioma: a rare and still unclear entity. *Laryngoscope* **99**: 1–10.

Margileth A. M. (1985) Cat scratch disease. Current concepts. *Hosp. Med.* **21**: 57.

Merriman T., Davidson P. M. & Myers N. A. (1991) The spectrum of cervical cystic hygroma. *Pediatr. Surg. Int.* (in press).

Muir I. F. K. (ed.) (1987) Other conditions of the face. In: *Plastic Surgery in Paediatrics*, pp. 93–104. Lloyd-Luke (Medical Books), London.

Muir I. F. K. & McKay K. A. (1987) The ear. In: Muir I. F. K. (ed.) *Plastic Surgery in Paediatrics*, pp. 82–92. Lloyd-Luke (Medical Books), London.

Myers E. N. & Cunningham M. G. (1988) Inflammatory presentations of congenital head and neck masses. *J. Pediatr. Infect. Dis.* **7**: S162–S168.

Nathanson L. K. & Gough I. R. (1989) Surgery for thyroglossal cysts: Sistrunk's operation remains the standard. *Aust. NZ J. Surg.* **59**: 873–875.

Wright J. E. (1989) Cervical lymphadenitis in childhood: which antibiotic agent? *Med. J. Aust.* **150**: 150–151.

17

The Umbilicus

After birth, the umbilical cord desiccates and separates, and the umbilical ring closes. Complications arise when this process is incomplete. The stump of the cord may become infected, or rarely, the visceral channels of embryonic life may persist, that is the urachus from the bladder and the vitello-intestinal (omphalomesenteric) duct from the ileum. The commonest abnormality is persistence of the abdominal defect through which the cord passed, and results in an umbilical hernia. The less common but more severe condition of exomphalos (syn. omphalocele) is discussed in Chapter 9.

UMBILICAL HERNIA

Involution of the umbilical vessels and Wharton's jelly in the linea alba normally is accompanied by contraction of the umbilical ring in the first few days after birth. When this does not occur, a central or 'true' umbilical hernia results; the peritoneum bulges into the defect, followed by a loop of bowel (Fig. 17.1).

Some degree of umbilical herniation is present in almost 20% of newborn babies, still more in premature infants or when there is any increase in intra-abdominal pressure, for example in ascites, Down syndrome or cretinism.

When the infant lies quietly, the umbilical skin merely looks redundant, but on crying or straining, bowel fills the hernia and the lesion enlarges to become tense and bluish beneath the thin shiny skin. The bowel can be reduced easily, often with an audible gurgle.

Most umbilical hernias close spontaneously. However, there are several practical points which must be explained to the parents:

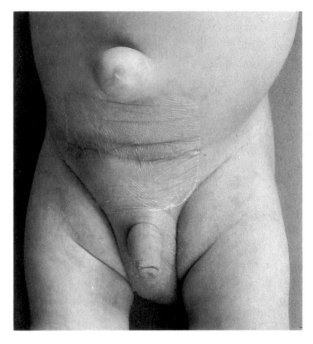

Fig. 17.1 Umbilical hernia in a baby with repaired inguinal hernias.

(1) The time of natural closure. In the first 3–4 months of life the bulge may actually increase a little, before getting smaller. Resolution usually occurs in the first 12 months, but may take up to 3 years

(2) The skin never ruptures, and the thin skin of the first 4 weeks gradually becomes thicker

(3) Strangulation is virtually unknown and it is safe to wait. The tenseness of the hernia when the infant cries is often interpreted incorrectly as causing pain; umbilical hernias probably are symptomless.

Treatment

The use of strapping does not induce closure when this would not otherwise have occurred spontaneously, and because strapping may cause complications it is contra-indicated.

Surgery should be considered if the hernia is still present after the age of 3 years.

If the neck of the sac is less than 1 cm in diameter at 12 months of age, eventual spontaneous closure is still likely, and surgery should be deferred until at least 3 years of age. Even if the neck is 2 cm or more in diameter at 12 months, and spontaneous closure is less likely, surgery is deferred until the third year.

PARA-UMBILICAL HERNIA

This is a defect in the linea alba separate from but adjacent to the umbilical cicatrix. Most are just above the umbilicus, rarely to one side or below it. The defect is a transverse elliptical slit with sharp edges, in contrast to the rounded shape and blunt edges of a central umbilical hernia. Spontaneous closure is unlikely and surgery is required in nearly all cases, as an elective procedure after the first year of life.

THE INFANT WITH A DISCHARGE FROM THE UMBILICUS

A discharge from the umbilicus may be pus, urine or faeces.

Purulent discharge

The commonest cause of a purulent discharge is a localized infection, and the rarest an abscess in a urachal or vitello-intestinal remnant.

Umbilical sepsis

Umbilical sepsis (omphalitis) is a dangerous infection which occurs in the neonatal period in the exposed stump of the cord. Consequently, an important aspect of preventive medicine is to keep the stump dry and dressed with antiseptics. The commonest causative organisms are *Staphylococci*, *Escherichia coli* and *Streptococci*. In minor infections the navel is red and swollen with a seropurulent discharge but responds well to local and systemic antibiotics.

There may be little superficial evidence of inflammation when infection has spread further, via lymphatics or the umbilical vessels. Drainage of abscesses and local and general antibiotics are required. Septicaemia and/or peritonitis result when organisms enter the bloodstream through the superficial vessels, or through the recently patent vessels in the umbilicus: the two umbilical arteries retain a lumen for some time after birth and provide a route of infection to the internal iliac arteries. An abscess along this pathway is more common than entry of micro-organisms into the circulation or into the peritoneal cavity.

Infection also can travel along the lumen of the umbilical vein to the portal vein and via the ductus venosus to the vena cava. Clinically overt infections in these structures are rare but serious, and latent infection can lead to thrombophlebitis and thrombosis of a segment of the portal vein. Recanalization and opening collaterals may lead to a cavernomatous malformation of the portal vein, and portal hypertension (Chapter 26).

Umbilical granuloma

An umbilical granuloma is an extremely common lesion which presents as a small mass of heaped cherry-red granulations, accompanied by a seropurulent discharge. It is granulation tissue produced in response to subacute bacterial colonization of the cord stump. If there is a definite stalk, it can be ligated without anaesthesia, but if it is soft, deep or too broad, topical application of silver nitrate will enable epithelium to cover the surface and is curative. Sometimes, a small area of ectopic bowel mucosa at the base of the umbilicus has a similar clinical appearance and is treated in the same way (see below).

Urinary discharge

Urinary discharge from the umbilicus results from a rare persistent communication through the urachus to the bladder (Fig. 17.2). Persistent urachus may occur in association with obstruction in the lower urinary tract, for example posterior urethral valves, and occasionally with imperforate anus.

The surgical treatment is excision of the urachal remnant after investigation and relief of any underlying anomalies.

A mass or abscess in the midline at or below the umbilicus also may develop from a partly obliterated urachus; drainage and excision are required.

Mucous or faecal discharge

Ectopic mucosa

Discharge of mucus from the umbilicus may be caused

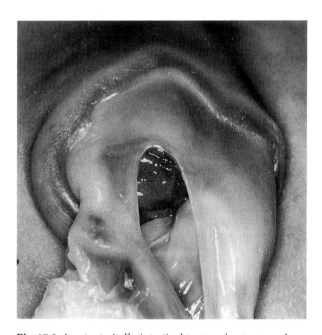

Fig. 17.2 A patent vitello-intestinal tract and patent urachus may look similar, and the diagnosis is made according to whether the discharge is urinary or faecal.

by a small sequestrated nodule of ectopic alimentary mucosa, which appears shiny, spherical, bright red, and situated in the depths of the umbilical cicatrix. Crusts form on the cicatrix and on the surrounding skin and a persistent vitello-intestinal (omphalomesenteric) tract may be suspected.

Careful inspection will show the 'pseudopolyp', and the application of silver nitrate on one or two occasions is all that is needed to remove the alimentary epithelium, which is replaced rapidly by normal skin.

Persistent vitello-intestinal duct

Persistence of the vitello-intestinal (omphalomesenteric) duct, a rare condition, produces a communication between the intestinal tract and the umbilicus, reflecting the embryonic communication between the yolk sac and the mid-gut which normally disappears at about the sixth week of fetal life. Persistence of part or all of this tract gives rise to a group of lesions which usually present in early infancy but on occasions not until some years later (Fig. 17.2).

A vitello-intestinal duct represents patency of the whole tract, and the contents of the ileum may discharge intermittently. Very rarely, when the channel is short and broad, the ileum may intussuscept through it onto the surface of the umbilicus as a Y-shaped segment of bowel, inside out, with two orifices.

A sinus or cyst is the result of partial obliteration of the duct; these may become infected, form an abscess, and discharge pus.

A vitello-intestinal band is the remnant of the duct and runs from the deep surface of the umbilicus to the ileum. It may cause no symptoms throughout life or it may, at any age, cause intestinal obstruction when a loop of bowel becomes entangled beneath it.

Meckel's diverticulum is the patent inner segment of the duct, and very rarely a band attaches it to the underside of the umbilicus. The presenting features and complications are described in Chapter 23.

All remnants of the vitello-intestinal duct are excised, which may necessitate a laparotomy to search for discontinuous segments of the tract.

FURTHER READING

Campbell J., Beasley S. W., McMullin N. D. & Hutson J. M. (1986) Umbilical swellings and discharges in children. *Med. J. Aust.* **145**: 450–453.

Lasaletta L., Fonkalsrud E. W. *et al.* (1975) The management of umbilical hernia in infancy and childhood. *J. Pediatr. Surg.* **10**: 405–409.

Rich R. H., Hardy B. E. & Filler R. M. (1983) Surgery for anomalies of the urachus. *J. Pediatr. Surg.* **18**: 370–372.

Shaw A. (1986) Disorders of the umbilicus. In Welch K. J. Randolph J. G., Ravitch M. M., O'Neill J. A. & Rowe M. I. (eds), *Pediatric Surgery*, 4th edn, Vol. 2, p. 731. Year Book, Chicago.

18

Vomiting in the First Months of Life

Vomiting is common in the first months of life, when the evaluation of its significance is particularly important. The temptation to disregard it must be resisted: it is a symptom, not a diagnosis, and its cause must be established (Table 18.1).

Vomiting is significant when it is:

(1) Bile-stained
(2) Persistent
(3) Projectile
(4) Blood-stained; that is, 'coffee grounds', flecked with altered blood
(5) Accompanied by loss of weight or failure to gain weight.

Vomiting most commonly is due to non-surgical conditions or feeding difficulties. Neonatal infections, for example septicaemia, meningitis or urinary tract infection, may present with a wide variety of clinical features including vomiting, convulsions, diarrhoea,

pallor, cyanosis and hypothermia. Gastroenteritis may be seen in bottle-fed babies, but is uncommon in fully breast-fed infants. In approximately 25% of those with the rare syndrome of congenital adrenal hyperplasia there is a salt-losing metabolic disturbance with severe vomiting, and genital abnormalities in females (Chapter 11).

Malrotation with volvulus usually presents in the first week or so of life but may occur at any age. The vomiting is bile-stained, and in any child with sudden onset of green vomiting the possibility of malrotation with volvulus must be entertained. An urgent barium meal will diagnose malrotation. If volvulus goes unrecognized the entire mid-gut may be lost from ischaemia and the child will die.

Strangulated inguinal hernias are common in infants and are easily diagnosed on examination. A hard, tender irreducible swelling at the external inguinal ring will confirm the diagnosis.

Table 18.1 Causes of vomiting at 1 month of age

Septic	Meningitis
	Urinary tract infection
	Septicaemia
	Gastroenteritis
Mechanical	Gastro-oesophageal reflux
	Pyloric stenosis
	Strangulated inguinal hernia
	Malrotation with volvulus (usually bile-stained vomiting)
Other	Congenital adrenal hyperplasia
	Overfeeding

PYLORIC STENOSIS

Pyloric stenosis is the commonest cause of vomiting requiring surgery in infants, and affects 1 : 450 children of whom 85% are boys.

Congenital hypertrophic pyloric stenosis is an important surgical condition in infancy because it is common, there is risk to life and permanent relief is obtained by a relatively simple operation. The aetiology remains obscure and is partly genetic. Almost 20% have a family history of pyloric stenosis.

Symptoms

The usual presentation is with severe vomiting, which commences between 3 and 6 weeks of age in an otherwise well baby. Pyloric stenosis is rare in infants younger than 10 days or older than 11 weeks.

The vomiting occurs after all feeds and is copious. The vomitus contains milk with some added gastric mucus and is practically never bile-stained. Occasionally, it may contain brown coffee-ground flecks of altered blood, reflecting the gastritis secondary to the gastric outlet obstruction. Often the vomiting is projectile and may occur well after the last feed. Initially, the child is active and hungry and a key feature is his readiness and ability to feed again immediately after vomiting. Later, with increasing dehydration and electrolyte imbalance he becomes weak, lethargic and listless, not unlike the clinical picture seen in a child with sepsis. He loses weight and looks scrawny. If untreated he may ultimately die of dehydration and metabolic alkalosis.

Signs

Peristaltic waves of gastric contraction indicate hypertrophy of the gastric muscle secondary to slowly progressive obstruction: their presence makes pyloric stenosis very likely. Palpation of the thickened pylorus in the epigastrium, however, confirms the diagnosis. The hypertrophied and thickened pylorus is traditionally called a 'pyloric tumour'. It feels like an olive or a small pebble and has been likened to the terminal segment of the little finger. It is relatively mobile. It is palpable most easily in the angle between the liver and the lateral margin of the right rectus abdominus muscle or in the gap between the two recti midway between the umbilicus and the xiphisternum (Fig. 18.1). It is felt most easily when the baby is relaxed and not crying, and when the stomach is empty. When difficulty is experienced in feeling the 'tumour', a nasogastric tube should be passed to empty the stomach.

Failure to palpate the pyloric tumour

If the initial palpation is not conclusive, further observation is necessary and a second examination is made a

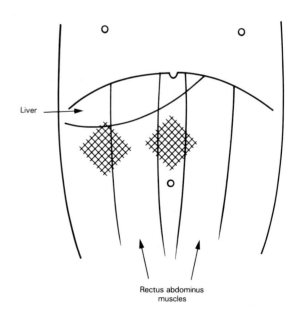

Fig. 18.1 Schema showing the surface markings of the pylorus.

few hours later. Other manoeuvres which may assist in the palpation of an elusive pyloric tumour are summarized in Table 18.2. When no tumour can be palpated, and septic causes of vomiting have been excluded, radiological investigation may be required. Real-time ultrasound may identify the hypertrophied pylorus (Fig. 18.2). A barium contrast meal performed under fluoroscopic control may show gastric outlet obstruction (Fig. 18.3) and may show other pathology, including gastro-oesophageal reflux. These investigations are required in a small minority of cases only.

The diagnosis may be delayed because vomiting has been attributed to pre-existing gastro-oesophageal reflux (which is extremely common in infants) or feeding problems. Often there is a history of several changes in feeding patterns before the diagnosis is made. However, the palpation of a tumour is the *sine qua non* of diagnosis and excludes all other causes. Other features, such as visible gastric peristalsis and the observation of projectile vomiting are supporting evidence but not in themselves diagnostic.

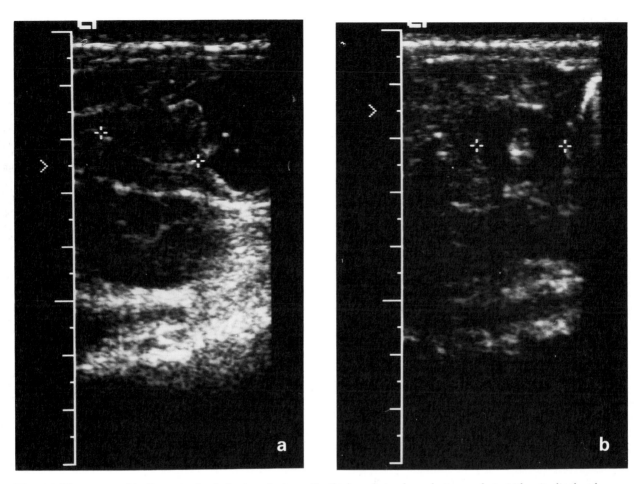

Fig. 18.2 Ultrasonographic diagnosis of pyloric stenosis shows the thickened circular pyloric muscle in (a) longitudinal and (b) transverse section.

Investigation

The history and clinical findings reveal the degree of dehydration. The extent of the electrolyte and acid–base imbalance must be determined to guide appropriate resuscitation before operation. Further estimations of the serum electrolytes and acid–base parameters after resuscitation should confirm complete correction of the electrolyte disturbance before surgery.

Treatment

Treatment involves correction of the fluid and electrolyte abnormality followed by pyloromyotomy, the Ramstedt operation. These infants should be resuscitated with 0.45% sodium chloride and supplementary potassium chloride in 5% dextrose. The rate is determined after estimation of the percentage dehydration, weight of the infant and maintenance requirements.

The Ramstedt operation involves splitting the hypertrophied pyloric muscle as far as the mucosa,

Table 18.2 Difficulty palpating pyloric tumour

(1) Is the baby relaxed? (Hard to feel pylorus through contracting anterior abdominal wall musculature.)
 Be patient
 Repeat examination
 Flex hips
 Wait until crying stops or infant asleep
 Allow infant to suck on dummy
 Palpate at commencement of feed
(2) Is the stomach empty?
 Put down nasogastric tube to empty stomach
(3) Is the diagnosis wrong?
 Consider septic causes
 Check hernial orifices
(4) Pyloric stenosis still suspected (e.g. because gastric peristalsis present)
 Barium meal
 Ultrasound

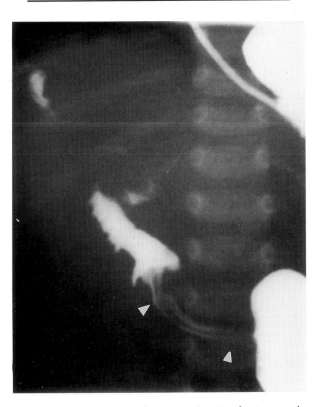

Fig. 18.3 Pyloric stenosis. The 'string sign' in a barium meal, that is the greatly narrowed pyloric canal (arrowheads) causing gastric outlet obstruction.

enabling it to bulge through the gap, thus providing a wider channel into the duodenum. The best results are obtained when the muscle split includes the distal 1–2 cm of antrum. Normal oral feeds can be commenced 24 h after operation. The babies rapidly regain their lost weight.

GASTRO-OESOPHAGEAL REFLUX

Incompetence of the sphincteric mechanism at the oesophagogastric junction causes vomiting in the neonatal period and tends to become less severe as the infant gets older. Vomiting occurs at any time during or between feeds and usually is neither projectile nor bile-stained, but if oesophagitis is present bleeding may occur as bright blood in the vomitus, or more commonly as 'coffee ground' flecks of altered blood.

Gastro-oesophageal reflux affects most infants and the diagnosis is made on clinical grounds.

Management

Because there is a natural tendency towards spontaneous improvement with age the initial treatment should be conservative, including putting the infant prone with the head of the cot elevated on blocks. Thickening of feeds and the use of mild antacids, Gaviscon and Maxalon also may be helpful.

In severe cases where there is evidence of oesophagitis, oesophageal stricture, anaemia, respiratory symptoms or failure to thrive, a barium swallow is advisable to confirm the presence of gastro-oesophageal reflux and to demonstrate any oesophageal stricture (Fig. 18.4).

Oesophagoscopy and oesophageal biopsy should be performed if haematemesis has occurred or when anaemia is present to assess the extent and severity of the peptic oesophagitis, or when a barium swallow shows evidence of oesophageal obstruction. Further information may be gained from 24 h pH monitoring and oesophageal manometry.

If the conservative regime fails, or there is an oesophageal stricture or if a large 'sliding' hernia is present, surgery to control the reflux is indicated. This

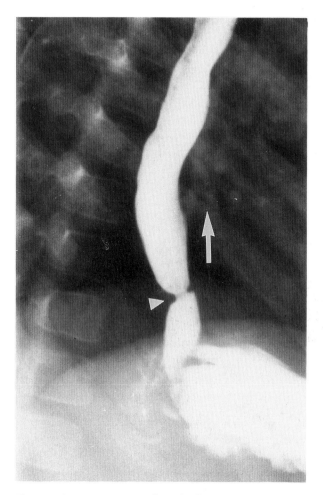

Fig. 18.4 Severe gastro-oesophageal reflux with an oesophageal stricture secondary to reflux oesophagitis (arrowhead). The contrast can be seen to flow freely up the oesophagus (arrow).

involves plication of the fundus of the stomach around the lower oesophagus (Nissen fundoplication). The oesophageal hiatus is repaired at the same time. Oesophageal strictures secondary to reflux normally resolve spontaneously once the reflux has been eliminated.

FURTHER READING

Beasley S. W., Hudson I., Hok Pan Yuen & Jones P. G. (1986) Influence of age, sex, duration of symptoms and dehydration on serum electrolytes in hypertrophic pyloric stenosis. *Aust. Paediatr. J.* **22**: 193–197.

Fonkalsrud E. W., Ament M. E. & Berquist W. (1985) Surgical management of the gastroesophageal reflux syndrome in childhood. *Surgery* **97**: 42.

Hutson J. M. & Beasley S. W. (1988) Non bile-stained vomiting in infancy. In: *The Surgical Examination of Children* pp. 71–76. Heinemann Medical, Oxford.

Jolley S. G., Halpern C. T., Sterling C. E. & Feldman B. H. (1990) The relationship of respiratory complications from gastroesophageal reflux to prematurity in infants. *J. Pediatr. Surg.* **25**: 755–757.

Meyers W. F., Roberts C. C., Johnson D. G. & Herbst J. J. (1985) Value of tests for evaluation of gastroesophageal reflux in children. *J. Pediatr. Surg.* **20**: 515–520.

Ohhama Y., Tsunoda A., Nishi T., Yamada R. & Yamamoto H. (1990) Surgical treatment of reflux stricture of the esophagus. *J. Pediatr. Surg.* **25**: 758–761.

Rasmussen L., Anderson O. P. & Pedersen S. A. (1990) Intestinal malrotation and volvulus in infancy. *Pediatr. Surg. Int.* **5**: 27–29.

19

Intussusception

In intussusception, one segment of the bowel passes onwards inside the adjacent distal bowel. Once this telescoping phenomenon becomes established, intestinal obstruction follows. Intussusception represents one of the commoner surgical emergencies in the first 2 years of life.

AETIOLOGY

In 90% of episodes there is no obvious cause, although in older children there is more likely to be a lesion at the lead point of the intussusceptum, for example a Meckel's diverticulum, a polyp or a duplication cyst.

In idiopathic intussusception, which usually affects infants, it is possible that a submucosal plaque of lymphoid tissue in the distal ileum (Peyer's patch) may become oedematous, possibly as the result of a viral infection, and become the apex of the intussusception. The apex moves through the ileocaecal valve into the colon and occasionally may reach the anus.

INCIDENCE

The peak incidence is in infants 4–7 months old, and 70% of patients are between 3 and 12 months of age. Boys are affected more frequently than girls.

CLINICAL FEATURES (TABLE 19.1)

Symptoms

Pain is the most important symptom (85%) and is typically a colicky pain which lasts 2–3 min during which the infant screams and draws up his knees.

Table 19.1 Presenting features of intussusception

Vomiting
Abdominal colic
Pallor
Lethargy
Abdominal mass
Rectal bleeding

Spasms occur at intervals of 15–20 min. The infant becomes pale, clammy, exhausted and lethargic between spasms. After 12 h or so, the pain becomes more continuous.

Vomiting, the most frequent symptom, usually occurs once or twice in the first hours, and then reappears once the intestinal obstruction is fully established.

Signs

The children look pale and lethargic and are intermittently aroused by a spasm of severe pain. A mass (sometimes described as being 'sausage-shaped') is palpable in more than half the infants and is usually found in the right hypochondrium, although it may be anywhere between the line of the colon and the umbilicus (Fig. 19.1). The intussusception mass is felt most easily early in the course of the disease, before abdominal distension and increasing abdominal tenderness conceal it.

A normal or loose stool is often passed at or soon after the onset of symptoms. In about half the patients a bloody and mucousy stool is passed ('red currant jelly'), formed by the diapedesis of red cells through the congested mucosa of the intussusceptum. Blood may be identified on the glove following rectal examination in

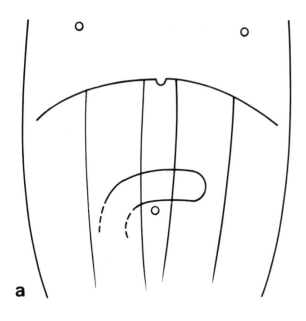
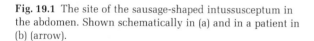
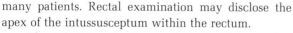

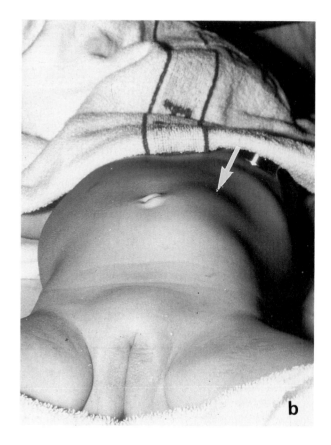

Fig. 19.1 The site of the sausage-shaped intussusceptum in the abdomen. Shown schematically in (a) and in a patient in (b) (arrow).

many patients. Rectal examination may disclose the apex of the intussusceptum within the rectum.

The infant is pale, limp and tired and has tachycardia. If there is delay in diagnosis, the infant will become dehydrated, listless, febrile, have abdominal distension and look ill. These are late signs and the diagnosis should be made before they appear.

Differential diagnosis

Wind colic is common in the first 3 months of life but rarely lasts more than an hour and usually is not accompanied by vomiting. Persisting severe colic for more than 1–2 h should arouse suspicion of an intussusception, particularly if accompanied by vomiting.

Gastroenteritis

Colic and the passage of blood and mucus in severe cases of gastroenteritis may mimic intussusception, except that the volume of diarrhoea is greater. In intussusception the small loose stools passed early in the course of the disease simply represent evacuation of the colon distal to the obstruction. Persistent vomiting and pain without diarrhoea is unlikely to be gastroenteritis.

A strangulated inguinal hernia may present with abdominal pain, vomiting and distension, but is recognized easily on examination.

Investigations

A plain X-ray of the abdomen may be normal, show non-specific abnormality or be that of a small bowel obstruction with air-fluid levels in dilated small bowel. Occasionally, the apex of the intussusceptum can be seen.

An air or barium contrast study will not only confirm the diagnosis, but also will be therapeutic.

TREATMENT

Enema reduction of intussusception should be attempted in most cases, unless there is clinical evidence of dead bowel as demonstrated by peritonitis or septicaemia. Gas (air or oxygen) is more effective and probably safer than barium and is the medium of choice if available (Fig. 19.2). Successful enema reduction is slightly less likely if there is a long duration of symptoms (> 24 h), age extremes (< 3 months or > 24

months) or when there is an established small bowel obstruction with air–fluid levels on X-ray.

Technique of gas enema reduction

The infants should be resuscitated with intravenous fluids and kept warm. A Foley catheter is inserted into the rectum and the balloon inflated. The buttocks are strapped tightly together. Gas (usually oxygen from the wall supply) is introduced into the colon through the catheter, the pressure being controlled by a manometer (Fig. 19.3). Under continuous fluoroscopic control progress of the reduction is monitored (Fig. 19.4). Sudden filling of the small bowel with gas suggests reduction is complete. The infant can be fed within hours of the procedure.

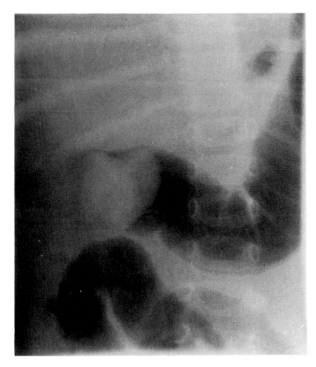

Fig. 19.2 Gas enema showing end of intussusceptum, which confirms the diagnosis of intussusception (reproduced with permission from Phelan *et al.* 1988).

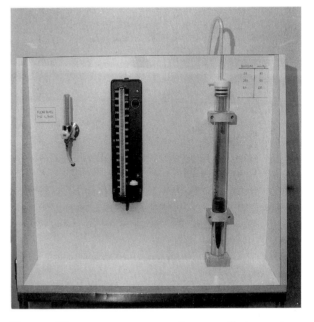

Fig. 19.3 The oxygen enema apparatus currently in use at the Royal Children's Hospital uses oxygen from the wall supply. There is an overflow valve so that the pressure cannot rise above a predetermined level (reproduced with permission from Phelan *et al.* 1988).

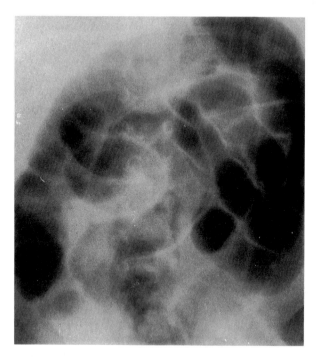

Fig. 19.4 Air enema showing complete reduction of the bowel and gas filling the small bowel (reproduced with permission from Phelan *et al.* 1988).

Surgery

Surgery is indicated when the enema fails to reduce the intussusception, where there is peritonitis clinically or where there is strong evidence of a pathological lesion at the leadpoint, for example circumoral pigmentation of Peutz-Jegher's syndrome. A laparotomy is performed through a transverse right supra-umbilical incision. The intussusception is reduced manually and resection may be required if there is gangrene or for a lesion at the leadpoint, for example Meckel's diverticulum or polyp.

RECURRENT INTUSSUSCEPTION

Recurrence of intussusception occurs in about 7% of patients. It is more likely after enema reduction than surgery. It usually occurs within 2 or 3 days of the first reduction. Recurrent intussusception is treated the same way as a first episode, except in a child more than 2 years of age. The possibility of a lesion at the leadpoint should be considered.

FURTHER READING

Auldist A. W. (1970) Intussusception in a children's hospital: 203 cases in 7 years. *Aust. NZ J. Surg.* **40**: 136–143.

Beasley S. W. (1988) Annotation. Can the outcome of intussusception be improved? *Aust. Paediatr. J.* **24**: 99–100.

Hutson J. M. & Beasley S. W. (1988) Colic. In: *The Surgical Examination of Children*, pp. 77–84. Heinemann Medical, Oxford.

Ong N-T. & Beasley S. W. (1990) Progression of intussusception. *J. Pediatr. Surg.* **25**: 644–646.

Ong N-T. & Beasley S. W. (1990) The leadpoint in intussusception. *J. Pediatr. Surg.* **25**: 640–643.

Phelan E., de Campo J. F. & Malecky G. (1988) Comparison of oxygen and barium reduction of ileocolic intussusception. *Amer. J. Radiol.* **150**: 1349–1352.

Sparnon A. L., Little K. E. T. & Morris L. L. (1984) Intussusception in childhood: A review of 139 cases. *Aust. NZ J. Surg.* **54**: 353–356.

— 20 —

Appendicitis

In this chapter, the presentation and management of appendicitis, the commonest abdominal emergency in children, is discussed. Other less common abdominal emergencies, some of which may mimic appendicitis, are described at the end of the chapter.

The knowledge that delay in diagnosis of appendicitis is dangerous has probably been a major factor in reducing its morbidity in children. As a rule, all abdominal pain in childhood lasting 3–4 h or more should be regarded as evidence of a potential abdominal emergency until proven otherwise. Likewise, diarrhoea lasting more than 24 h should suggest the possibility of a pelvic, retrocaecal or retroileal appendicitis, and even in gastroenteritis, diarrhoea does not preclude the possibility that appendicitis has supervened. Only a minority of children presenting with these features are found to have a genuine surgical cause. Where there is a high index of suspicion of appendicitis the child must be reassessed frequently with early referral to a paediatric surgeon.

THE INTERPRETATION OF ABDOMINAL PAIN IN CHILDREN

The presence of significant abdominal pain in small children tends to be recognized late by parents and professionals alike, largely because of the young child's inability to voice his symptoms adequately, and partly because the pain of appendicitis may not be dramatic in this age-group.

In the infant the observation of unnatural immobility, refusal to be cuddled, wanting to be left untouched and reluctance to be examined, all suggest movement exacerbates the pain, as in peritonitis.

If abdominal pain is persistent, observation must be continued and re-examination repeated until there are definite signs which indicate surgery, or until the pain has subsided. In most children whose pain is subsiding, operation should be deferred if the physical signs are not completely diagnostic.

ASSESSMENT OF PHYSICAL FINDINGS

Examination of the older cooperative child is straightforward, whereas in a young, sick and frightened child it requires great skill. The examination must be unhurried and gentle, and performed with warm hands, with the examiner seated beside the child. Useful assessment can sometimes be made if the child is asleep when first seen or if the abdomen is palpated from behind with both hands while the mother cuddles the child's front against her. However, with a continually crying child, adequate assessment is difficult and re-examination must be undertaken a short time later. Failure to acknowledge inadequate examination is likely to result in serious diagnostic delay.

Abdominal tenderness

Localized tenderness is found in conditions ranging from excess flatus, an overloaded colon or inflamed lymph nodes, to acute appendicitis and strangulated gut; so that this finding alone is an inadequate basis for operation.

In children, localized tenderness can be elicited by direct palpation over any distended or inflamed loop of gut. This is a particular feature of the solitary distended loop in intestinal obstruction, but can also be observed in gastroenteritis. Irritated or inflamed visceral peritoneum will produce tenderness by direct, rather than by reflex, pathways.

Localized tenderness in the right iliac fossa, without guarding or a strongly suggestive clinical history may be due to causes other than appendicitis. Although localized tenderness is often the earliest sign of appendicitis, children requiring operation soon develop guarding to support the diagnosis, whereas tenderness due to non-surgical conditions subsides in 1–2 days.

Guarding

Children with local or general peritonitis rarely display the board-like rigidity so often found in adults. More often there is a variable degree of involuntary increased muscle resistance, referred to as 'guarding'. Small differences in resistance in the lower and upper abdomen, or between right and left sides, may be significant when the findings are consistent.

There are no pathognomonic symptoms or signs of appendicitis itself, but when signs of peritonitis are localized to the right iliac fossa, appendicitis is likely.

Acute appendicitis may be missed when it presents with signs of local peritonitis other than in the right iliac fossa; the interposition of other tissues between the appendix and the anterior abdominal wall in pelvic, retrocaecal and retroileal appendicitis delays the appearance of abdominal signs until relatively late, and even then they may be atypical.

In retrocaecal appendicitis, the signs are high on the right side, whereas in pelvic appendicitis, or in retroileal appendicitis, the signs are more central or may even be predominantly left-sided.

A palpable mass

Excluding faecal masses and symptomless masses in the loin (Chapter 25), the commonest mass in the abdomen in childhood is an appendiceal abscess, particularly in children under 5 years of age, in the mentally retarded or when the appendix is in an unusual position.

Rectal examination

When appendicitis has been diagnosed on the basis of the history and anterior abdominal signs, a rectal examination is not indicated. However when: (i) the signs are equivocal; (ii) ovarian pathology is suspected; (iii) low and diffuse tenderness suggests pelvic appendicitis; or (iv) the duration of symptoms or the passage of blood, mucus or diarrhoea suggests a pelvic collection, rectal examination is mandatory.

The lateral position is traditional in small children, but more information may be obtained when the digital examination is performed with the child in the dorsal position, combined whenever possible with bimanual palpation. Rectal palpation causes some stretching of the anal canal and sphincters, and pain from this source may be misinterpreted as pelvic or peritoneal tenderness.

The use of an enema

When the differential diagnosis includes constipation in a child with equivocal abdominal symptoms and signs, an enema may prove both diagnostic and therapeutic. There is no evidence that an enema is disadvantageous in early acute appendicitis.

Signs arising in other systems

Infections in the ear, the tonsils or the respiratory passages may be accompanied by abdominal pain and vomiting and may simulate an abdominal emergency. Measles or chicken-pox may produce abdominal signs, as can a wide range of viral infections, by causing mesenteric lymphadenitis. Acute appendicitis can co-exist with other conditions, so that the finding of pneumonia, tonsillitis, or generalized lymphadenopathy should not divert attention from any abdominal signs which also may be present.

Similarly, gastroenteritis may progress to appendicitis, so that even a well-established and undoubted diagnosis of gastroenteritis should be subject to review.

Special diagnostic difficulties can be presented by the abdominal crises of diabetic acidosis, Henoch-Schönlein purpura, and various haematological disorders, including haemophilia, in all of which surgical intervention generally is contra-indicated.

Repeated observation and re-examination for the development of peritoneal signs is essential.

ACUTE APPENDICITIS

The mortality of acute appendicitis in children is less than 0.2%, due to early diagnosis and the management of fluids and electrolytes before and after operation.

Clinical diagnosis

The abdominal findings are the crucial factors on which the diagnosis and the decision to operate is made. The value of history lies in arousing suspicion that an abdominal emergency is present, and in determining its most likely cause.

The clinical diagnosis is determined by the presence of objective signs of local or general peritonitis. However, acute appendicitis is not only the commonest abdominal emergency, but also the greatest imitator, and it may appear in a variety of guises (Table 20.1).

Differential diagnosis

A perforated appendix is the only common cause of general peritonitis in childhood. In most children with an appendical abscess, there are signs of local or generalized peritonitis. Occasionally, however, an appendical mass may be present with little or no constitutional upset or localized signs of peritoneal irritation.

In acute appendicitis, mild pyuria (20–50 white blood cells/mm^3) may be seen and is due to an inflamed appendix adjacent to the ureter or the bladder. Conversely, acute pyelonephritis may be present without pus cells or bacteria in the bladder, and this must be distinguished from high retrocaecal appendicitis, in which tenderness and rigidity often extend into the loin.

Infections in the lower urinary tract, particularly those associated with vesicoureteric reflux, can mimic appendicitis in the right iliac fossa, but do not exhibit the guarding typical of peritoneal irritation. In pelvic appendicitis, the child may complain of low abdominal pain during micturition.

Peritonitis in the young child

Peritonitis is a frequent complication of appendicitis which may be difficult to recognize in infants and young

Table 20.1 The variety of presentations of acute appendicitis

Presentation and differential diagnosis

Local tenderness in the right iliac fossa
  Simple colic
  'Bilious attack'
  Gastroenteritis
  Acute constipation
  Mild mesenteric adenitis
  Urolithiasis
  Deep iliac lymphadenitis

Localized peritonitis (most often in right iliac fossa)
  Severe mesenteric adenitis
  Primary peritonitis
  Meckel's diverticulitis
  Ruptured luteal cyst, that is the 'apoplectic ovary'
  Torsion of an ovarian cyst or ovary
  Torsion of the omentum
  Suppurating deep iliac lymph nodes

Generalized peritonitis
  Primary peritonitis
  Perforated Meckel's diverticulum

An inflammatory mass
  Intussusception
  Duplication of the gut
  Ectopic kidney
  Retroperitoneal masses (Chapter 25)

Intestinal obstruction
  Adhesive bowel obstruction
  Internal hernia
  Meckel's band

'Gastroenteritis' (from retroileal or pelvic appendix)
  Gastroenteritis

'Urinary tract infection'
  Urinary tract infection
  Acute pyelonephritis

children. Tenderness may be diffuse rather than localized, and rigidity may be absent, even when there is advanced general peritonitis. More often, a lesser degree of involuntary muscular rigidity or 'guarding' is encountered. Differences between the right and left sides or between the lower and upper abdomen, are highly significant.

As localized peritonitis progresses, the signs become more definite but paradoxically, as the peritonitis becomes more generalized and the abdomen more distended, the signs may appear to diminish. In this situation, abdominal distension and reluctance on the child's part to allow palpation of the abdomen are signs of great significance.

Even without distension, however, the persistence of pain, with or without accompanying diarrhoea, demands careful assessment, rectal examination and re-examination of the abdomen.

Treatment

The management involves:

(1) Adequate pre-operative intravenous correction of fluid and electrolyte deficits

(2) Surgical removal of the appendix

(3) Irrigation of the peritoneal cavity to remove pus and contaminated free peritoneal fluid; and

(4) Effective perioperative antibiotic treatment.

Fluid and electrolyte deficits are replaced by intravenous infusions, and if there is marked abdominal distension and vomiting, the bowel is decompressed by nasogastric suction. A dehydrated, toxic child, with severely depleted fluid and electrolytes is a poor candidate for anaesthesia or operation. Obstruction of the airways by inhaled vomitus, unexpected cardiac arrest and prolonged 'surgical shock' with peripheral circulatory collapse, are less likely following fluid resuscitation.

Antibiotics are given to reduce the incidence of septic complications of appendicitis and peritonitis. Peritonitis is a polymicrobial infection caused by bowel organisms, so that a wide spectrum of antibacterial activity is necessary. A combination of an anti-aerobic with an anti-anaerobic agent is more effective than either alone.

Wound infection results from intra-operative inoculation by peritoneal contaminants. To be prevented, an effective concentration of an appropriate antibacterial agent must be present at the time of intra-operative inoculation; this can be achieved by instillation or pre-operative systemic antibiotics.

The aim of surgery is to remove the appendix and perform intraperitoneal toilet.

ABDOMINAL PAIN OF UNCERTAIN ORIGIN

This represents a substantial group of children (Table 20.1) in which the final diagnosis remains in doubt. 'Indigestion', wind pains, acute constipation, 'gripes', and other minor disturbances of bowel function, are impossible to establish as objective diagnoses but are labels which tend to be attached to a number of children.

Perhaps the most troublesome condition is mesenteric adenitis ('non-specific viral infection'), because of the difficulty in distinguishing some cases from acute appendicitis. The combination of high fever, minimal abdominal tenderness in two or more areas (which may vary), the absence of guarding and failure of the signs to progress, suggest mesenteric adenitis.

ABDOMINAL EMERGENCIES IN MENTALLY RETARDED CHILDREN

Acute appendicitis is the commonest condition. Impaction, ulceration or perforation of the alimentary canal by an ingested foreign body is more frequent than in children of normal intelligence.

The degree of difficulty in diagnosis is dependent on the severity of the retardation. In the most severely affected children, with hyperkinesia, hypertonia, inability to speak and a high threshold of pain, there may be few symptoms, and abdominal signs, for example tenderness or rigidity may be difficult to detect or evaluate. Distension and the absence of bowel sounds, although late developments, are usually present when attention is first drawn to the abdomen. Vomiting, fever and tachycardia also may be present.

As in normal children less than 5 years of age, appendicitis in retarded children usually has progressed to a local abscess or to spreading peritonitis by the time the diagnosis is made. A palpable mass on rectal examination, signs of intestinal obstruction from involvement of a loop of small bowel in the wall of an appendical abscess or signs of paralytic ileus, are common.

The delay in diagnosis leads to an increase in the incidence of complications and consequently an increase in the mortality.

INTESTINAL OBSTRUCTION

In children who have not had a previous abdominal operation, the cause of the obstruction may be a volvulus (Chapter 7), Meckel's band or diverticulum (Chapter 23), a duplication (Chapter 7), or, very rarely, an internal hernia.

A more common cause is strangulation of an inguinal hernia which, if looked for, presents few problems in diagnosis or management.

Most cases of obstruction in older children are due to bands or adhesions following a previous abdominal operation, most commonly appendicectomy. Recurrent pain, accompanied by vomiting, generally causes these patients to present early. Clinical evidence of distended loops of gut, either visible and palpable, or fluid levels in an X-ray of the abdomen, will confirm the diagnosis.

Obstruction is less obvious and more likely to be overlooked: (i) in the early postoperative period when pain is difficult to interpret and delay in recovery from paralytic ileus may mask the presence of an early fibrinous obstruction from adhesions; (ii) in children in whom vomiting alone is the presenting feature of a high small bowel obstruction in which pain and abdominal distension may be absent.

Treatment

All oral fluids are withheld, the stomach is aspirated by a nasogastric tube, and intravenous fluid and electrolytes are commenced. Some children respond promptly to this regimen and the symptoms and signs subside within a few hours.

Continuing or increasing volumes of aspirate or persistent localized abdominal tenderness are sufficient grounds for laparotomy, preferably before a rising pulse rate and severe pain suggest impending strangulation of a loop of bowel.

MECKEL'S DIVERTICULUM

It is the commonest cause of major gastrointestinal bleeding in childhood (Chapter 23). It may also be suspected before operation in intestinal obstruction in a child who has not undergone a previous abdominal operation. Its other manifestations are indistinguishable clinically from appendicitis and the true diagnosis only becomes apparent at operation.

PAEDIATRIC GYNAECOLOGIC EMERGENCIES

In menarchal or pubertal girls, a gynaecologic disorder may be unsuspected or present signs which are not recognized.

This group of conditions includes the exaggerated intraperitoneal bleeding at the normal time of ovulation (mittelschmerz bleeding) or rupture of a small luteal cyst. Tubal menstruation, torsion of the ovary, acute salpingitis and primary peritonitis are all uncommon and rarely diagnosed unless they come to operation.

If carefully sought for by bimanual palpation in the dorsal position, differences in the size and degree of tenderness of the tube and ovary on each side can be detected, for pelvic peritoneal tenderness in the pouch of Douglas often is more marked than the abdominal signs in the hypogastrium. Typically, extreme tenderness in the pelvis contrasts with the relative absence of abdominal signs.

Distinction between rupture of a follicular or luteal cyst and acute pelvic appendicitis can be difficult. Pelvic ultrasound can detect ovarian cysts 1 cm diameter or less with accuracy and save many of these children from unnecessary exploration. However, in all cases with abdominal peritonism or a palpable mass, including a painful pelvic swelling, exploration is necessary.

FURTHER READING

Auldist A. W. (1967) Acute appendicitis in children less than 5 years of age. *Aust. Paediatr. J.* **3**: 144–150.

O'Rourke M. G. E., Wynne J. M. *et al.* (1984) Prophylactic

antibiotics in appendicectomy: a prospective double blind randomized study. *Aust. NZ J. Surg.* **54**: 535–541.

Puri P., Guiney E. J. & O'Donnell B. (1985) Effects of perforated appendicitis on subsequent fertility. *Br. Med. J.* **288**: 25.

Wright J. E. (1982) Appendicitis in childhood: Reduction in wound infection with preoperative antibiotics. *Aust. NZ J. Surg.* **52**: 127–129.

Tsuji M., McMahon G., Reen D. & Puri P. (1990) New insights into the pathogenesis of appendicitis based on immunocytochemical analysis of early immune response. *J. Pediatr. Surg.* **25**: 449–452.

21

Recurrent Abdominal Pain

Recurrent abdominal pain is one of the commonest problems seen in paediatric practice. The child usually has frequent, short-lived but severe episodes of abdominal colic, which are felt in the central abdominal region. The attacks last a few minutes and only interrupt the child's play or school work momentarily. Sometimes, the pain is brought on by stress, for example pressure with school work or domestic upsets; it is real and can be compared to the stress-induced headaches or indigestion which adults suffer. In others it is likely to be related to constipation (Chapter 22) or in adolescent girls to gynaecological problems. Parents bring their child to the doctor because they fear he/she has an underlying disease, for example cancer, appendicitis or 'twisted bowel'. It is important for the doctor to exclude these less common causes for pain, and then reassure the family that the pain has no known long term significance.

HISTORY

The nature and characteristics of the pain provide the key features of the history. Most commonly, recurrent abdominal pain is felt around the umbilicus, whereas surgical pain tends to be localized, for example loin pain with hydronephrosis.

Recurrent abdominal pain colic certainly hurts the child, but surgical pain is often more severe and persistent, and may wake the child from sleep or make him vomit. Stress-induced pains rarely occur at night and are not associated with vomiting.

Vomiting not only indicates the severity of pain but also, when bile-stained and associated with severe episodic pain, indicates the possibility of malrotation and volvulus.

Recurrent abdominal pain seems to affect the child on most days and scarcely a week goes by without some symptoms. Surgical pain may be absent for months, only to come on with a severe episode. The duration of recurrent abdominal pain is often short—minutes—and interferes only briefly with normal activities. It is probable that in some patients constipation contributes to the painful episodes, although this is not always easy to prove.

The family and social histories are important. When stress is contributing to the pain, it will be found usually within the family. Difficulties at school may relate to a child trying to live up to the parents' and teachers' expectations, which are beyond the reach of the child. This applies to children at both ends of the class list.

Sometimes, when one asks the question: 'How does your child get on at school?', the answer is that there is no problem because the child always comes first in his or her subjects. The parents may not realize the pressure the child is under to keep performing at this level.

PHYSICAL EXAMINATION

In most patients with recurrent abdominal pain examination reveals no abnormality. Occasionally, an abdominal mass is felt, for example the faecal masses of constipation or a hydronephrotic kidney. The height and weight of the child should be recorded on a growth chart, since weight loss in association with recurrent pains suggests inflammatory bowel disease (Chapter 24).

SPECIAL INVESTIGATIONS

In the majority of children, special investigation is not helpful, though it may be useful to allay specific parental anxieties. Of all investigations, the abdominal ultrasound is the most useful and the least invasive: the kidneys, bladder, ovaries, gall bladder, liver, spleen and pancreas can all be examined. Investigation should be reserved for patients with a possible surgical cause of the pain. The return on the investigation of recurrent abdominal pain is not particularly good, but occasionally a child is treated as recurrent abdominal pain for many years before a hydronephrosis is diagnosed on ultrasound.

TREATMENT

Following exclusion of significant pathology, recurrent abdominal pain is treated by reassurance, identification of the stress factors (if any) and helping the family to understand the possible link between the stress and the child's symptoms. It is hard to 'cure' the pain, but if the family understands the pathology, they can live with the symptoms.

It is important to uncover any possible hidden fears the family may have. For example, a relative may have died recently of cancer, and the parents may fear the child has a tumour. These underlying fears must be dispelled by demonstrating to the parents' satisfaction that the child is free of these problems. Tranquilizers have been used for children with recurrent abdominal pain, but they do not treat the underlying problem.

Constipation may be a factor aggravating recurrent abdominal pain. It is a simple matter to use laxatives to clear the bowel in these children, and in some this may be helpful in reducing the colic.

Some parents worry that their child has 'chronic appendicitis'. While laparotomy and appendicectomy are performed sometimes in a highly selected group of the more severely affected, the results are variable and if the selection is poor, the symptoms are worsened. The best results are obtained in those previously well children who have multiple episodes of right iliac fossa pain and tenderness which settle spontaneously. These children have recurrent bouts of pain over a few months, unlike those with stress-induced pain, in whom the symptoms are very long-standing.

The management of children with recurrent abdominal pain is a test of clinical acumen and counselling skills. The cases presenting for surgical opinion are usually more severe and it is important to exclude any underlying 'surgical' cause. A thorough clinical history and physical examination is the basis of diagnosis in these children. Extensive, traumatic or invasive investigations rarely are indicated and an ultrasound examination probably gives the best return.

FURTHER READING

Apley J. (1975) *The Child with Abdominal Pains*, 2nd edn. Blackwell Scientific Publications, Oxford.

Paediatric Handbook (1991) Royal Children's Hospital, Melbourne.

22

Constipation and its Sequelae

Constipation is a common problem in infancy and childhood, and may be the direct cause of abdominal pain, soiling, fissures and rectal prolapse. When constipation is chronic, treatment may be required: an understanding of its pathophysiology reveals that treatment must be prolonged and persistent, and that an 'occasional dose of laxative' is not adequate.

THE PATHOPHYSIOLOGY OF CONSTIPATION

The normal rectum is empty most of the time, except when a mass reflex of the colon conveys faeces into the rectum once or twice each day. The distension thus produced stretches the muscles and stimulates pressure receptors to initiate the afferent arc of the defaecation reflex.

The urge to defaecate is felt, and the efferent arc—when reinforced by removal of cortical inhibition—causes contraction of the rectum and relaxation of the sphincters; evacuation is then completed with the aid of contraction of the abdominal wall musculature. The whole process is initiated by stimulation of the stretch receptors in the wall of the rectum, which is collapsed and empty until faeces enter it.

In acute constipation of short duration, for example following appendicectomy in a child with previously normal bowel habits, the rectum retains its tone and defaecation is readily produced by the stimulation of a laxative, a suppository or an enema. An enema is particularly effective because a large volume of fluid causes distension and fires the defaecation reflex when the tone in the rectal wall is normal.

This is not the case in chronic constipation, for the rectum is not empty and its wall is chronically over-stretched, so additional oncoming faeces neither reach nor stretch the rectum further. The sensory receptors are dulled and the rectal wall is flaccid and unable to contract effectively. When the stool is not evacuated soon after it enters the rectum, water is absorbed and the stool becomes harder. The harder the stool, the more difficult and painful is its passage; it often splits the anal mucosa (anal fissure), further diminishing the child's willingness to defaecate. And so the cycle commences again (Fig. 22.1).

Even temporary accumulation of faeces in the rectum potentially may serve as the starting point of the vicious circle described above.

The essential step of treatment is to empty the rectum, and to keep it empty as often as possible, for weeks or months, until colonic and rectal tone returns. The oncoming stool will initiate the reflex and provide the 'urge' which makes training possible.

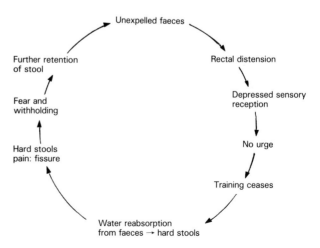

Fig. 22.1 Constipation. The cylical nature of the causative factors.

PREDISPOSING FACTORS

There are a number of factors which contribute to constipation (Table 22.1), the most common of which is 'holding back'. Constipation begins most frequently in the toddler age-group just as toilet training is beginning, at a time when the acquisition of receptivity and response is most vulnerable. A minor episode of pain on defaecation caused by a hard stool, for example due to dehydration during a febrile illness, may start the sequence of constipation and rectal distension (Fig. 22.1).

A temporary minor illness, such as measles or an operation, for example appendicectomy; and the combined effect of recumbency, fever, a degree of dehydration, abdominal pain and possible shyness in asking for assistance, may go unheeded, and contribute to the development of constipation. Prolonged recumbency in chronic illness, for example leukaemia or Perthes' disease, is another cause.

Breast-fed babies often become constipated on weaning to artificial feed. In older children, there may be insufficient intake of cellulose fibre to promote peristalsis, low intake of fresh fruit and vegetables and inadequate fluid consumption.

Organic causes of obstruction, for example anal stenosis or Hirschsprung's disease, are obvious but less common causes of retained faeces. Neural lesions, for example myelomeningocele, spinal trauma, tumours or infections, may interfere with the mobility of the bowel and with the reflex arcs. Mentally retarded children and those with severe emotional or neurotic disorders also may suffer chronic constipation.

PREVENTION

Prevention is possible by reasonable supervision, with special attention to the following points:

(1) The selection of a normal and appropriate diet (see below)

(2) A rational plan of toilet training with rewards rather than punishments

(3) The establishment of normal defaecation following minor illnesses, after operations and on weaning from breast feeding.

TREATMENT

Mild constipation

In babies with constipation, the intake of cow's milk should be reduced and Maltogen added to the milk.

In older children, the bland diet of low fibre and refined manufactured foods makes constipation a common problem in our community. Common sense alteration to the diet should be advised, although it is hard to change cultural dietary habits. Laxatives (e.g. Senokot) soften the stool and may stimulate bowel activity; and most are well tolerated in children.

Severe constipation

This is associated with faecal impaction and rectal inertia. In very severe cases the anal sphincters lose their tone and the bowel requires invasive mechanical emptying.

Suppositories and disposable enemas offer stimulation for rectal emptying and work well for those at the less severe end of the spectrum. Severe constipation is a serious problem and treatment should be established in

Table 22.1 Predisposing factors in chronic constipation

```
'Holding back'
    commencement of toilet training
    anal fissure
Concurrent minor illness
Prolonged recumbency
Dietary factors
    at time of weaning
    low fibre and fluid intake
Organic causes
    anal stenosis (rare)
    Hirschsprung's disease
    spinal lesions, for example spina bifida
Psychogenic causes
    severe mental retardation
    emotional disturbance
```

hospital by experienced paediatric staff. The very severely affected require bowel washouts and occasionally manual disimpaction under general anaesthesia. Once the bowel is emptied the parents can continue treatment with simpler means (diet, laxatives, suppositories) at home for the weeks or months it takes for bowel function to return. Occasionally, biofeedback techniques are required to re-establish rectal function.

THE SEQUELAE OF CONSTIPATION

Colonic inertia

Colonic inertia is the name given to the extreme form of constipation when there is no underlying organic lesion such as Hirschsprung's disease (Chapter 7) or a neural lesion (Chapter 10). In these conditions too, accumulation of faeces may occur, adding the features of colonic inertia to the initial disease. 'Colonic inertia' is not a specific disease but a convenient term to describe the result of prolonged chronic constipation produced by any one or a combination of the predisposing factors. Such is the severity and duration of the constipation that a diagnosis of Hirschsprung's disease may be entertained; but there are several distinguishing points:

(1) The symptoms of colonic inertia date from the toddler age rather than the neonatal period
(2) A barium enema shows that the retained faeces extend into the anal canal and down to the external sphincter
(3) A suction rectal biopsy shows that normal ganglion cells are present in the rectum, the final and absolute criterion when X-rays have been equivocal.

Faecal soiling ('spurious' incontinence)

Chronic constipation is by far the most common cause of soiling. The presence of constipation may not be immediately apparent, because soft faeces are passed, but in fact they escape around an impacted faecal mass, and

through the relaxed anal sphincters. The diagnosis is made obvious when the hard faecal mass is felt on rectal digital examination and in the abdomen and pelvis on examination of the abdomen.

The term, 'encopresis', is reserved for cases in which there is no constipation, and no neurological basis, that is it is entirely a functional abnormality of psychological origin. When constipation and behavioural problems coexist it is often difficult to determine which predominates or came first. The tension and frustration surrounding an incontinent child with colonic inertia inevitably add to the problems. Whatever its associations, it is important that the constipation should be treated on its own merits.

Abdominal pains

Constipation can cause abdominal pain of several types and in several sites, usually central but also in either iliac fossa (Chapter 21). In some instances the colic is one of the most severe encountered, and the first thoughts of the parents are of appendicitis; but colic in constipation may cause the child to roll around in bed, whereas this is rare in acute appendicitis.

In constipation colic, the bowel sounds are accentuated, and the abdomen is resonant and lax, although there may be tenderness in the left iliac fossa or over the colon loaded with faeces. Not infrequently, at a further examination 1–2 h later, all the pain and tenderness have gone and there are no signs of any abnormality in the abdomen. A final diagnosis should not be made until the accumulated faeces have been evacuated.

Other sequelae of constipation include rectal bleeding (Chapter 23); anal fissure and rectal prolapse (Chapter 19).

FURTHER READING

Sarahan T., Weintraub W. H., Coran A. G. & Wesley J. R. (1982) The successful management of chronic constipation in infants and children. *J. Pediatr. Surg.* **17**: 171–174.

23

Bleeding from the Alimentary Canal

Haemorrhage, large or small, can occur from any part of the alimentary canal and at any age. Sometimes the haemorrhage is important in its own right, in that the amount of blood lost threatens the life of the child. On other occasions, it is an important sign of other medical or surgical pathology.

Alimentary tract bleeding may present with a variety of symptoms, according to the level and rate of haemorrhage. Bleeding into the alimentary tract may be 'occult' and present as iron-deficiency anaemia or it may be seen as blood passed per rectum; in this instance, it may be as melaena (dark changed blood) or as bright red bleeding (Table 23.1).

If bleeding occurs into the oesophagus, stomach or duodenum, it may present as either 'coffee grounds' in the vomitus or as the vomiting of frank blood.

'COFFEE GROUNDS' VOMITING

A small amount of blood mixes with the gastric contents, is denatured and changes to a brown colour. When vomited, these flecks of blood may have the appearance of coffee grounds. It is seen in a variety of conditions:

Pyloric stenosis

Obstruction of the pylorus results in gastritis and small amounts of blood mix with the gastric contents and may be vomited. Hypertrophic pyloric stenosis, which occurs in approximately 1 : 600 infants, causes vomiting at about 1 month of age. Cardinal clinical features are projectile vomiting, visible gastric peristalsis and a pyloric 'tumour' palpable in the epigastrium (Chapter 18).

Reflux oesophagitis

Acid reflux into the lower oesophagus sometimes causes ulceration of its mucosal surface. Small vomits occur after meals and when lying flat, often with epigastric discomfort. Initial treatment of this common condition includes thickening of the feeds, administration of antacids and posturing the baby prone with the head elevated. Surgical treatment occasionally is necessary for complications (e.g. oesophageal stricture), and consists of fundoplication (Chapter 18).

Non-specific gastritis

This condition may be due to a viral infection, and usually responds to non-specific measures.

Mallory-Weiss syndrome

This can occur in any child who vomits or retches continually, and is thought to be due to small splits

Table 23.1 Vomiting of blood

'Coffee grounds'	Pyloric stenosis
	Reflux oesophagitis
Frank blood	Oesophageal varices
	Peptic ulcer
Others	Nose bleeds
	Nasogastric tube ulceration
Rare causes	Aneurysm of bed of tonsil
	Foreign body perforation of aorta

occurring in the upper gastric mucosa. Fortunately, it responds to medical treatment if the vomiting can be stopped.

HAEMATEMESIS

The vomiting of frank blood means that there has been significant loss of blood into the stomach.

Oesophageal varices

Oesophageal varices are the result of portal hypertension and, in children, this occurs in two main groups:

(1)   Extrahepatic portal hypertension, where thrombosis of the portal vein in the neonate results in 'cavernous malformation' of the portal system;

(2)   Intrahepatic portal hypertension due to: cirrhosis of the liver, caused by biliary atresia; inborn errors of metabolism, such as α_1-antitrypsin deficiency; chronic viral hepatitis; or cystic fibrosis.

Oesophageal varices may bleed torrentially, and many require tamponade with a Sengstaken-Blakemore tube followed, if necessary, by surgical treatment. Surgery consists of direct injection of the varices with sclerosants at endoscopy, oversewing the varices, or creating a shunt to join the portal system to the systemic venous system, bypassing the liver and aiming to lower the pressure in the portal system. In practice, the shunt operations are very difficult in patients with extrahepatic portal hypertension, as there is no normal portal vein; so this form of surgery has not been very effective. In patients with intrahepatic portal hypertension and a normal portal vein, shunts are technically easier, but more dangerous for the patient because the blood from the portal bed then bypasses the abnormal liver with the effect of worsening liver function.

Peptic ulcer

Peptic ulcer disease is rare in children, but a 'stress ulcer' may occur in a child of any age with severe burns,

cerebral tumour, head injury or other forms of severe stress. In all these conditions, there tends to be an increased production of gastric acid with resultant diffuse ulceration of the gastric lining or more localized ulceration in the duodenum. Peptic ulceration also may occur as a complication of drug treatment, for example after administration of steroids. In adolescents who develop peptic ulceration the aetiology is the same as in adults. There may be a strong family history of ulcer disease.

Treatment

For a bleeding peptic ulcer, the treatment is:

(1)   Adequately resuscitate the patient with blood replacement

(2)   Treatment of the cause, for example, in peptic ulceration administer antacids or H-2 antagonists

(3)   Surgery to the bleeding point that is uncontrolled by other measures.

IRON-DEFICIENCY ANAEMIA

Iron-deficiency anaemia in children is caused by poor dietary intake, but can be due to reflux oesophagitis or one of the other causes mentioned in Table 23.2.

Table 23.2 Occult bleeding in children causing iron-deficiency anaemia

Reflux oesophagitis
Haemangioma of bowel
Polyps
Inflammatory bowel disease

RECTAL BLEEDING

Rectal bleeding in children can be considered under various distinct clinical groups (Table 23.3).

Table 23.3 Rectal bleeding in children

Neonatal
    Necrotizing enterocolitis
    Volvulus with ischaemia
    Haemorrhagic disease of the newborn
    Gastroenteritis
    Anal fissure
    Maternal blood
Ill child with an acute abdominal condition
    Intussusception
    Gastroenteritis
    Henoch-Schönlein purpura
Major haemorrhage from the gastrointestinal tract
    Oesophageal varices
    Peptic ulcer—gastric erosions
               —duodenal ulcer
    Meckel's diverticulum
    Tubular duplications
Small amount of bright blood in well child
    Fissure
    Polyps
    Unrecognized prolapse
    Haemorrhoids
    Idiopathic
Chronic illness with diarrhoea
    Crohn's disease
    Ulcerative colitis
    Non-specific colitis

Neonatal bleeding

There are two important surgical conditions and several important medical conditions which lead to rectal bleeding in children:

Necrotizing enterocolitis (Chapter 7)

This is an important condition that has become more common with the advent of the modern neonatal nursery which cares for extremely premature babies. Most babies with necrotizing enterocolitis respond to supportive treatment consisting of adequate ventilatory care, support of their circulation, resting the gastrointestinal tract and the administration of antibiotics. Some patients require surgery for full-thickness necrosis of

the intestine, as revealed by free intraperitoneal gas on X-ray or by continued clinical deterioration despite intensive supportive care.

Volvulus neonatorum with ischaemia (Chapter 7)

Volvulus of the mid-gut occurs at any age, but is more likely in the neonatal period. In the presence of malrotation, the attachment of the mid-gut is a narrow mesentery which allows easy twisting of the entire mid-gut. The first sign results from obstruction of the lumen of the bowel with bile-stained vomiting; but the most serious event which may occur is ischaemia of the mid-gut, due to obstruction of the vessels in the twisted mesentery. Bleeding from the bowel is a late sign, and very urgent surgical treatment is necessary at this stage if there is to be any hope for the baby.

Non-surgical causes

Haemorrhagic disease of the newborn is due to Vitamin K deficiency and is prevented by routine administration of Vitamin K_1. Gastroenteritis may occur in the neonatal period, resulting in blood mixed with diarrhoea. An anal fissure may occur at any age, and in the neonate is common after a rectal examination. The baby may swallow maternal blood, either during delivery or from a cracked nipple.

A small amount of blood in a well child

A small amount of fresh blood may be passed in a well child. This is by far the most common clinical group, and the cause of the bleeding may often be distinguished on the history alone. (Fig. 23.1)

Anal fissure

Anal fissure occurs at any age and usually is due to constipation (Chapters 22 and 27). The child passes a large, hard stool which splits the anus, usually in the midline, either posteriorly or anteriorly. The child complains of pain on defaecation and there is bright blood on

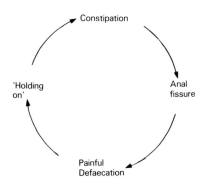

Fig. 23.1 The cycle of anal fissure. The treatment is to break the cycle.

the surface of the stool or immediately following it. The fissure can be seen by gently parting the anus. Rectal examination causes severe pain. The fissure heals quickly, and even when a fissure is not seen, the history may be quite diagnostic. Sometimes a 'sentinel pile', a mound of oedematous skin just external to the fissure, is visible. Anal fissures in children almost always respond to adequate treatment of the constipation. Local applications of anaesthetic agents achieve little, and surgical operations on the anal sphincter are rarely indicated in children.

Polyps

Juvenile polyps are relatively common in children and should be suspected when there is no constipation or no pain on passage of a stool (Chapter 27).

Rectal prolapse

Prolapse of the rectum is easily diagnosed on the history or by direct observation (Chapter 27). Sometimes, the rectal prolapse may become congested or traumatized, bleed and then reduce spontaneously; the parents observe the bleeding without knowing its cause. Rectal prolapse may occur with malabsorption or chronic diarrhoea, straining with constipation, and occasionally, as the presenting symptom of cystic fibrosis.

Haemorrhoids

Symptoms from haemorrhoids are rare in children but do occur. The presence of a venous abnormality of the rectum should be considered. In older children, haemorrhoids may cause bleeding and can be treated conservatively. In some children no cause for rectal bleeding can be found.

An ill child with an acute abdominal condition

In these children, the symptom of bleeding is not important in its own right, but points to another significant condition.

Intussusception

Intussusception presents with vomiting, colic, pallor and lethargy. In 50% of patients the stools are blood-stained, the typical 'red-currant jelly stool' (see Chapter 19).

Gastroenteritis

Patients with severe gastroenteritis often have vomiting, colic and blood mixed with the stool. The separation of these patients from those with intussusception can be difficult in the child under 2 years (see Chapter 19)

Henoch-Schönlein purpura

This condition causes arthralgia and a typical rash over the extremities. Submucosal haemorrhages in the bowel with abdominal pain and passage of blood rectally also occur. Henoch-Schönlein purpura needs to be distinguished from intussusception.

Chronic illness with diarrhoea

Crohn's disease may occur anywhere in the bowel and should be suspected in a patient with a chronic illness, unexplained fever, weight loss, bowel symptoms and chronic blood loss in the stools (Chapter 24). In patients with ulcerative colitis the diarrhoea is more prominent, and again it may contain blood. In non-specific colitis there is usually involvement of only the lower part of the large bowel with less general symptomatology.

Major haemorrhage per rectum

In these patients the haemorrhage is enough to cause anaemia or to require acute transfusion. The causes range from oesophageal varices and peptic ulcer (as discussed under the heading of vomiting) to Meckel's diverticulum and tubular duplications.

Meckel's diverticulum

Meckel's diverticulum occurs in 2% of the population, and in a small proportion of these patients ectopic gastric mucosa forms part of the lining of the diverticulum (Fig. 23.2). Acid produced by the gastric mucosa causes ulceration of the adjacent small bowel mucosa. The bleeding usually presents as painless 'brick-red' stools with associated anaemia. The patient may require transfusion, but the bleeding usually stops spontaneously without the need for emergency surgery. The

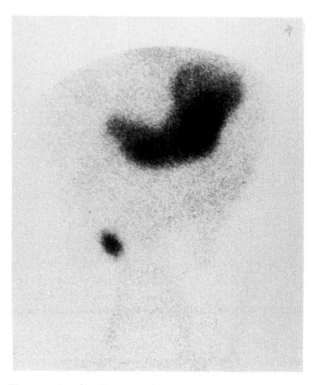

Fig. 23.3 A technetium scan showing ectopic gastric mucosa in a Meckel's diverticulum.

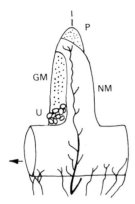

Fig. 23.2 Meckel's diverticulum. A composite diagram showing ectopic pancreas (P) and gastric mucosa (GM). An ulcer (U) lies in the adjoining normal ileal mucosa (NM). The site of attachment of a vitello-intestinal (omphalomesenteric) band is indicated at the tip.

definitive investigation is surgery, but a technetium scan may show the ectopic gastric mucosa (Fig. 23.3). A Meckel's diverticulum may result in a variety of other complications (Table 23.4)

Table 23.4 Complications of Meckel's diverticulum

(1)	Bleeding
(2)	Intussusception from an inverted diverticulum
(3)	An associated fibrous band causing a small bowel obstruction
(4)	Diverticulitis (rare in children)
(5)	Peptic ulceration with ileal perforation
(6)	Strangulation of diverticulum by its own band
(7)	Strangulation of diverticulum in an inguinal hernia

Tubular duplications

These are less common than a Meckel's diverticulum. Tubular duplications of the small bowel occur in the mesenteric side of the bowel and communicate proximally or distally with the bowel. They may be lined by gastric mucosa and cause bleeding when adjacent small bowel mucosa becomes ulcerated. Like a Meckel's diverticulum, they can be demonstrated by a technetium nuclear scan.

FURTHER READING

Beasley S. W., Auldist A. W., Ramanujan T. M. & Campbell N. T., (1986) The surgical management of neonatal necrotising enterocolitis, 1975–1984. *Pediatr. Surg. Int.* **1**: 201–217.

Cull D. L., Rosario V., Lally K. P., Ratner I. & Mahour G. H. (1990) Surgical implications of Henoch-Schönlein purpura. *J. Pediatr. Surg.* **25**: 741–743.

Hutson J. M. & Beasley S. W. (1988) Gastro-intestinal bleeding. In: *The Surgical Examination of Children*, pp. 202–207. Heinemann Medical, Oxford.

Previtera C. & Guglielmi M. (1990) Limitations and dangers of the Sengstaken-Blakemore tube in the treatment of haemorrhage from gastric varices. *Pediatr. Surg. Int.* **5**: 422–424.

Tsang T-M., Saing H. & Yeung C-K. (1990) Peptic ulcer in children. *J. Pediatr. Surg.* **25**: 744–748.

24

Inflammatory Bowel Disease: Crohn's Disease and Ulcerative Colitis

There has been a dramatic increase in the incidence of Crohn's disease throughout the world in the past 15–20 years. The increased incidence has occurred in all age groups, including children. About 20% of patients present before the age of 20 years. On the other hand, the incidence of ulcerative colitis in childhood has remained relatively static.

Crohn's disease can involve any part of the gastro-intestinal tract from the oral cavity to the anus. The pathological changes are similar regardless of the segment of gut involved. The inflammatory process involves the entire gut wall and the diagnostic feature is the presence of granulomas on histology. Perianal disease is common.

Ulcerative colitis is characterized by chronic inflammation of colonic and rectal mucosa. Disease limited to the rectum is uncommon in children, in whom more severe proximal disease is more likely than in adults.

The aetiology of inflammatory bowel disease remains unknown. Factors which have been implicated include infection, immune mechanisms and psychological disturbance.

CLINICAL FEATURES

Crohn's disease

There is great variability in the mode of presentation and symptomatology of Crohn's disease. This variability can lead to considerable delay between the onset of symptoms and diagnosis. While most of the paediatric patients are in their teenage years, a small number present under 10 years of age and occasionally less than 5 years.

The most common presentation is recurrent pain associated with weight loss. Often there is no change in bowel habit, although diarrhoea with or without blood loss can occur in a similar fashion to that seen in ulcerative colitis. In the adolescent a striking feature is growth failure with delayed onset of puberty. The onset of Crohn's disease may be heralded by development of extraintestinal symptoms or persistent or recurrent perianal disease. An uncommon presentation is that of acute abdominal pain, mimicking acute appendicitis.

Ulcerative colitis

As with Crohn's disease, most paediatric patients with ulcerative colitis present in the second decade; however, a few patients present under the age of 5 years. The usual symptomatology is gradually increasing diarrhoea with blood and mucus. Commonly, there is associated weight loss, fever and pallor.

Extraintestinal symptoms may antedate bowel symptoms. Growth failure and delay in pubertal development may occur with ulcerative colitis, but perianal disease is less common than with Crohn's disease. Acute toxic megacolon is rare.

Extraintestinal symptoms

Inflammatory bowel disease in children is frequently associated with involvement of other organ systems. These include arthritis and arthralgia, erythema nodosum, pyoderma gangrenosum, uveitis, liver disease and urinary tract calculi. The frequency and nature of these manifestations are similar in ulcerative colitis and Crohn's disease and can occur before, during or after the development of intestinal symptoms.

INVESTIGATIONS

Full blood examination

A low haemoglobin reflects iron-deficiency anaemia. In Crohn's disease with ileal involvement folic acid and Vitamin B_{12} absorption may be compromised and this can result in megaloblastic anaemia. The ESR is elevated when the disease is active.

Faecal microscopy and culture

Microbiological tests should include careful exclusion of enteric pathogens including *Salmonella*, *Shigella*, *Helicobacter*, *Yersinea* and *Giardia*. All these organisms can be responsible for chronic diarrhoea.

Liver function tests

These are required to exclude associated liver disease.

Endoscopy and biopsies

The most accurate assessment of patients with suspected inflammatory disease is provided by 'top and tail' endoscopy under general anaesthesia. This involves combined assessment by gastroscopy and colonoscopy, together with serial punch biopsies of the gut mucosa.

Patients with Crohn's disease often demonstrate inflammation involving the proximal gastrointestinal tract. In addition, Crohn's disease in childhood commonly affects the colon. Combined endoscopy provides a thorough assessment of the extent of disease as well as absolute confirmation of the diagnosis by demonstration of granulomas in the biopsy specimens.

In Crohn's disease the inflammation is typically segmental, unlike ulcerative colitis where inflammation is diffuse and extends for varying distances proximally in the colon. The degree of inflammation varies from normal mucosa macroscopically to severe ulceration with blood and pus in the intestinal lumen. In some instances, even when the macroscopic appearances at endoscopy are normal, multiple biopsies will show diagnostic histological features. A tissue diagnosis may be made from biopsies of perianal lesions. Periodic endoscopic review is employed to assess activity of disease and guide decisions concerning continuing therapy.

Radiology

Crohn's disease

In Crohn's disease, a barium meal and careful follow-through is important to assess the presence of inflammation in the small intestine. Most commonly, abnormalities are demonstrated in the terminal ileum and caecum. There may be stricture formation or displacement of bowel loops by an inflammatory mass (Fig. 24.1).

Ulcerative colitis

In ulcerative colitis barium enema has been largely superseded by colonoscopy. Typical radiological features of ulcerative colitis include a 'saw tooth' outline or marked mucosal irregularity associated with ulceration. With more advanced disease the colon becomes narrow, rigid and devoid of haustration (Fig. 24.2). There may be pseudopolyp formation or stenosis.

TREATMENT

The aims of treatment are to provide symptomatic relief, maintain adequate nutrition, abort acute attacks and minimize the frequency of relapses.

Medical treatment

The medical treatment of both forms of inflammatory bowel disease is similar. High doses of oral steroids are

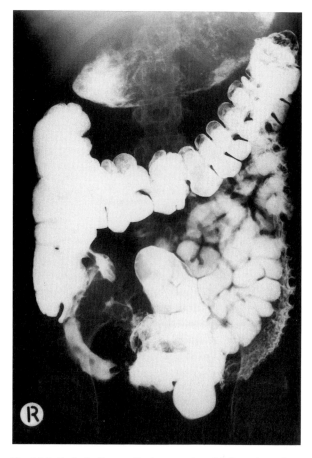

Fig. 24.1 Crohn's disease. Barium meal and follow-through showing irregular, inflamed terminal ileum and colon.

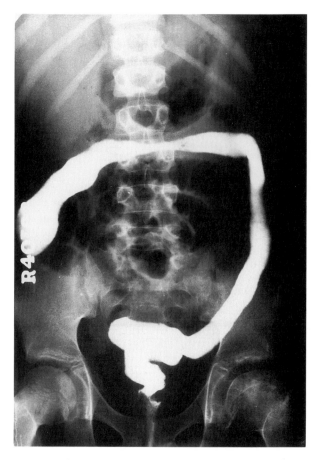

Fig. 24.2 Ulcerative colitis. Featureless colon with a sawtooth outline on barium enema.

used to induce a remission. Prednisolone in a dosage of 2–3 mg/kg (maximum 60 mg/day) is given for 4 weeks with subsequent gradual reduction and cessation by 8 weeks. Sulfasalazine is introduced up to a dose of 1 g twice daily to prevent relapses when the prednisolone dosage is reduced to 20 mg/day.

In Crohn's disease it may be necessary to continue low dose prednisolone (5 mg/day). Metronidazole is used in the treatment of perianal disease. In ulcerative colitis the prophylactic use of sulfasalazine is well supported by clinical trials, but in Crohn's disease its

efficacy is uncertain. Immuran is occasionally used in resistant cases.

Nutrition

Children with inflammatory bowel disease fail to grow because of the disease, not the treatment, and the reason the disease influences growth relates to its effect on appetite and caloric intake. High caloric dietary supplements and elemental diet may be beneficial when anorexia leads to inadequate uptake.

Total parenteral nutrition may be necessary in the severely diseased patient who cannot eat. Also, it may be useful in the patient who has an enteric fistula or obstruction prior to surgical treatment.

Surgical treatment

Surgery has an important role in the management of both forms of inflammatory bowel disease.

SURGERY IN CROHN'S DISEASE

Although surgery cannot cure Crohn's disease, it has an important role in the management of complications.

Perianal disease

Perianal disease is the commonest indication for surgical intervention. The development of a perianal abscess may necessitate drainage. Suppuration is usually associated with a fistula-in-ano, which should be excised.

More extensive suppuration may result in the formation of an ischiorectal abscess with pararectal extension, and has the potential to damage the sphincter anatomy; it may require faecal diversion (colostomy) as well as adequate drainage.

Intestinal complications

Intraperitoneal inflammatory masses, intestinal fistulae and strictures may require resection, the aim being to preserve as much intestine as possible.

Delayed growth and sexual development

Surgical intervention may be required for failed medical treatment with growth failure, delay in sexual development and steroid dependency. If there is localized obstructive disease, intestinal resection or a localized 'plasty' may be helpful, in contrast to the situation where there is widespread disease and poor physical development, where surgical intervention is not an option and the prognosis is poor.

Acute abdomen

Occasionally, laparotomy is necessary as a diagnostic procedure to exclude acute appendicitis.

SURGERY IN ULCERATIVE COLITIS

Improvements in medical treatment, with more aggressive use of steroids, have produced better control of this disease. Many children have remissions lasting several years, to the extent that the diagnosis subsequently is questioned. A small proportion of patients continue to have recurrent relapses and may require surgery.

In ulcerative colitis the disease can be cured by total colectomy. The indications for surgery are as follows:

(1) Failed medical treatment—usually associated with growth failure, delayed puberty and steroid dependency

(2) Toxic megacolon (rare)

(3) Prophylaxis against cancer.

Risk of cancer

Absence of symptoms is not necessarily an indication of quiescent or inactive disease, or of healing. Surveillance by regular colonoscopy and biopsy is indicated after 10 years of disease to assess the degree of dysplasia. The risk of developing cancer as a complication of ulcerative colitis in childhood is low.

The surgical options for the treatment of ulcerative colitis include:

(1) Total colectomy with permanent ileostomy

(2) Total colectomy with an ileal reservoir

(3) Subtotal colectomy with ileostomy. This is performed in the expectation that an ileorectal anastomosis may be possible subsequently, as in patients in whom rectal involvement is less severe.

(4) 'Soave' pull-through procedure—a sphincter preserving procedure. The success of this procedure

depends on minimal rectal involvement, an unlikely occurrence where colectomy is considered for severe disease.

FURTHER READING

Barnes G. L., Campbell P. E., Chow C. W. & Naidoo L. S. (1980) Colectomy and cancer in Melbourne children with ulcerative colitis. *Med. J. Aust.* **ii**: 84–87.

Davidson P. M., McLain B. I., Beasley S. W. & Stokes K. B. (1991) Peri-anal disease in childhood Crohn's disease: its frequency, characteristics and prognostic significance. *Pediatr. Surg. Int.* (in press).

Davidson P. M., McLain B. I., Stokes K. B. & Beasley S. W. (1991) Crohn's disease: the Melbourne experience. *Pediatr. Surg. Int.* (in press).

McLain B. I., Davidson P. M., Stokes K. B. & Beasley S. W. (1990) Growth after gut resection for Crohn's disease. *Arch. Dis. Child.* **65**: 760–762.

Raine P. A. M. (1984) BAPS collective review of chronic inflammatory bowel disease. *J. Pediatr. Surg.* **19**: 18–32.

25

The Child with an Abdominal Mass

The following points need to be considered when making a clinical diagnosis in a child with a mass in the abdomen:

(1) 'The site' of the mass and its precise characteristics, that is size, consistency and mobility, to determine the probable organ of origin

(2) The age of the patient and a knowledge of the most likely pathological process arising in that organ at that age

(3) The length of history and the type of symptoms (e.g. fever and tenderness may suggest an infection).

In more difficult cases, these considerations may not lead to a diagnosis but rather to a short list of two or three possible causes; the most useful and relevant investigations to reach the correct diagnosis with expedition, economy and the least distress to the patient then can be selected.

NORMAL AND ABNORMAL MASSES

The most common abdominal masses in infancy and childhood are the liver, which normally extends below the right costal margin until 3 or 4 years of age; faeces in the colon; a full bladder (Table 25.1). In addition, there are three pathological conditions which are sufficiently common to warrant special consideration as a

group which present as a mass in the loin: hydronephrosis, Wilms' tumour of the kidney and abdominal neuroblastoma.

They have certain features in common:

(1) They arise most frequently in infants and toddlers, that is between 12 months and 3 years of age

(2) At this age the abdomen is normally protruberant and tends to conceal the mass, which is often quite large when first detected

(3) General or local symptoms are frequently minimal or absent. The mass itself is usually the presenting feature, and typically is discovered by the mother while drying the child's abdomen after a bath.

The mass may extend downward toward the iliac fossa or forward, across to the other side, or it may straddle the midline. As a general rule it is only slightly tender and is so large that it may not move with respiration. When the mass is centred on the midline in the upper abdomen, a primary neuroblastoma is the most likely cause, particularly if the child is less than 4 years of age. Massive hepatic metastases (from a neuroblastoma) and a primary hepatoblastoma are other possibilities.

Investigations

The basic investigations are a plain abdominal X-ray and an abdominal ultrasound. The plain film of the abdomen may show calcification within the mass, more commonly in neuroblastoma (Fig. 25.1) than in Wilms' tumour, and not at all in hydronephrosis.

Abdominal ultrasound will determine whether a mass is 'cystic' or 'solid'. Cystic masses include hydronephrosis, polycystic kidneys, multilocular or simple renal cysts and a dilated kidney from severe vesi-

Table 25.1 The more common normal and abnormal masses in children

Normal	Abnormal
Liver	Hydronephrosis
Faeces	Wilms' tumour
Bladder	Neuroblastoma
(lower pole of kidneys)	

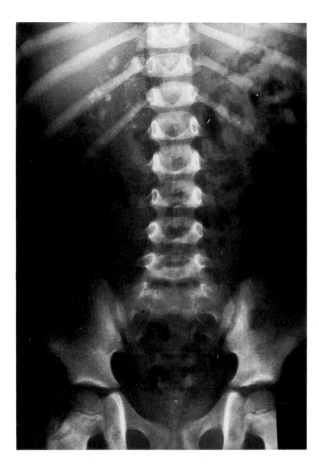

Fig. 25.1 Neuroblastoma showing calcification in the right paravertebral region.

coureteric reflux. Ultrasonography indicates the size, position and extent of a solid tumour and gives an indication of blood vessel involvement (e.g. extension of a Wilms' tumour into the inferior vena cava). Lymph node metastases within the abdomen and metastases within the liver may be demonstrated. A nuclear scan of the kidneys will demonstrate function of a hydronephrotic kidney or one involved by tumour, as well as the presence or absence of function of the contralateral kidney. In abdominal tumours other than Wilms' tumours, a more extensive assessment may be necessary, including abdominal computerized tomography (CT) scan or magnetic resonance imaging and, on occasions, angiography to determine its vascular supply. Intravenous pyelography is rarely necessary, except in the absence of a skilled ultrasonographer. The management of hydronephrosis is described in Chapter 33.

NEUROBLASTOMA

This is one of the common malignant tumours of early childhood. It arises from fetal neural crest cells, and the adrenal gland is the commonest site of origin (Fig. 25.1); the tumour may also arise in the adjacent retroperitoneal sympathetic plexus on the posterior abdominal wall, the mediastinum, the pelvis and, less commonly, in other sites.

Early metastases are found frequently and may be in the bone marrow, the cortex of long bones, the skull, regional or distant lymph nodes or the liver. The numerous sites of origin and the occurrence of early distant metastases account for the variety of presenting features, including a rubbery lymph node in the neck or in the axilla (lymph node metastases); paraplegia of rapid onset (spinal involvement); a nodule in the skull or proptosis and periorbital ecchymoses or pain and tenderness in the long bones (bone metastases); fever, loss of weight and energy; fleeting pain in the limbs; failure to thrive with or without anaemia (bone marrow involvement); diarrhoea caused by tumour metabolites (e.g. vasoactive intestinal peptide).

In view of the highly malignant nature of neuroblastoma, it is a paradox that in a small number of cases, the tumour may regress completely with a spontaneous cure. This only occurs if there is a small primary tumour with bone marrow, liver, lymph node or skin metastases; and never if there is cortical bone disease. Almost all children in this group are under 1 year of age. In 65–75% of cases, disseminated disease is present already when the diagnosis is made.

Diagnostic criteria

When an abdominal mass is suspected to be a neuroblastoma, the diagnosis can be confirmed by:

(1) A marrow biopsy for metastatic neuroblastoma, present at diagnosis in 65–75% of patients

(2) A 24 h collection of urine for biochemical analysis for tumour catecholamine metabolites (VMA, MHMA, [3-methoxy-4-hydroxymandelic acid], dopamine, adrenalin, noradrenalin)

(3) Biopsy of either the abdominal tumour or other sites of suspected metastases, for example lymph nodes.

The diagnosis is confirmed when neuroblastoma cells are identified within the bone marrow or in a biopsy specimen. When tumour metabolites in the urine are elevated significantly and neuroblastoma cells are seen in bone marrow, a laparotomy can be avoided. A chest X-ray should be performed pre-operatively to look for paravertebral extension of the tumour and mediastinal involvement. The MIBG scan highlights active metastases when meta-iodo benzyl guanidine is incorporated into functioning neuroblastoma tissue.

Treatment

Complete surgical excision of an abdominal neuroblastoma is not always possible and non-resectability is indicated by retroperitoneal extension of tumour encasing the aorta and inferior vena cava. If a small localized tumour is found, it should be removed. Treatment for large primary tumours and metastatic neuroblastoma involves intensive combination chemotherapy and reassessment after 3–6 months with surgical removal of the residual tumour, if feasible. Finally, high dose chemotherapy is given with autologous bone marrow rescue. In rare cases, radiotherapy may be used.

The prognosis is poor with less than 10% of children surviving when metastases are present at diagnosis.

WILMS' TUMOUR

Wilms' tumour or nephroblastoma of the kidney, arises from primitive embryonic cells and produces a mixed histological picture of epithelial structures, resembling tubules and a variety of mesenchymal tissues, including striated muscle fibres. This mixture of features is reported as 'favourable' histology, indicating its good prognosis. So-called unfavourable histology Wilms' tumour or sarcomatous Wilms' tumour are probably not true Wilms' tumours and represent a much poorer prognostic group.

If a bilateral Wilms' tumour is present, often seen in younger children, there may be an underlying genetic defect and chromosomal analysis should be performed, looking for an abnormality on chromosome 11. There may be an increased risk of recurrent primary tumours.

Clinical features

A Wilms' tumour usually presents as a smooth mass in the loin which reaches, but seldom crosses, the midline and extends downwards into the iliac fossa and upwards under the costal margin. A right-sided Wilms' tumour may extend upwards beneath, and sometimes behind, the liver which, if pushed downwards, can present as hepatomegaly. On the left side, a Wilms' tumour may be mistaken for an enlarged spleen.

Haematuria, often following minor trauma, is the mode of presentation in some children but does not indicate a poor prognosis. Clinical examination of the child should always include a blood pressure measurement, as this may be elevated.

Investigation

Ultrasonography provides detailed information of the site, size and extent of the tumour (Fig. 25.2a; Table 25.2). Ultrasonography also identifies renal vein and inferior vena cava involvement. This information must be ascertained prior to surgical excision of the tumour. The liver is examined for the presence of metastases and a chest X-ray excludes the presence of pulmonary metastases. A CT scan is employed on occasions (Fig. 25.2b).

Treatment

The kidney is removed if possible. In stage 1 tumours, adjuvant chemotherapy is given for a period of 3

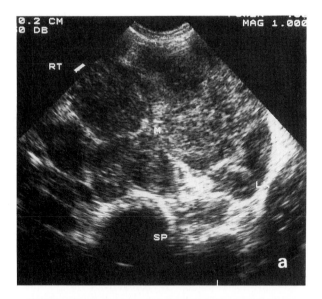

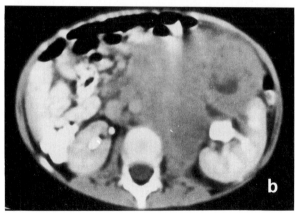

Fig. 25.2 (a) Ultrasound showing a large Wilms' tumour arising from the left kidney (LK). (b) CT scan showing the same tumour in cross-section as in (a).

Table 25.2 Staging of Wilms' tumour

Stage	Tumour spread
I	Confined to kidney and removed completely
II	Microscopic local disease after excision
III	Macroscopic residual disease after excision
IV	Distant metastases

months. In stage 2 tumours, two-agent chemotherapy will be used for 12–15 months, and in stage 3 tumours, three-agent chemotherapy is used for 12–15 months, with radiotherapy as an occasional adjunct. If the tumour is very large, chemotherapy may be used initially to 'shrink' the tumour prior to surgical removal. In stage 4 tumours, chemotherapy is the mainstay of treatment.

Two rare causes of a renal mass, mesenchymal hamartoma and multilocular cyst of the kidney, cannot be completely excluded by investigations or on their macroscopic appearance at operation, and are removed with the kidney.

Prognosis

Wilms' tumour, in contrast to neuroblastoma, usually has a good outcome. In stage 1 with 'favourable' histology the cure rate is greater than 95%. Even in unfavourable circumstances, for example with pulmonary metastases, the results are better than 50% 5 years' survival. Late occurrence locally, or as pulmonary metastasis, is very rare after 1 or 2 years, but careful follow-up with abdominal ultrasound and chest X-ray is required, particularly in the first 12 months of treatment.

LIVER TUMOURS

Hepatoblastoma is the most common malignant tumour presenting as a right upper quadrant mass in children less than 1 year of age. Alternative diagnoses include arteriovenous malformation, which may be accompanied by thrombocytopenia, and mesenchymal hamartoma; both of which are benign liver tumours. Elevation of serum α-fetoprotein—a tumour marker—is highly suggestive of hepatoblastoma. Accurate pre-operative assessment is necessary with imaging techniques including ultrasonography, CT scan and angiography. Surgical resection of the lesion, either locally or by lobectomy, remains the mainstay of treatment for all primary liver tumours. Chemotherapy has been shown to improve survival for malignant tumours and is used as adjuvant therapy.

FURTHER READING

Brown T. C. K., Davidson P. M. & Auldist A. W. (1988) Anaesthetic considerations in liver tumour resection in children. *Pediatr. Surg. Int.* **4**: 11–15.

Davidson P. M. & Auldist A. W. (1988) Surgical anatomy and operative techniques for elective hepatic resection in children. *Pediatr. Surg. Int.* **4**: 7–10.

de Campo J. & Phelan E. (1988) Imaging of liver tumours in childhood. *Pediatr. Surg. Int.* **4**: 1–6.

Grosfeld J. L. (1991) Neuroblastoma: a 1990 overview. *Pediatr. Surg. Int.* **6**: 9–13.

Hata Y., Naito H., Sasaki F. *et al.* (1990) Fifteen years' experience of neuroblastoma: a prognostic evaluation according to the Evans and UICC staging systems. *J. Pediatr. Surg.* **25**: 326–329.

Jacobs A., Delree M., Desprechins B. *et al.* (1990) Consolidating the role of *1-MIBG-scintigraphy in childhood neuroblastoma: five years of clinical experience. *Pediatr. Radiol.* **20**: 157–159.

Othersen H. B. Jr, DeLorimer A., Hrabovsky E., Kelalis P., Breslow N. & D'Angio G. J. (1990) Surgical evaluation of lymph node metastases in Wilms' tumor. *J. Pediatr. Surg.* **25**: 330–331.

Stevenson R. J. (1985) Abdominal masses. *Surg. Clin. North Am.* **65**: 1481–1504.

26

Spleen, Pancreas and Biliary Tract

THE SPLEEN

A number of haematological diseases may require splenectomy during the course of their treatment, which are discussed below. The management of splenic trauma is outlined in Chapter 38.

Spherocytosis

In spherocytosis the red cells are abnormally spherical and are destroyed in the spleen. This tends to result in:

(1) Chronic anaemia
(2) Episodic haemolytic jaundice
(3) A tendency to form pigment gallstones.

These complications can be controlled by splenectomy, but unless they are severe, splenectomy is delayed until at least the age of 7, because of the risk of postsplenectomy sepsis. About 2 weeks before elective splenectomy, the patient is immunized with multivalent pneumococcal vaccine. After splenectomy, long term oral penicillin is administered.

Idiopathic thrombocytopenic purpura

This is a common condition which usually resolves spontaneously. In children with a persistently low platelet count, steroids or γ-globulin infusions may improve the platelet count. However, in selected patients not responding to this treatment, splenectomy is required and usually improves the platelet count.

Thalassaemia

In thalassaemia major, a homozygous condition, the production of abnormal haemoglobin results in chronic haemolytic anaemia. In the past, chronic anaemia, blood transfusions and subsequent increasing iron stores have resulted in the patient developing a very large spleen, producing the added problem of secondary hypersplenism. The enlarged spleen tends to destroy all cellular elements in the blood.

Adequate transfusions help keep the children healthy and their spleens small. Regular parenteral desferrioxamine chelates excess iron liberated from haemolysed red cells and maintains normal serum iron levels. Splenectomy is no longer required in this condition.

Sickle cell anaemia

The presence of abnormal haemoglobin S results in an abnormally shaped red cell during hypoxia. These 'sickle cells' tend to flow through small vessels slowly, causing ischaemia in the organ involved. Splenic infarcts occur.

Splenectomy is usually contra-indicated as a higher haemoglobin tends to be associated with increased 'sickling' of the red cells.

THE PANCREAS

Pancreatitis

Pancreatitis in children is rare, but may occur following trauma, mumps, other viral infections or choledocholithiasis. Many cases have no identifiable cause. In the absence of a definitive history of blunt abdominal trauma, other underlying causes must be considered, for example biliary tract stones. The treatment is usually conservative, with pain relief, rest of the alimentary tract and intravenous fluids—and treatment of the cause, if applicable.

Pseudocyst

Damage to the pancreas may result in accumulation of pancreatic fluid in the lesser sac or adjacent to the pancreas. Treatment is non-operative in the first instance, and change in the size of the 'cyst' can be followed by ultrasound while the patient and his alimentary tract are rested. After several weeks it may be necessary to drain the pseudocyst into the stomach (or occasionally externally).

Hyperinsulinism (causing hypoglycaemia)

Excessive production of insulin may occur in several situations:

(1) In babies of diabetic mothers as a temporary response to high sugar levels

(2) β cell hyperplasia, a condition of unknown aetiology in which there is excessive production of insulin, which usually settles down with drug treatment (Diazoxide). Extensive pancreatectomy is only necessary occasionally

(3) Beckwith-Weidemann syndrome, a condition of newborn babies which is characterized by exomphalos;

organomegaly (large tongue and abdominal organs); hemihypertrophy; low blood sugar from excessive insulin production

(4) Islet cell tumours are a rare cause of hypoglycaemia but can be cured if the tumour (usually benign) is localized and excised.

THE BILIARY TRACT

Gallstones

In children, gallstones are seen in the following circumstances:

(1) Pigment calculi in babies: in all newborn babies, there is an increased load of pigment associated with the change from a high fetal haemoglobin to a lower, newborn level. Occasionally, this results in pigment stone formation in the gall-bladder

(2) Pigment calculi in haemolytic anaemia: in spherocytosis and thalassaemia, the high pigment load may produce gallstones

(3) Congenital obstructive abnormalities of the bile duct or choledochal cysts are more likely to form stones

(4) Cholesterol stones in adolescents, in which there is often a family history.

The ways in which a child with gallstones may present are summarized in Table 26.1.

Treatment

Treatment involves cholecystectomy and removal of stones in the common bile-duct.

Choledochal cysts

Choledochal cysts have many forms, but usually represent cystic enlargement of the common bile-duct. (Fig. 26.1) The presenting symptoms and signs are those of pain, jaundice, an upper abdominal mass and fever. Occasionally prenatal ultrasound reveals a cystic lesion in the abdomen, which can be treated postnatally before symptoms arise.

Table 26.1 Presentation of the child with gallstones

(1) Biliary colic: pain from a stone in the neck of the gall-bladder or in the common bile-duct

(2) Cholecystitis: chemical or bacterial inflammation of the gall-bladder usually associated with cystic duct obstruction

(3) Obstructive jaundice: dark urine and pale stools, due to a stone obstructing the common bile-duct

(4) Pancreatitis

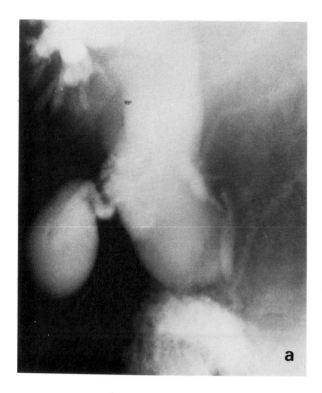

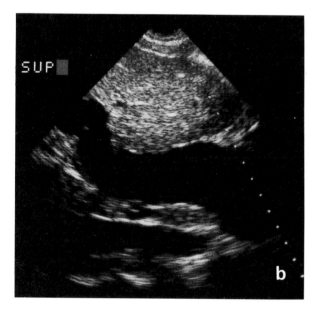

Fig. 26.1 Contrast X-ray (a) and ultrasound (b) of biliary tract showing the massive tubular dilatation of a choledochal cyst.

Treatment

Treatment is by excision of the cyst and drainage of the proximal bile-duct into the bowel by a choledocho-jejunostomy anastomosis to a Roux-en-Y loop of jejunum. Older treatments by drainage into the duodenum or direct drainage of the cyst into a Roux-en-Y jejunal loop proved to have an excessively high incidence of cholangitis and have been abandoned.

Biliary atresia

Biliary atresia presents with obstructive jaundice in the first weeks of life. The baby has persisting jaundice, pale stools and dark urine.

The cause of biliary atresia is unknown, but an accepted theory is that there is viral damage to the extrahepatic duct system, often accompanied by damage to the liver itself.

Diagnosis

Diagnosis is by history, clinical examination and liver biopsy (the most helpful test). Nuclear medicine scan shows decreased bile flow (e.g. HIDA scan). The diagnosis is confirmed at laparotomy where an operative cholangiogram shows an absent or incomplete biliary tree.

The disease must be distinguished from both metabolic disease (e.g. galactosaemia and α_1-antitrypsin deficiency) and from neonatal hepatitis caused by viral hepatitis, cytomegalovirus or syphilis.

Treatment

Biliary atresia is treated by hepatic porto-enterostomy. At operation the remnant of the common hepatic duct is dissected to the porta hepatis where a mass of fibrous tissue is found at the confluence of the hepatic ducts. This area is excised and joined to a Roux-en-Y jejunal loop.

Despite the absence of visible ducts, this operation is successful in up to 50% of patients. The earlier the hepatic porto-enterostomy, the better the results. Liver transplantation provides the only hope for the others.

FURTHER READING

Baesl T. J. & Filler R. M. (1985) Surgical diseases of the spleen. *Surg. Clin. North Am.* **65**: 1269–1286.

Hall R. J. & Karrer F. M. (1990) Biliary atresia: perspective on transplantation. *Pediatr. Surg. Int.* **5**: 94–99.

Miyano T., Ohya T., Kimura K., Shimomura H., Yamataka A. & Suruga K. (1990) Indications for the Kasai operation: experience with 103 Suruga II modifications. *Pediatr. Surg. Int.* **5**: 82–86.

Sawyer S. M., Davidson P. M., McMullin N. & Stokes K. B. (1989) Pancreatic pseudocysts in children. *Pediatr. Surg. Int.* **4**: 300–302.

Stewart B. A., Hall R. J., Karrer F. M. & Lilly J. R. (1990) Long-term survival after Kasai's operation for biliary atresia. *Pediatr. Surg. Int.* **5**: 87–90.

27

Anus, Perineum and Female Genitalia

ANAL FISSURES

These are confined mostly to infants and toddlers in whom the passage of a large stool splits the anal mucosa. There is a sharp pain and a few drops of bright blood on the surface of the stool. On other occasions, there may be painful defaecation without bleeding: there is no obvious fissure and the pain is produced by the large stool stretching the anus.

When the area is examined, the fissure often has already healed, an indication of its superficial nature and its rapid healing. When still present, it is visible usually anteriorly or posteriorly.

Treatment

The condition is of no consequence in itself and treatment is directed to the underlying constipation. No local treatment is required since the mucosal tear heals so rapidly.

After relief of constipation, crying on defaecation may continue for several weeks because the child associates defaecation with pain and reacts accordingly. The emotional tension built up around the act is more difficult to treat than the fissure itself and can be the forerunner of the whole vicious circle of constipation (see Chapter 22).

PERIANAL ABSCESS

This is fairly common in infants and arises from infection in the anal glands, which open into the crypts of the anal valves. Although the abscess almost always presents superficially, the fistulous tract passes through the lowest fibres of the internal sphincter to open at the level of the anal valves.

Treatment

Treatment involves identification and laying open of the fistula and drainage of the abscess (Fig. 27.1). Failure to deal with the fistula will result in recurrent infection.

Sometimes young children may develop a superficial subcutaneous abscess in the buttock or near the anus, which is often secondary to a nappy rash and involves infection with skin organisms. Simple drainage and antibiotics are curative.

RECTAL PROLAPSE

Rectal prolapse is not uncommon in toddlers and is an alarming experience for the parents (Fig. 27.2), but in most cases disappears spontaneously after a few weeks or months without residual damage.

Aetiology

In only a small minority is there an organic cause:

(1) Paralysis of anal sphincters in myelomeningocele or sacral agenesis (but even in these conditions it is surprisingly infrequent)

(2) Marasmic, undernourished, hypotonic infants are seen rarely in this community, but are recognized as possible candidates for prolapse

(3) In ectopia vesicae there is a high incidence of prolapse

(4) Following anoplasty or rectoplasty for imperforate anus or rectum, there may be redundant rectal mucosa which may resemble a rectal prolapse.

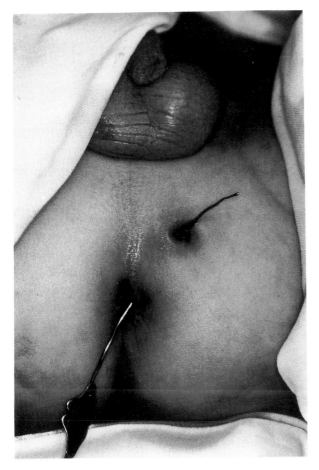

Fig. 27.1 In perianal abscess there is a fistulous tract which runs from the abscess to the anus at the level of the anal valves. The tract is displayed by the lacrimal probe.

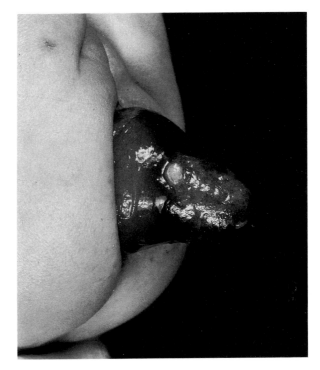

Fig. 27.2 Rectal prolapse. The mucosa is congested and oedematous and may bleed.

The two common predisposing factors are:

(1) Straining at stool by a child with constipation. Less frequently, diarrhoea as part of a malabsorption syndrome (e.g. cystic fibrosis or coeliac disease) may contribute

(2) Explosive or reluctant defaecation: a healthy child occasionally develops a prolapse because the act is precipitate and little time is permitted for moulding of the stool by the muscles of the pelvic floor. Alternatively, the parents' ill-advised training may demand prolonged attempts to defaecate, producing excessive straining in the absence of constipation.

Clinical features

Most children with prolapse have normal anatomy. The prolapse rolls out painlessly only during defaecation and usually returns spontaneously; manual replacement is required infrequently. The mucosa may become abraded while it is prolapsed and cause some bleeding, but this tends to be minimal.

Differential diagnosis

A rectal polyp may prolapse (see below), and this can be identified by observation, digital palpation or proctoscopy.

(157)

The apex of an intussusceptum can appear at the anus. This is a rare event and is accompanied by its own clinical features (Chapter 19).

External haemorrhoids do not occur in childhood, but congestion of the submucosal venous plexus during straining at stool sometimes produces a bluish sessile bulge.

Treatment

Constipation is the commonest cause and treatment for at least several weeks is required (Chapter 22). When there is no constipation, the possibility of a malabsorption syndrome should be investigated.

A common error is to squat the child on a pot on the floor, which stretches the pelvic floor and the anal sphincters to the maximum disadvantage. A potty-chair or an inset for an adult seat enables the child to sit with support for the pelvic floor; and a reasonable time limit should be set.

Strapping the buttocks is required occasionally when the prolapse fails to return after defaecation.

Rarely, it is necessary to inject a sclerosant into the submucous plane of the rectum to cause fibrosis and contraction of the rectal wall. This is reserved for the few stubborn cases which fail to respond to conservative measures; 0.5 mL of 5% phenol in almond oil is injected into the submucosa at three equally spaced points, 2 cm above the anal valves. Even more rarely, a suture may be inserted into the subcutaneous tissues around the anus (Thiersch operation) and tied while a finger is held in the anus. This is applicable in certain neurogenic lesions and in severe hypotonia, but is contra-indicated in ordinary constipation. The extensive operations for rectal prolapse performed in adults are never justified in infants and children.

RECTAL POLYP

A rectal polyp is a benign hamartomatous lesion and a relatively common cause of rectal bleeding. Bright bleeding is produced painlessly at the end of defaecation and is typically intermittent over long periods. Occasionally the polyp prolapses through the anus (Fig. 27.3).

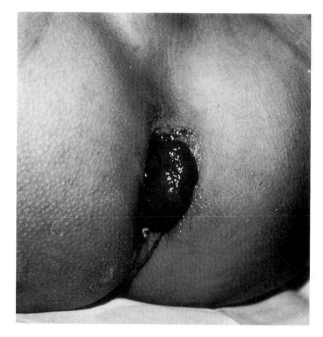

Fig. 27.3 Prolapse of a benign rectal polyp through the anus.

The polyp is almost always within reach of an examining finger. The diagnosis is discussed in the section on rectal bleeding (Chapter 23).

Treatment

On the rare occasions that the polyp presents through the anus, the base can be ligated without anaesthesia. Otherwise, under general anaesthesia, the polyp can be located through a proctoscope and withdrawn to demonstrate its stalk, which is transected with diathermy or transfixed with a suture-ligature. Higher lesions can be similarly removed through a colonoscope. Recurrence is rare and malignancy unknown.

MULTIPLE POLYPOSIS

This is a rare familial condition with malignant potential seen in adults, and even more rarely in children. It should be considered when more than three polyps are identified, and when there is a family history of multiple polyposis. Colonoscopy and a double contrast barium enema are indicated. In children, major fluid and electrolyte losses may ensue and the colon should be removed.

The Peutz-Jeghers' syndrome

This is an even rarer condition which has gained prominence because of the external evidence of its existence—the presence of pigmented freckles on the mucocutaneous margins of the lips and the anus. Polyps are found anywhere in the gastrointestinal tract, especially in the jejunum, and give rise to massive bleeding, intussusception or intestinal obstruction. The polyps may become malignant, but this is less common than in familial polyposis of the colon.

POSTANAL DIMPLE (COCCYGEAL DIMPLE)

Many babies have a small shallow pit in the skin over the coccyx which is of no significance. Occasionally, it is narrow and deep and may become infected, in which case it should be excised.

A simple benign coccygeal dimple is not to be confused with a sacral sinus which, although rare, is potentially more dangerous. The sacral sinus lies over the sacrum, not the coccyx, and is associated with an underlying spina bifida occulta (Chapter 10). The depths cannot be seen and there is likely to be a small track which communicates directly with the spinal theca or with an intraspinal dermoid cyst. This track is a source of recurrent meningitis and the child should be referred to a neurosurgeon for treatment.

SACROCOCCYGEAL TERATOMA

A teratoma arising from and attached to the tip of the sacrum or the front of the coccyx occurs in 1 : 40 000 births, and slightly more frequently in females (Fig. 27.4). It is usually obvious at birth and may be so large as to cause obstetrical difficulties. Occasionally the

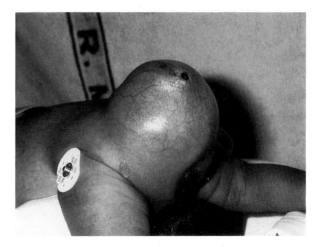

Fig. 27.4 Sacrococcygeal teratoma of medium size; note the distortion of the perineum and anal canal, and a small ulcer on the surface of the tumour. The prognosis for faecal continence after operation, however, is excellent.

swelling is in the pelvis and does not protrude from the perineum.

The tumour is a mixture of solid and cystic areas arising from all embryonic layers. The incidence of malignancy varies—from 5 to 35%—and is of the type known as an endodermal sinus or yolk-sac tumour. Malignant degeneration is less likely when a teratoma is removed immediately after birth.

Management

Even very small lesions over the coccyx should be referred to a tertiary paediatric centre for excision at birth. Differential diagnosis includes other rare tumours (chordoma or ganglioneuroma) or an anterior sacral meningocele. Computerized tomography scan or magnetic resonance imaging may be required to determine the degree of intrapelvic tumour. Excision is undertaken in the first few days of life if the infant has no other developmental anomalies which might have priority. In spite of gross stretching of the pelvic floor, its nerve supply and the anal canal, the structures will recover completely after careful surgery without any long term neural deficit or lack of function.

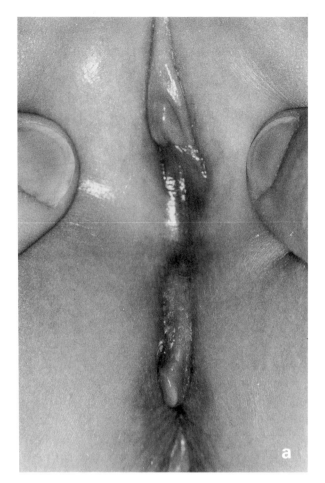
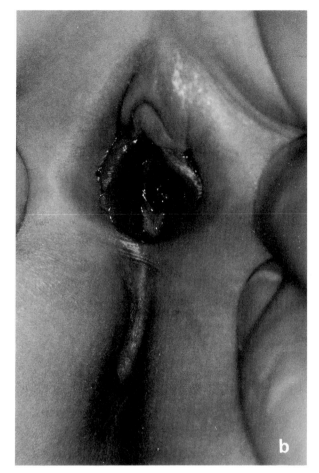

Fig. 27.5 Adherent labia minora (labial adhesions). The normal labia majora have been flattened by lateral traction to display the line of fusion (a). Following separation the introitus is fully visible (b).

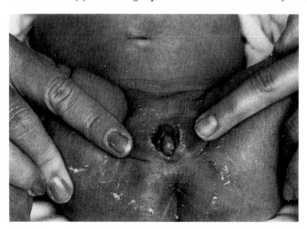

Fig. 27.6 Imperforate hymen causing mucocolpos in a newborn infant.

Prognosis

Local malignant recurrence is uncommon, but more likely if:

(1)   The tumour is uniformly solid and devoid of cysts

(2)   When operation is not undertaken until after the age of 1 month.

The large benign teratoma presents at birth and could hardly be overlooked; it is removed in the neonatal period. However, a small malignant teratoma may escape diagnosis until a rapid increase in size brings it to notice later in the first year of life.

THE FEMALE GENITALIA

Developmental anomalies are rare in girls: the commonest abnormality, adhesion of the labia minora, is probably caused by ulceration of the labia (nappy rash) with secondary adhesion during re-epithelialization.

Labial adhesions

This is a common condition which may cause discomfort on micturition but is more often discovered on routine examination (Fig. 27.5). There is a delicate midline adhesion of the two labia minora which partially closes the posterior introitus, overlying the opening of the urethra, and may extend as far anteriorly as the clitoris.

Congenital absence of the vagina is diagnosed frequently in error, causing the parents much unnecessary anxiety. Labial adhesions never present at birth.

Treatment

In infants and young children, the fused labia can be separated by exerting gentle lateral traction on the labia minora without anaesthesia or by sweeping them apart with the blunt end of a thermometer. In older children the labia may require separation under anaesthesia. Because of the tendency for the adhesions to recur, the mother should separate the labia daily for 2 weeks and apply petroleum jelly to the introitus to help prevent recurrent adhesion.

Imperforate hymen

This is a rare condition, which presents either at birth (the vagina secretes mucus which accumulates beneath the bulging imperforate hymen to form a mucocolpos; Fig. 27.6) or at puberty when apparent primary amenorrhoea, haematocolpos or even haematometrocolpos may be the presenting features, with cyclic attacks of abdominal pain. During childhood the condition is usually symptomless, except for possible urinary symptoms such as 'wetting', or dysuria when the cystic swelling distorts the urethra.

Treatment at birth is removal of a circular disc of membrane to provide drainage.

Vaginal discharge

The chief symptom is vulval irritation, but in some cases the discharge itself may be the only complaint. A profuse offensive or blood-stained discharge suggests the present of a foreign body. Small objects may be successfully removed by irrigation using a soft rubber catheter or instrumental removal under anaesthesia, through a miniature vaginoscope.

The possibility of sexual abuse must be considered, and where suspected, the discharge should be sent for microbiological examination (Chapter 36).

FURTHER READING

Ein S. H., Mancer K. & Adeyemi S. D. (1985) Malignant sacrococcygeal teratoma—endodermal sinus, yolk sac tumor—in infants and children: a 32 year review. *J. Pediatr. Surg.* **20**: 473–477.

Fowler R. (1967) The anatomy and treatment of rectal prolapse in childhood. *Aust. Paediatr. J.* **2**: 90–98.

Smith E. D. (1976) Pelvic malignancies. In: Jones P. G. & Campbell P. E. (eds) *Tumours of Infancy and Childhood*, Chapter 21. Blackwell Scientific Publications, Oxford.

Stephens F. D., Smith E. D. & Paul N. W. (1988) *Ano-rectal Malformations in Children*. A. R. Liss, New York.

Whalen T. V., Mahour G. H., Landing B. H. & Woolley M. M. (1985) Sacrococcygeal teratomas in infants and children. *Am. J. Surg.* **150**: 373–375.

28

Undescended Testes

DEFINITIONS

Undescended testis

An undescended testis, is one which cannot be made to reach the bottom of the scrotum. It represents the second most common problem in paediatric surgery after indirect inguinal hernia. Most undescended testes have no recognizable primary abnormality, but become secondarily dysplastic if they do not reside in the scrotum. In the vast majority, the cause of maldescent is unknown, but is likely to be from a mechanical rather than a hormonal defect.

In a few patients there is a small, ill-formed and relatively immobile testis with a short spermatic cord. Most are located near the pubic tubercle, some are in the inguinal canal or even higher, in the abdomen. Some of those in the canal can be manipulated through the external ring, but when palpation ceases, they return to an impalpable position. Many of these are primarily dysplastic.

Retractile testis

A true undescended testis has to be distinguished from a retractile testis that can be manipulated to the bottom of the scrotum regardless of the position in which it is first located. A retractile testis will remain in the scrotum for some time after manipulation. It is a normal size and there is a history that it is present in the scrotum on some occasions, such as during a warm bath. All normal prepubertal boys have retractile testes which lie in a bilocular space: the lower loculus lines the scrotum and the upper portion is the so-called 'superficial inguinal pouch' between the external oblique aponeurosis and the membranous layer of the abdominal fascia. The position of the testis is controlled by the cremaster muscle which regulates the testicular temperature by retracting the testis out of the scrotum when cold; it also protects the testis from trauma. Cremasteric contraction is absent in the first few months after birth and is maximal between 2 and 8 years.

Ascending testis

An 'ascending' testis is one that is in the scrotum in infancy, but where the spermatic cord fails to elongate at the same rate as body growth, the testicular position becomes progressively higher during childhood. On occasions, there is a history of the testis descending into the scrotum some weeks after birth. This anomaly is thought to be intermediate between normal and undescended testes.

Impalpable testis

An impalpable testis is uncommon (<10%) and agenesis is rare (approximately 2% of all impalpable testes). A fully descended but grossly hypoplastic testis may be impalpable and only identified by exploration.

EXAMINATION

The examination of the testis should take place in warm and relaxed surroundings, and is begun by placing one finger on each side of the neck of the scrotum to pull the scrotum up to the pubis and to prevent the testes from being retracted out of the scrotum by the other

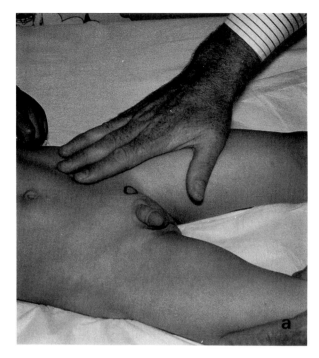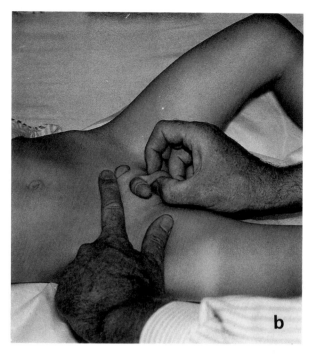

Fig. 28.1 Examination to locate the position of the testis. The fingers of one hand push the testis towards the neck of the scrotum (a), while the other hand 'snares' the testis at the top of the scrotum to see whether it can be pulled right to the bottom of the scrotum (b).

examining hand. Each side of the scrotum is then palpated for a testis; if it is not there, the fingertips of the left hand are placed just medial to the anterior superior iliac spine and moved firmly towards the pubic tubercle (Fig. 28.1a), where the right hand waits to capture the testis if it appears (Fig. 28.1b). Its range of movement is determined carefully, for the diagnosis depends on this. The precise diagnosis of a palpable testis is made by determining how far it can be manipulated into the scrotum.

More than two-thirds of undescended testes are located in the 'superficial inguinal pouch' (i.e. they are palpable in the groin) (Fig. 28.2). The testes are normal in size and have a good length of spermatic cord, which makes them deceptively mobile. The cause of mal-descent is probably mechanical. Rarely, the testis may migrate to a truly ectopic position, such as the

perineum, the base of the penis (prepubic) and the thigh (femoral).

SEQUELAE OF NON-DESCENT

The higher temperature of the extra-scrotal testis causes testicular dysplasia with interstitial fibrosis and poor development of the seminiferous tubules. A testis in the inguinal region is more liable to direct violence as it overlies the pubic tubercle. Torsion occasionally occurs in undescended testes; but it is more often found in those which are fully descended.

The risk of seminoma arising in an undescended testis in later life is five to 10 times greater than in a normal testis. It is uncertain whether orchidopexy early in life will prevent the development of tumours, but at least it makes early detection more likely.

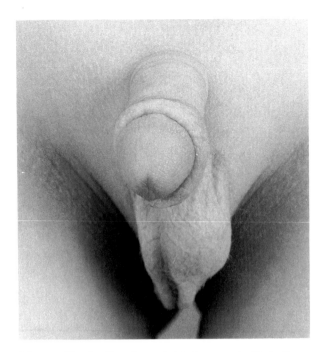

Fig. 28.2 Nearly all undescended testes are palpable in the groin. Here the right testis is too high to be seen at the neck of the scrotum.

TREATMENT OF UNDESCENDED TESTES

The object of treatment is to preserve normal spermatogenesis and prevent dysplasia, which could lead to malignancy. Hormone function at puberty (i.e. testosterone output) is normal regardless of treatment. The production of spermatozoa is adversely affected in undescended testes from the age of 1 or 2 years onwards, and to a degree proportional to the length of time the testis remains undescended beyond this age. A few testes may descend fully at puberty, but they are poorly developed and spermatogenesis is deficient.

The best time for orchidopexy is at about 1 year of age, as shown by evidence of subsequent biopsies and sperm counts. Orchidopexy usually is performed as a day surgery procedure.

Exploration for the uncommon impalpable testis is worthwhile, for in about 50% a useful testis can be brought down, and in the other 50% there is either no testis present (testicular agenesis or intrauterine testic-

ular torsion) or a useless and potentially neoplastic testis is removed. Gonadotrophic hormones are ineffective except for borderline retractile testes. A coexistent indirect inguinal hernia is almost universal but usually latent; when it becomes apparent clinically, herniotomy is necessary regardless of the boy's age, at which time orchidopexy is performed.

Absent testes

Rarely the testis is absent or excised because of torsion (and necrosis), tumours or dysgenesis. Together these conditions account for 1–2% of boys with undescended testes. These boys have psychological problems and suffer significant embarrassment in the locker room. The use of prosthetic testes should be considered when psychological problems arise, but ideally insertion of a prosthesis should be delayed until adolescence when adult-sized implants can be accommodated in the scrotum.

VARICOCELE

A varicocele is an enlargement of the veins of the pampiniform plexus in the spermatic cord and usually appears in boys over 12 years of age, at or before the onset of puberty. The mass of veins is visible and palpable when the patient is standing, and feels like 'a bag of worms'. There is sometimes a small secondary hydrocele. The varicosities empty when the boy lies down, and clinical examination should always include getting the boy to stand up. It is usually on the left side and symptomless, though a dragging ache may develop when the varicocele is large.

The problem of varicocele relates to the effect of the varicocele on spermatogenesis, because a unilateral collection of veins warms both testes and, by raising their temperature several degrees, causes oligospermia.

Treatment

The optimal temperature for spermatogenesis (and the normal scrotal temperature) is 33°C, 4°C below body temperature. Relative infertility cannot be assessed until late adolescence, but secondary atrophy of the testis is well-recognized and if the affected testis is significantly smaller than the other then early operation is indicated.

High ligation of the spermatic veins, or ligation of the cremasteric veins, which anastomose freely with the spermatic veins, should prevent recurrence in most patients.

Very rarely, a varicocele develops as the result of obstruction of the renal veins by a renal or perirenal tumour, for example Wilms' tumour or a neuroblastoma, almost always on the left side, in a boy less than 5 years of age. The tumour can usually be palpated as an abdominal mass.

FURTHER READING

Cendron M., Keating M. A., Huff D. S., Koop C. E., Snyder H. McC. III & Duckett J. W. (1989) Cryptorchidism, orchiopexy and infertility: critical long-term retrospective analysis. *J. Urol.* **142**: 559–562.

Cywes S., Louw J. H. & Retief P. J. M. (1979) Results and fertility after orchidopexy for undescended testes. *Z. Kinderchir.* **26**: 328.

Das S. & Springer A. (1990) Controversies of perinatal torsion of the spermatic cord: a review, survey and recommendations. *J. Urol.* **143**: 231–233.

Edler J. S. (1988) The undescended testis: hormonal and surgical management. In: Resnick M. I. (ed.) Urologic Surgery, *Surg. Clin. North Am.* **68**: 983–1005.

El-Gohary M. A. (1984) Boyhood varicocele: an overlooked disorder. *Ann. R. Coll. Surg. Engl.* **66**: 35.

Fenton E. J. M., Woodward A. A., Hudson I. L. & Marschner I. (1990) The ascending testis. *Pediatr. Surg. Int.* **5**: 6–9.

Fonkalsrud E. W. & Mengel W. (1981) *The Undescended Testis.* Year Book Medical, Chicago.

Fonkalsrud E. W. (1985) The role and timing of surgery for cryptorchidism. *Aust. NZ J. Surg.* **54**: 431–434.

Hadziselimovic F. (1977) Cryptorchidism. Ultra structure of normal and cryptorchid testis development. *Advances in Anatomy, Embryology and Cell Biology*, Vol. 53, Fasc. 3.

Hutson J. M., Williams M. P. L., Attah A., Larkins S. & Fallat M. (1990) Undescended testes remain a dilemma despite recent advances in research. *Aust. NZ J. Surg.* **60**: 429–439.

Koff W. J. & Scaletscky R. (1990) Malformations of epididymis in undescended testis. *J. Urol.* **143**: 340–343.

Scott J. E. S. (1982) Laparoscopy as an aid in the diagnosis and management of the impalpable testis. *J. Pediatr. Surg.* **17**: 14–16.

Thorup J. & Cortes D. (1990) The incidence of maldescended testes in Denmark. *Pediatr. Surg. Int.* **5**: 2–5.

Wright J. E. (1989) Testes do ascend. *Pediatr. Surg. Int.* **4**: 269–272.

29

The Inguinoscrotal Region

In children, more surgical conditions occur in the inguinoscrotal region than in any other part of the body. Accurate diagnosis is easier, because the area is readily accessible to inspection and palpation, but depends on a knowledge of the normal anatomy of the area and of the many conditions which may occur.

The inguinoscrotal region cannot be regarded as being isolated from the rest of the body, for symptoms and signs can arise here in diseases primarily located elsewhere, and vice versa; for example blood or meconium in the tunica vaginalis from intraperitoneal haemorrhage or meconium peritonitis or torsion of the testis presenting with pain referred to the abdomen.

A careful examination of each organ, the contiguous areas, and the whole patient, is necessary to avoid diagnostic errors. The prepuce is retracted, if this can be accomplished easily, and the urethral meatus is inspected. The testis, epididymis and vas deferens are examined separately and the region of the external ring is examined for evidence of an inguinal hernia.

Abnormalities apparently confined to the groin can also provide clues to more general conditions affecting the whole child; for example balanitis in a hitherto unrecognized diabetic and ambiguous genitalia in disorders of the adrenal glands.

Table 29.1 Causes of acute scrotum in children

(1)	Torsion of one of its appendages, that is, the appendix testis (hydatid of Morgagni)	60%
(2)	Torsion of the testis	30%
(3)	Epididymo-orchitis	< 10%
(4)	Idiopathic scrotal oedema	< 10%
	As per Clift and Hutson (1989).	

THE 'ACUTE SCROTUM'

There is a group of conditions which cause a painful or enlarged scrotum (Table 29.1). There are wide variations in the speed of onset, the rate of progression of the local signs, and the severity of pain.

Torsion of the testis

Even though it is not the most common cause of an acute scrotum, it is certainly the most important. The term is actually a misnomer, as it is the spermatic cord which undergoes torsion, obstructing the spermatic vessels. It most often occurs in a fully descended testis and is a surgical emergency because of the high incidence of necrosis of the testis if the cord is not untwisted promptly.

Two kinds of torsion occur:

(1) Intratunical (or 'intravaginal'), the most common, is made possible by an abnormally high investment of the cord by the tunica vaginalis (Fig. 29.1a), but also because the normal vertical fixation by the non-peritonealized strip of the epididymis is lacking (Fig. 29.1b, d). The predisposing abnormality is almost always present on the opposite side as well, and this testis should be fixed to prevent torsion at the time of surgery. Rarely, torsion occurs between the testis and the epididymis, which are connected by a thin sheet of tissue.

(2) Extratunical (or 'extravaginal') torsion (Fig. 29.1c) is rare and confined to the neonate in whom there is a plane of mobility in the areolar tissue outside the tunica. The testis is always necrotic by the time the diagnosis is made.

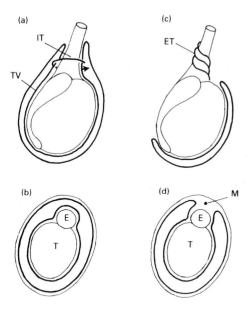

Fig. 29.1 Torsion of the testis: (a) intratunical torsion (IT) of the terminal portion of the cord within an abnormally high investment by the tunica vaginalis, which (b) completely invests the testis and epididymis. (c) Extratunical torsion (ET) of the cord above a normal tunica vaginalis which has (d) a normal mesorchium (M) preventing intratunical torsion. (Reprinted from *Arch. Dis. Childh.* 1962, **37**: 215, by permission of the Editor and Publishers.)

An undescended testis, too, may undergo torsion—particularly when an accompanying hernial sac completely invests the cord—but it would appear torsion of an undescended testis is less common than torsion of a fully descended testis. The true incidence is obscured by the phenomenon known as 'testis redux': when a fully descended testis undergoes torsion, the apparent length of the spermatic cord is shortened and it may be misdiagnosed at operation as torsion of an undescended testis, or clinically, as a strangulated hernia if it is located over the pubic tubercle.

Clinical signs

The onset is usually sudden, with pain in the testicle and/or abdomen, nausea or vomiting. Sometimes the onset is more gradual, without severe pain, and the diagnosis will be delayed if only the more acute form is accepted as typical.

A previous history of similar but short-lived, even momentary pain is suggestive of episodes of incomplete and spontaneously resolving torsion. A horizontal 'lie' of the testes when the child stands indicates the possibility of torsion involving the epididymis and the testis, and should be taken as an indication for exploration and orchidopexy.

The swollen testis and epididymis are exquisitely tender (unless already necrotic) and may be partially obscured by overlying scrotal oedema and an effusion into the tunica (reactive hydrocele). The amount of swelling depends on the time that has elapsed and the rate of progression. The hydrocele and the exquisite tenderness may make precise palpation of the testis difficult.

Treatment

Urgent exploration of the scrotum is arranged to untwist the testis and epididymis and to anchor ('pex') both it and the contralateral testis to prevent subsequent torsion. If the testis is completely necrotic, it should be removed.

Torsion of an appendage

Torsion of an appendage (e.g. 'hydatid of Morgagni') is the commonest cause of the acute scrotum in the prepubertal boy. The vestigial remnants are attached to the testis or the epididymis, and are present in 90% of the male population (Fig. 29.2). Recurrent attacks also occur, sometimes very frequently, and the boy may present with a suggestive history, but few acute signs. A small tender lump at the upper pole of the testis is diagnostic.

Clinical signs

The boy complains of severe pain in his scrotum. A blue-black spot may be seen through the skin of the scrotum near the upper pole of the testis: palpation of it causes extreme pain, whereas palpation of the testis

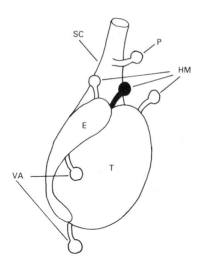

Fig. 29.2 Torsion of the testicular appendages. The commonest appendage is also the one most often twisted (black). Others less commonly present are (P) the paradidymis attached to the spermatic cord (SC), the appendix of the epididymis (E), and the superior and inferior vas aberrans (VA). (HM, 'hydatids of Morgagni') (Reprinted from *Arch. Dis. Childh.* 1962, **37**: 218, by permission of the Editor and Publishers.)

itself causes no discomfort. The epididymis is nontender and not enlarged. It may be impossible to distinguish from testicular torsion once a secondary hydrocele has developed.

Treatment

Where torsion of the testis cannot be excluded on clinical examination, urgent exploration is mandatory and at operation the appendix testis is removed. If the tender 'pea' of a twisted testicular appendage is palpable, surgical excision of it provides immediate relief of symptoms and prevents recurrence.

Epididymo-orchitis

It is common practice to refer to inflammatory conditions in the scrotum as 'epididymo-orchitis', even though the epididymis alone is usually affected.

Infection may be blood-borne, or may be carried by retrograde flow along the vas deferens from infections in the urinary tract, in which case the common organism is *Escherichia coli*. Predisposing factors include trauma, abnormalities of the urinary tract or urethral instrumentation, for example an indwelling catheter which may have been inserted months previously. Often no cause can be identified and a virus is suspected.

Clinical signs

The usual findings are dysuria, pain in the scrotum of subacute onset, swelling and tenderness. A lax secondary hydrocele is common, and bilateral signs, while uncommon, are particularly suggestive of epididymitis. Examination of the urine may show pyobacteriuria. The seminal vesicles may be involved and should be examined by rectal examination, as should the prostate and urethra.

Boys with epididymo-orchitis due to urinary organisms should have a renal ultrasound and micturating cysto-urethrogram 1–3 months after the epididymitis has subsided; this is to identify anomalies of the lower urinary tract before irreversible damage to the kidneys has occurred.

Differential diagnosis

The clinical picture can mimic torsion of the testes so closely that in most if not all children the diagnosis should be made only after exploration of the scrotum. True acute orchitis is very uncommon, but may occur in mumps or septicaemia. The testis is larger and harder than in epididymo-orchitis. Mumps orchitis is extremely rare prior to puberty. Infiltration of the testis is rare also, but does occur occasionally in leukaemia or with a primary neoplasm (embryonic adenocarcinoma, seminoma or a benign tumour of the interstitial cells of Leydig).

Treatment

Treatment of epididymitis consists of rest, antibiotics (e.g. Septrin, Furadantin), a high fluid intake and alkalinization of the urine. Severe or repeated infections may lead to an abscess or progressive destruction of the testis, but sterility is rare when only one side is affected.

Idiopathic scrotal oedema

In this condition, there is a rapidly developing oedema of the scrotum which may then spread to the inguinal region, penis and foreskin or on to the perineum.

The scrotum is symmetrically swollen, pale pink or red, and there is slight discomfort rather than acute pain.

Careful palpation reveals non-tender testes which are normal in size. The oedema subsides in 1–2 days, but may occasionally recur some weeks later. There may be a history of allergy or of playing out of doors at the onset; a bite from an insect or a spider is a probable cause in some, but as a rule the history is inconclusive.

Differential diagnosis

It can be distinguished from other causes of the 'acute scrotum' by the complete absence of tenderness in the epididymis and testis, and by the spread of oedema beyond the confines of the scrotum.

The spread of infection from an unobtrusive streptococcal pustule in the perineum can produce a swathe of slightly reddened skin and subcutaneous oedema which extends beside or across one-half of the scrotum. A tender enlarged inguinal node at or near the external inguinal ring assists in diagnosis of perineal lymphangitis.

A toddler who sustains a straddle injury or sits on a toy with a sharp projection may injure the urethra, causing superficial extravasation of urine. Pain on voiding and progressive oedema of the perineum, scrotum and suprapubic region, are suggestive of urethral injury which is confirmed on urethrography (Chapter 38). An indwelling catheter and urinary antibiotics may be required.

Fat necrosis of the scrotum

This extremely rare condition presents with tender, usually bilateral, comma-shaped small lumps within the scrotal wall of stout boys. Trauma may be responsible, but usually a history of swimming in very cold water is obtained—pointing to cold injury as the cause. Treatment is supportive, as the necrotic fat gradually absorbs. If doubt exists, exploration is required.

Management of the acute scrotum

As a general rule, an urgent exploration is required in all cases of acute scrotum in which the possibility of testicular torsion cannot be completely excluded.

Unless there is a history of recurring urinary tract infections, a known developmental anomaly of the renal tract or significant pyobacteriuria, the diagnosis of epididymitis or orchitis should be avoided and the scrotum should be explored.

A midline scrotal incision has advantages: when torsion of the testis is found it can be untwisted and fixed, and exploration and fixation of the opposite testis can be done through the same incision.

INGUINAL LYMPHADENITIS

The superficial inguinal lymph nodes drain the lower limbs, the perineum, the buttocks and the perianal region—all common sites of minor coccal skin infections in the 'napkin area' in infants. Infections often reach the inguinal nodes, which become enlarged and may form an abscess after the initial focus has disappeared. Occasionally, MAIS infection in pre-school children involves these nodes. The axilla, neck and spleen should be examined for evidence of a generalized lymphadenopathy.

In children under 5 or 6 years of age, one or more of the superficial inguinal nodes are situated above the inguinal ligament just lateral to the pubic tubercle, and an abscess here may be mistaken for a strangulated inguinal hernia. Treatment is along the usual lines, including incision and drainage when necessary.

Deep external iliac adenitis

The next proximal relay of the nodes of the femoral canal is a group on the brim of the pelvis around the external iliac artery. For no apparent reason an infection may pass inconspicuously through the more superficial inguinal nodes to form an abscess in an extraperitoneal plane on the front of the external iliac artery and the iliopsoas muscle.

Clinical features

These are vague; general signs of toxaemia and fever are variable, and the hip may be held in slight flexion. The abscess is at first too deep to palpate clearly, and the diagnosis may be delayed until the abscess is large enough to appear above the inguinal ligament.

On the right side it may resemble an appendiceal abscess, but a distinguishing point is that a deep iliac abscess is contiguous with the the inguinal ligament, whereas in an appendiceal abscess there is a gap between the two. The absence of vomiting and bowel disturbance is also helpful.

Treatment

Extraperitoneal drainage is required and pus is often present even when fluctuation cannot be detected clinically because of the thickness of the intervening tissues.

INGUINAL HERNIAS

The testis descends into the scrotum during the seventh month *in utero* through a tube of peritoneum, the processus vaginalis (Fig. 29.3a). This begins to obliterate shortly before birth and closure is normally completed during the first year of life, leaving only the tunica vaginalis surrounding the anterior part of the testis (Fig. 29.3b).

Failure of obliteration of the processus vaginalis accounts for several clinical conditions in infancy and childhood: hernia, hydrocele and encysted hydrocele of the cord.

A hernial sac may extend from the internal inguinal ring and remain completely patent and continuous with the tunica vaginalis—the so-called inguinoscrotal hernia (Fig. 29.3c). More commonly, there is a so-called 'incomplete sac' proximal to an obliterated segment which

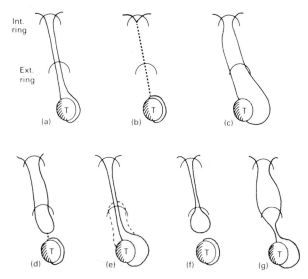

Fig. 29.3 Hydroceles and hernial sacs. (a) The anatomy at term, showing testis (T) and sites of internal and external inguinal rings. (b) Normal consequences of spontaneous closure of the processus, leaving tunica vaginalis around the testis. (c) 'Infantile', 'congenital' or 'complete' hernia; the fundus is continuous with the tunica vaginalis, common in infancy, with the spermatic cord in a 'mesentery' on the inner aspect of the sac. (d) Incomplete hernia, separate from the tunica vaginalis, the most commonly encountered variety. (e) 'Communicating' hydrocele: the processus is patent (2–4 mm in diameter) allowing peritoneal fluid to collect in the tunica surrounding the testis; fluctuations in size indicated by interrupted lines. (f) 'Encysted' hydrocele of the cord: same as (e) but fluid collects in a 'cyst' (part of the processus) separate from the tunica. (g) Combined indirect inguinal hernia (sac) and a distal hydrocele of the tunica.

intervenes between the sac and the tunica vaginalis (Fig. 29.3d). This accounts for the the vast majority of inguinal hernias in children.

A hydrocele in childhood is a collection of the lubricating fluid which is formed by the serosa of the peritoneal cavity; the fluid trickles down a narrow processus and collects in the space between the tunica vaginalis and the testis (Fig. 29.3e).

An encysted hydrocele of the cord develops in the same way; the peritoneal fluid collects in a loculus of the processus at some point along its course in the spermatic cord. This loculus usually retains its communication with the peritoneal cavity (Fig. 29.3f).

Combined abnormalities: multiple spaces or cysts develop along the processus, and it is not uncommon to find a proximal hernial sac communicating through a narrow tract with a distal hydrocele (Fig. 29.3g).

The higher incidence of abnormalities on the right side may be because the right testis descends later than the left and the processus on the right side is therefore more likely to remain patent. The higher incidence of hernias in premature babies is because the normal postpartum intra-abdominal pressures applied in immature infants make it more difficult for the processus to close spontaneously.

In girls, the canal of Nück undergoes the same obliteration as the processus vaginalis in boys. Statistically the obliteration is more likely to be complete, with a lower total incidence of hernias but a higher incidence of bilateral hernias.

Indirect inguinal hernia

Nearly all inguinal hernias in children are indirect, with an incidence of 1 in every 50 live male births. This is the commonest condition requiring surgery during childhood and there is a high familial incidence.

Some 12% of indirect inguinal hernias occur in girls, in whom they appear at any age, spread more evenly throughout childhood than in boys. In boys the greatest incidence is in the first year of life, especially the first 3 months (Fig. 29.4): 60% are on the right side, 25% on the left, and 15% bilateral. The sac usually contains loops of small bowel, and sometimes omentum. In girls, the ovary is often palpable in the sac and may be difficult to reduce.

Diagnosis

The child's mother reports that there is an intermittent swelling overlying the external inguinal ring. It is usually painless but on occasions may cause discomfort. It is often present when there is an episode of crying or straining, and in infants is seen during nappy changes. It may reach the bottom of the scrotum, as in the case of a 'complete' sac, and there is an impulse on crying, straining or coughing.

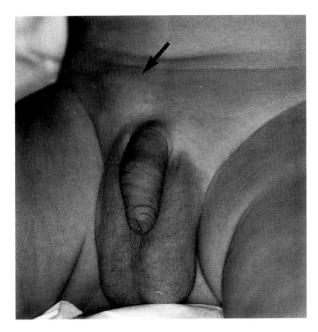

Fig. 29.4 Right indirect inguinal hernia in an infant (arrowed).

When the history is suggestive but the hernia is not producible during examination, the index finger can be rolled transversely across the spermatic cord at the point where it lies on the pubic crest; when there is a hernial sac the spermatic cord is thickened in comparison with the side on which no swelling has been seen, and the 'rustle' of contiguous layers of peritoneum represents the empty hernial sac.

One source of confusion between the history and the clinical signs arises when the parents mistake a retractile or an undescended testis in the superficial inguinal pouch for a hernia, and the site of the reported swelling should be precisely indicated and the concurrent presence of a testis in the scrotum documented. If doubt still exists, a further examination is made a few days later.

In infants and younger children, no attempt should be made to insert the index finger through the external ring in search of an impulse on straining. The opposite side should always be examined, and both testes confirmed descended in the scrotum.

Differential diagnosis

The primary distinction to be made is between a hernia and a hydrocele; the latter is cystic, brightly translucent and irreducible, with no impulse on coughing, crying or straining, and its upper pole is identifiable.

Femoral and direct inguinal hernias are rare but should be kept in mind; a retractile or undescended testis may mislead the unwary, and in young children, an inguinal lymph node may be situated above the inguinal ligament close to the external inguinal ring.

Treatment

Surgery is necessary in all cases because of the danger of strangulation, which occurs most commonly in the first 6 months of life. Operation should be performed as soon as practicable, unless there is an intercurrent condition which requires attention, for example a skin infection or bronchitis.

A herniotomy is performed through an incision in the transverse inguinal skin crease, and is a relatively simple operation in experienced hands, even in the newborn. Herniorrhaphy is contraindicated as it may disturb the normal anatomy of the inguinal canal. Recurrence does not occur.

Exploration on the opposite side is usually undertaken in boys under 1 year of age, in whom a significant contralateral sac is present in more than 50% of cases. In 75% of girls of any age, a sac is found on the opposite side. Ligation of a latent contralateral sac will prevent the not uncommon appearance of a hernia on the other side after a unilateral operation with the requirement for a second admission to hospital. Contralateral exploration adds little to the time and nothing to the risk of operation.

Strangulated inguinal hernia

This, the only significant complication of an indirect inguinal hernia, is common in infancy but somewhat less common in older children. A loop of small bowel becomes trapped in the hernial sac, and although the blood supply is not compromised immediately in most cases, a hernia which is even temporarily irreducible should be considered as being potentially strangulated. The obstruction in the sac is at the external inguinal ring, unlike in adults where the obstruction is often at the internal ring.

Strangulated hernias are seen more often in infants under 6 months of age, such that about 30% of infants with an inguinal hernia initially present with a strangulated hernia.

Clinical features

The infant cries lustily and cannot be pacified; when the mother changes the nappies and a swelling in the groin is noted—perhaps for the very first time. There is a tense, tender swelling which extends to the external inguinal ring, and no impulse on crying. Local pain is later replaced by generalized colicky abdominal pain, vomiting, abdominal distension and constipation when complete intestinal obstruction supervenes—but this is not as a rule established until at least 12 h after the onset. With gross delay in diagnosis there may be redness and induration overlying the lump, or signs of peritonitis.

Differential diagnosis

The differential diagnosis includes an encysted hydrocele of the cord, which may appear suddenly—but the swelling is not tender, the cyst moves readily with the cord and abdominal signs and symptoms are lacking.

Absence of a testis in the scrotum on the affected side may point to torsion of an undescended testis or of a descended testis which has been elevated out of the scrotum with torsion.

Lymphadenitis or a local inguinal abscess, or funiculitis (a rare type of inflammation in the spermatic cord) may be so confusing in young children as to warrant exploration to clarify the diagnosis.

Secondary effects

In the first few years of life the testicular vessels can be severely compressed by a tense, strangulated hernia, especially when the vessels lie in a mesentery in the wall of the sac, a common anatomical finding in this age group. Some degree of atrophy of the testis develops in 15% of baby boys after an episode of irreducibility and strangulation. For this reason, early reduction is as important for the testis as for the imprisoned bowel. Occasionally, in infant girls the ovary can be strangulated inside the sac.

Treatment

A strangulated hernia may reduce spontaneously *en route* to the hospital, but more often than not persists. Reduction of a strangulated hernia by taxis should be attempted forthwith, and the attempt repeated after sedation if initially unsuccessful.

The tips of the fingers of one hand are applied to the fundus of the hernia while the fingertips of the other hand are cupped at the external ring. Gentle pressure is exerted initially to disimpact the hernia from the external ring, and then the contents of the hernia are reduced along the line of the inguinal canal. Nothing seems to be accomplished for a minute or two, and then the bowel suddenly gurgles and returns to the abdomen. Taxis is a manipulative trick, not a matter of force, and if necessary can be attempted several times. A distressed child can be sedated with chloral hydrate 15 mg/kg. There is virtually no chance of producing reduction-en-masse, and in over 90% of cases, taxis is successful. When it is successful, the patient should not return home until herniotomy has been performed, usually after 24 h, to give time for oedema of the sac and its investing tissue to subside.

When taxis is unsuccessful, immediate operation is necessary and herniotomy is performed. The friable sac is difficult to handle and the surgery is best performed by a paediatric surgeon. In exceptional cases, the bowel is gangrenous and a segmental excision with anastomosis may be necessary. The need for resuscitation before operation will be obvious from the clinical findings.

Direct inguinal hernia

Direct inguinal hernias are rare in paediatric practice, forming less than 1% of inguinal hernias. They are occasionally seen in premature infants who develop bronchopulmonary dysplasia after prolonged ventilation, and in teenage children with cystic fibrosis. Repair of the posterior wall of the inguinal canal medial to the epigastric vessels is required.

Femoral hernia

Femoral hernias are equally rare. The diagnosis is made clinically when the swelling is below the inguinal ligament and lateral to the pubic tubercle.

As in adults, femoral hernias are more common in females, and the diagnosis is usually made between 5 and 10 years of age. The hernia is usually small and irreducible, for most of it is composed of a fibro-fatty investment of the fundus. The hernia can be repaired easily from below the inguinal ligament.

HYDROCELES

Almost all hydroceles in infancy and childhood communicate via a patent processus with the peritoneal cavity (Fig. 29.3), which is the source of the fluid. Much less common is the development of an 'acute' hydrocele secondary to some affliction of the testis or epididymis, for example torsion, infection or trauma.

Clinical signs

A hydrocele is a painless cyst containing peritoneal fluid which has tracked down a narrow but patent processus vaginalis. It is situated in front of the testis, is brightly translucent and cannot be emptied by pressure because of a 'flap valve' at its junction with the processus. When the hydrocele is lax, the testis within it can usually be palpated with ease, or, when the hydrocele is tense, its shadow can be demonstrated by transillumination.

The upper limit of the hydrocele is clearly demonstrable, that is the palpating fingers 'can get above it', except in the unusual variety shown in Fig. 29.3e. The interrupted line shows the upper portion of the hydrocele located in the canal. There is no impulse on crying or straining.

Hydroceles in infants

Unilateral or bilateral hydroceles are quite common in the first few months of life. They are often large, lax, nearly always symptomless and have a strong tendency to close and absorb spontaneously. Virtually all will have disappeared by the age of 1 year and surgery is only required if the hydrocele persists beyond about 2 years.

An encysted hydrocele of the cord is a loculus of fluid located above and separate from the tunica vaginalis (Fig. 29.3d). These do not require surgery in infancy, and may be considered a variant of the natural process of obliteration. After 2 years of age or after observation for a year, operation to close the communication with the peritoneal cavity may be required.

Hydroceles in older children

In boys more than 2 years of age, there is often a diurnal variation in its size. It is small or absent in the mornings and at its biggest in the late afternoon, when it may cause a dragging ache. These changes reflect the narrow communication with the peritoneal cavity along which the fluid returns during recumbency and reaccumulates by the effect of gravity during the day. Despite the patency of the processus, the fluid can almost never be expelled by pressure.

A hydrocele in this age group rarely disappears spontaneously and surgery is required. The processus is transfixed and divided at the internal inguinal ring (i.e.

herniotomy). The whole sac need not be removed but the fluid in it can be released.

FURTHER READING

Cartiledge J. McP. (1968) Strangulated inguinal hernia in the neonatal period. *Aust. Paediatr. J.* **4**: 196.

Clift V. L. & Hutson J. M. (1989) The acute scrotum in childhood. *Pediatr. Surg. Int.* **4**: 185.

Cox J. A. (1985) Inguinal hernia of childhood. *Surg. Clin. North Am.* **65**: 1331–1342.

Das S. & Singer A. (1990) Controversies of perinatal torsion of the spermatic cord: a review, survey and recommendations. *J. Urol.* **143**: 231–233.

Hutson J. M. & Beasley S. W. (1988) Inguinoscrotal lesions. In: *The Surgical Examination of Children* pp. 35–54. Heinemann Medical, Oxford.

Ong T. H. & Solomon J. R. (1973) Fat necrosis of the scrotum. *J. Pediatr. Surg.* **8**: 919.

Puri P., Guiney E. J. & O'Donnell B. (1984) Inguinal hernia in infants: the fate of the testis following incarceration. *J. Pediatr. Surg.* **19**: 44–46.

Rowe M. I. & Lloyd D. A. (1986) Contralateral exploration. In: Welch K. J., Randolph J. G., Ravitch M. M., O'Neill J. A. & Rowe M. I. (eds) *Pediatric Surgery*, 4th edn, pp. 784–787. Year Book Medical, Chicago.

Solomon J. R. (1967) The practice and implications of contralateral exploration in children with unilateral inguinal hernia. *Aust. NZ J. Surg.* **37**: 125.

Thomas E. W. G. & Williamson R. C. N. (1983) Diagnosis and outcome of testicular torsion. *Brit. J. Surg.* **70**: 213.

Wright J. P. & Vassy L. E. (1984) The diagnosis and treatment of the acute scrotum in children and adolescents. *Am. Surg.* **190**: 664.

30

The Penis

THE PREPUCE AND GLANS PENIS

The prepuce (foreskin) is lightly adherent to the glans in the first few days of life, but becomes more densely adherent during the first year.

Forcible retraction of the prepuce should be avoided until spontaneous separation occurs. This is usually in infancy, but it may take 5 years or even longer. The normal process of separation of preputial adhesions is by the build-up of shed skin cells from the inner aspect of the foreskin (smegma). This sebaceous deposit of white cheesy material builds up under the foreskin to lift it off the glans, the discharge of this material is often mistaken for infection.

Accumulations of smegma may produce a yellowish bulge in the preputial skin (Fig. 30.1), and may be mistaken for a sebaceous cyst or even a tumour!

Care of the normal foreskin

The normal foreskin needs no special care. If the foreskin is healthy, it need not be retracted and does not have to be more specially cleaned than any other part of the body. If there is phimosis, the foreskin cannot be retracted and there will be problems with hygiene.

Three abnormal conditions arise in the prepuce:

Phimosis

Phimosis (Fig. 30.2) is stenosis of the preputial orifice, caused by ill-advised forceful retraction, recurrent balanitis or an incomplete circumcision. Ammoniacal dermatitis (nappy rash) also is a common cause of

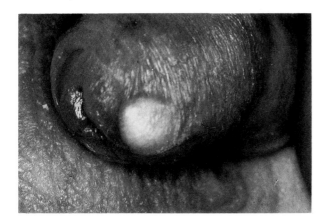

Fig. 30.1 Accumulation of smegma beneath the foreskin appears as a yellowish bulge at the level of the coronal groove.

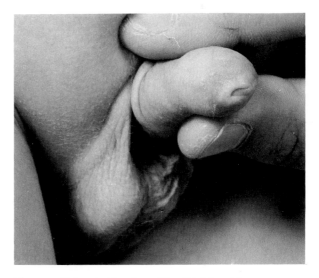

Fig. 30.2 Phimosis. Scarring of the distal foreskin causes stenosis of the opening.

phimosis. The space between the foreskin and glans penis cannot be cleaned adequately and the accumulation of smegma and urine leads to further attacks of balanitis. Phimosis may be treated by local application of steroid cream or by circumcision. Ballooning of the foreskin on micturition is a sign of urinary obstruction requiring circumcision.

Paraphimosis

This occurs in older children, when the foreskin has been pulled behind the glans but cannot be returned to its normal position because the tight foreskin causes oedema and swelling of the glans penis and adjacent foreskin (Fig. 30.3). Paraphimosis is extremely painful and micturition is difficult. It is likely to occur if there is a mild degree of phimosis already present, but in many children the foreskin is normal. Digital replacement of the retracted prepuce is required and may require a general anaesthetic because of the extreme pain produced.

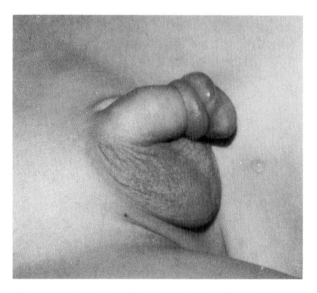

Fig. 30.3 Paraphimosis. The penis is red, swollen and painful. The foreskin has been retracted behind the glans and is compressing the shaft, causing oedema and venous congestion.

Balanitis

Balanitis is an infection of the foreskin, usually with contaminated urine pooling between the foreskin and glans. This may be acute, subacute or chronic, and occurs when the prepuce has not been, or cannot be, retracted often because of phimosis. It is most common in the preschool years when the foreskin is still partially adherent to the glans. Topical or systemic antimicrobial treatment is required to avoid severe inflammation.

Circumcision

The occurrence of any of these conditions may be an indication for circumcision. However, the local application of steroid ointment may cause rapid resolution of phimosis, reducing the need for circumcision.

Apart from surgical indications and theological considerations, circumcision for social reasons is a controversial matter and one largely of individual preference. The pendulum of opinion has swung back and forth in Western countries, and circumcision is now performed less frequently than previously.

The commonest reason given for circumcision is to facilitate cleanliness and for convenience, in that no retraction of the prepuce is required. Carcinoma of the prepuce is rare and occurs only in the elderly, and as such should not enter into the discussion. There is a slightly increased risk of urinary tract infection in uncircumcised infants.

Against circumcision is the view that it is unnecessary, and carries a significant morbidity and mortality, albeit very small, from anaesthesia, haemorrhage and infection. There is also the incidence of meatal stenosis, which virtually only occurs in the circumcised.

Circumcision in the newborn period is undesirable, where it is performed in a non-operating theatre situation, with inadequate asepsis and without anaesthesia. The lack of anaesthetic engenders haste, and hence the greater possibility of inadequate technique (haemorrhage, poor planning of the level of excision of skin and accidental amputation of the tip of the glans) and most importantly, the risk of serious infection (septicaemia and meningitis) at an age when an infant's immune systems are poorly developed.

Beyond the neonatal period, these risks largely can be avoided—with proper anaesthesia, careful technique in an operating theatre with full asepsis. Operation at 6 months of age or older, under these conditions, can be performed safely. An informed and detailed consultation with the parents should be held before going ahead with circumcision.

Meatal stenosis

This is an acquired lesion in the circumcised child. The cause is scarring following abrasion and ulceration of the exposed tip of the glans by the irritation of a dry dressing or nappy in the immediate post-circumcision period; its incidence can be reduced by the application of Vaseline on the glans after circumcision. Less commonly, it may result from chemical irritation by the urine (ammoniacal dermatitis) and, rarely, by direct trauma during circumcision. Only very rarely is there any significant obstruction to the passage of urine, even when the meatus is minute and the stream is needle-fine; retention and vesical back pressure are almost unknown.

Meatal ulceration predisposes to meatal stenosis by scarring unless it heals rapidly. The usual presenting symptom of a meatal ulcer is pain. The infant or toddler screams as voiding commences and a drop of blood appears at the end of micturition or on the napkin. This can be distinguished from haematuria on the history of pain and the presence of a tiny scab or ulcer in the meatus.

Treatment

An anaesthetic ointment provides temporary relief, but seldom a cure; a generous meatotomy, allowing for some subsequent decrease in the size of the orifice, is curative. Instructions should be given to eliminate ammoniacal dermatitis by boiling the nappies and drying them in direct sunlight (UV radiation). A simpler but more expensive solution is to use disposable nappies at night.

HYPOSPADIAS

In hypospadias the urethra opens on the ventral aspect of the penis, at a point proximal to the normal site (Fig. 30.4). This is one of the commonest congenital abnormalities of the male genitalia, occurring in 1 in 300 male births. There are various degrees of severity, depending on how far back the urethral meatus lies on the undersurface of the penis or in the perineum (Table 30.1).

Chordee is a coexistent deformity which may be marked in the more severe cases, and is the result of relative deficiency of ventral skin (compared with normal dorsal penile skin) and adherence between skin and deeper tissues. It causes a ventral curvature of the shaft and becomes much more marked during erection.

There is a deficiency in the ventral segment of the prepuce producing an unsightly dorsal hood of redundant skin (Fig. 30.4). The ventral skin raphe may wander away from the midline to one side. At the normal site of the urethral orifice there is a shallow groove in the glans, and in the floor of the groove, or just proximal to it in the midline, there are usually one or more minute sinuses lined by epithelium.

Another, less common, anomaly which resembles hypospadias is a chordee deformity without hypospadias, in which the urethra opens at or near the tip of the glans and is associated with a gross chordee, a condition aptly named by the French *hypospadie sans hypospadie*.

The disabilities of hypospadias are: the stream of urine may be deflected downwards or splash and drip

Table 30.1 Features of hypospadias

(1) Proximal ventral opening of urethra:
—glandular
—penoglandular
—penile
—penoscrotal
—scrotal
—perineal
(2) Chordee (ventral curvature of penile shaft)
(3) Dorsal hood of prepuce
(4) ? Position of testes

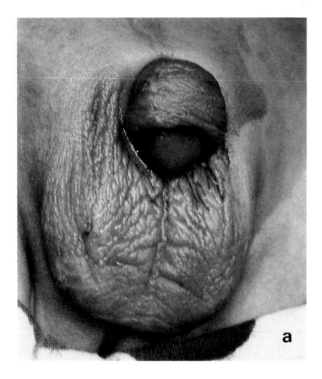
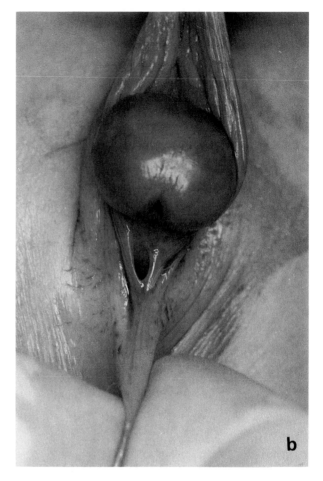

Fig. 30.4 Hypospadias. Incomplete fusion of the inner genital folds leads to a proximal urethral meatus, dorsal-hooded prepuce and chordee. The penis can look fairly normal (a) until the foreskin (dorsal hood) is pulled upwards revealing the proximal urethral meatus (here proximal to the corona) and chordee (b).

back along the shaft of the penis; boys with a peno-scrotal or perineal hypospadias must void in the sitting position; uncorrected chordee interferes with normal intercourse, and semen from a penoscrotal or perineal hypospadias may not be directed into the vagina. Inability to void normally while standing inhibits development of the 'male' body image and may cause the unfortunate boy to be ostracized during early school years.

Associated anomalies

In boys with hypospadias, one or both testes may be undescended. When both testes are absent from the

scrotum in a 'boy' with a perineal hypospadias, the appropriate gender of rearing should be determined as soon as possible by immediate referral for expert opinion (see Chapter 11).

The incidence of abnormalities in the urinary tract is relatively high in patients with severe degrees of hypospadias; in these, urological investigation may be indicated.

Treatment

In almost all repairs, the prepuce is required as a source of extra skin, such that no infant with hypospadias should be circumcised prior to repair.

The objectives of repair are to provide: a urethra of adequate length and calibre, opening at the tip of the glans; an unobstructed orifice directed forwards to prevent splashing; a penis which is straight enough to permit normal sexual intercourse and insemination.

By far the commonest type of hypospadias is penoglandular in which the meatus lies in or very close to the coronal groove. In most of these, chordee is present and operative correction is necessary. However, an orifice on the distal half of the glans, if unaccompanied by chordee, may need only minimal surgery—meatal advancement and glanduloplasty which commonly can be performed as a day case.

Surgery on the common coronal type of hypospadias with chordee achieves an orifice on the tip of the glans, a straight penis and the appearance of a 'normal' circumcised penis. One-stage and two-stage techniques are available, the choice being determined by the surgeon's preference and the degree of chordee. The existing urethra is mobilized and the ventral skin is transected to permit straightening of the ventral curvature. This invariably involves some movement of the urethral meatus back towards the perineum. At a later stage a urethroplasty is required to extend the urethra forward along the straightened shaft. Glandular hypospadias may be repaired as a day case at the age of 6 months. More severe cases requiring a urethroplasty are repaired at 1–2 years.

EPISPADIAS

In this condition the urethra opens at the base of the penis, on its dorsal aspect. It is part of the spectrum of lower abdominal wall defects in which ectopia vesicae is the most severe form (Chapter 9). Most boys with epispadias are incontinent of urine because the bladder neck is also deficient; epispadias as an isolated abnormality in a continent child is exceptionally rare, even rarer than ectopia vesicae itself, which occurs in 1 in 30 000 live births.

Apart from the problem of the repair of the urethra, using the same type of urethroplasty as in hypospadias, there are many of the same major difficulties that arise in ectopia vesicae.

FURTHER READING

Chatterjee S. (1989) Circumcision in India. Letter to the editor. *Pediatr. Surg. Int.* **4**: 236–237.

Coran A. G. (1989) Circumcision in the United States: medical and nonmedical attitudes. *Pediatr. Surg. Int.* **4**: 229–230.

Cywes S. (1989) Circumcision in South Africa. *Pediatr. Surg. Int.* **4**: 233–235.

Gonzales E. T. Jr, Veeruraghavan K. A. & Jehanne J. (1983) Management of distal hypospadias with meatal-based vascularized flaps. *J. Urol.* **129**: 119.

Hofmann V. & Kap-herr S. (1989) Circumcision in Germany. *Pediatr. Surg. Int.* **4**: 227–228.

King P. A., Caddy G. M., Cohen S. H. & Pacca L. E. (1989) Circumcision—Maternal attitudes. *Pediatr. Surg. Int.* **4**: 222–226.

Morgan W. K. C. (1965) The rape of the phallus. *J. Am. Med. Assoc.* **193**: 223.

Morgan W. K. C. (1967) Penile plunder. *Med. J. Aust.* **1**: 1102.

Report of the Ad Hoc Task Force in Circumcision (1975) *Pediatrics* **56**: 610–611.

Rickwood A. M. K. (1989). Circumcision of boys in England: current practice. *Pediatr. Surg. Int.* **4**: 231–232.

Smith E. D. (1981) Hypospadias. In: Holder T. M. & Ashcraft K. W. (eds), *Pediatric Surgery*, pp. 770–792. W. B. Saunders, Philadelphia.

31

Urinary Tract Infection

Urinary tract infections (UTI) are misdiagnosed commonly in children. Dysuria and the passage of cloudy urine are common symptoms in children with a febrile illness and do not necessarily reflect UTI. On the other hand, many children with UTI are symptomless or have unexplained fever, vomiting or even failure to thrive: in these patients the diagnosis may be overlooked.

DIAGNOSIS

The diagnosis of UTI can be made definitely when there is a pure culture of a urinary pathogen, in the presence of pyuria from an appropriately collected specimen. A high index of suspicion of UTI is needed in any unwell child.

There are considerable difficulties in collecting a mid-stream specimen of urine (MSSU) in infants and toddlers, but it should be possible to collect a clean mid-stream specimen in the older child.

A sample reagent strip to detect nitrites in the urine largely excludes UTI when negative. However, the presence of urinary nitrites does not prove UTI.

Suprapubic aspiration of urine

The most reliable technique of collecting urine is by suprapubic aspiration, which is the method of choice in infants up to about 18 months. This is because the bladder in infants is an intra-abdominal organ, making suprapubic needle aspiration of urine simple, quick and reliable. A 'bladder tap' should be performed in any sick infant to exclude UTI, particularly if a urine specimen obtained by other means is inadequate. In a 'septic workup', it is important to do the suprapubic aspiration first, as infants will void during painful procedures such as venepuncture or lumbar puncture.

A 10 mL syringe with a 23-gauge 4 cm needle is used for the procedure (Fig. 31.1). The child is nursed supine and restrained by an assistant. The suprapubic area is swabbed with skin disinfectant, and the needle introduced in the midline, 1 cm above the upper margin of the symphysis pubis. The needle should be introduced by aiming perpendicular to the floor: in the neonate, insert the needle about 2 cm; further in older infants. The needle is then withdrawn while aspirating on the syringe, until urine is drawn into the syringe. It

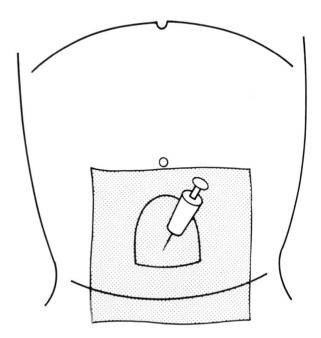

Fig. 31.1 The method of suprapubic aspiration for urine culture. The shaded area is the area of antiseptic skin preparation.

is sent for culture in a sterile container. Any pure culture is significant if collected by suprapubic aspiration.

Bag specimen of urine

In the neonate and infant, one sometimes has to rely on a bag specimen of urine, which may be contaminated from the surrounding skin or prepuce in the male, and from retrograde flow of urine into the vagina in the female. A pure culture of a urinary pathogen with a colony count of $>10^5$ organisms, and with more than 100 white blood cells per high-power field is highly suggestive of a UTI in a bag specimen.

Mid-stream specimen of urine

In a continent male child, the foreskin should be retracted until the urethral meatus is exposed, and the glans cleaned with soap and water using a soft flannel. The urine is collected mid-stream during continuous voiding, while keeping the foreskin retracted. The foreskin must be returned to its unretracted state following this procedure.

Similarly, in the older female child the labia should be parted, cleansed with a flannel, soap and water from the front to the back three times, and the child asked to void while holding the labia parted. The urine is collected in mid-stream during continuous voiding. Alcoholic preparations should not be used as these cause intense pain on delicate mucosa.

Pitfalls in diagnosis

The urine specimen may be clear in a child with early pyelonephritis, especially in the presence of upper tract obstruction. In this instance, the child should be treated empirically for pyelonephritis, and further specimens of urine should be taken during the course of treatment, as it is common for bacteriuria to be detected on the second or third day.

The child with an infected urinary calculus may culture more than one urinary pathogen.

Cloudy urine does not always signify UTI. In many instances, the cause of the cloudiness is simply precipitation of phosphate crystals when urine cools rapidly.

CLINICAL PRESENTATION

UTI can present a wide variety of features. Table 31.1 emphasizes the fact that UTI may present with vague symptomatology, and hence one must have a high index of suspicion for UTI in any child who is unwell, with no obvious cause.

The purpose of evaluating a child with a UTI is to exclude any underlying anatomical abnormality.

History

A good history is important, looking for previous UTI or any previous episodes of unexplained fever. Bed-wetting or voiding disorders do not necessarily indicate a urinary tract abnormality, except in a child who has been previously continent. On the other hand, a history of constant dribbling of urine is abnormal and requires investigation to exclude an ectopic insertion of a ureter. The family history is pertinent, as vesicoureteric reflux and duplex kidneys are known to be common among siblings.

Clinical examination

Many abnormalities can be diagnosed from the history and physical examination, prior to organ imaging. Radiological investigations often confirm clinical suspicions.

Table 31.1 Presentation of urinary tract infection

Infants	Older children
Pyuria of unknown origin	Abdominal pain
Septicaemia	Dysuria
Listlessness and lethargy	Pyrexia
Haematuria	Haematuria
Vomiting	Pyelonephritis
Failure to thrive	Dysfunctional voiding
Persistent neonatal jaundice	

After a general physical examination, the abdomen should be examined carefully for a renal mass or an overdistended or expressible bladder, which in a neonate is indicative of a neurogenic bladder. The perineum should be inspected carefully, and perianal sensation and anal tone assessed. Labial adhesions, phimosis, meatal stenosis (and even rarities such as a prolapsing ureterocele in a female) can be diagnosed on inspection. A 'urological examination includes a neurological examination', as a neurogenic bladder is an important cause of UTI. The lower limbs are examined for signs of muscle wasting, sensory loss and orthopaedic deformities (e.g. talipes), which suggest the possibility of a neurological abnormality. The bony spine is inspected and palpated for occult forms of spina bifida or sacral agenesis. An overlying patch of abnormal skin (e.g. pigmented naevus, hair, haemangioma, lipoma or sinus) may indicate the presence of a serious spinal lesion. Measurement of the blood pressure is essential because hypertension in a child with a UTI indicates significant renal pathology.

INVESTIGATIONS

The incidence of urinary tract abnormality in children with one proven UTI is at least 30%, and higher in the first year of life. It is mandatory to investigate all children after one documented UTI. It cannot be overstated that adequate documentation of UTI is important, and a clinical diagnosis of 'UTI' without urine culture is inadequate. A micturating cystourethrogram and a renal ultrasound are the primary investigations, although there are a number of additional investigations which may be indicated in certain circumstances. For example, a plain abdominal X-ray may identify a renal or ureteric calculus (as most urinary calculi in children are radio-opaque).

Micturating cystourethrogram

A micturating cystourethrogram (MCU) is performed by the insertion of a small catheter into the bladder, filling the bladder and screening the patient during voiding to detect abnormalities. While a nuclear MCU is an excellent investigation to exclude vesicoureteric reflux, it is not appropriate as a first investigation, because it will not demonstrate abnormal anatomy such as posterior urethral valves, para-ureteric diverticula, and trabeculation of a neurogenic bladder.

The only investigation which can exclude local anatomical abnormalities is a radiological MCU. In the male child it is mandatory to examine the urethra during voiding to exclude outlet obstruction from posterior urethral valves.

All children under 1 year should be investigated early in the illness, as urinary obstruction is a common cause of UTI in this age-group. It is appropriate to perform an MCU immediately on these children, provided there is adequate antibiotic cover.

Renal ultrasound

This is an accepted preliminary investigation to exclude urinary obstruction. It can be presumed that any significant obstruction will produce proximal dilatation, which is manifested as hydronephrosis, hydroureter or both. A good ultrasound investigation should detect any dilatation within the collecting system. It must be remembered, however, that an ultrasound examination gives no information on the function of the kidneys.

If the ultrasound shows obstruction to the upper tracts, an emergency percutaneous nephrostomy should be considered to drain the infected urine. This is minimally invasive, and similar to draining an abscess, provides immediate relief of symptoms, and may save the kidney.

Ultrasound is valuable in the diagnosis of double systems and ureteroceles. Renal size and the status of the renal parenchyma are also measured. Ultrasound is a good study for children as there is no ionizing radiation involved and there is no need for painful injections.

Intravenous pyelogram

This is a good investigation for delineating anatomy and overall function. In specific circumstances, where knowledge of the anatomy is essential (e.g. in the management of urinary calculi, duplex systems and ureteroceles) it is the investigation of choice. An intravenous pyelogram not only will outline the renal anatomy and position of the calculus, but also show obstruction caused by it. It is of limited usefulness in the neonate, because of the poor concentrating ability of the immature neonatal kidney. Likewise, in the poorly functioning or very dilated system, dilution of the contrast medium will lead to poor definition of the anatomy. Other disadvantages include the high radiation dose and the lack of quantitation.

Antegrade and retrograde pyelograms

These are invasive investigations and are reserved for those conditions in which it is essential to define the anatomy. They need general anaesthesia in most children. An antegrade pyelogram can be performed in conjunction with a percutaneous nephrostomy when drainage of an obstructed system is required.

Nuclear isotope imaging

Nuclear imaging of the renal tracts is useful for assessment of renal function, but does not give good anatomical information. There are two main renal isotope scans available, the DTPA and the DMSA scans.

The DTPA scan is an excretory scan that measures relative renal function, glomerular filtration rate and excretion rate. It is also a measure of obstruction, as this causes a delay in excretion. It is unreliable in the neonate, until about 6 weeks post-term, due to the immaturity of the neonatal kidney. Dehydration may interfere with assessment of obstruction as low urine flow causes delayed excretion.

The DMSA scan is a more useful test in the neonatal period. DMSA is taken up by functioning renal cortical tissue, but does not give any indication of the excreting or concentrating ability of the kidney. It is useful in determining renal damage in reflux-associated nephropathy, and whether there is any functioning renal tissue in the neonate with gross hydronephrosis.

In general, the choice of which 'second-line investigation' is best left to the attending urologist or paediatrician to decide.

THE MANAGEMENT OF URINARY TRACT INFECTION

In the child who is not toxic, it is reasonable to obtain a urine specimen and wait for cultures before commencing antibiotics. If a child is unwell, a suprapubic aspirate is performed and treatment started while waiting for the results of urine culture. It is best to admit these children to hospital. Any child under 1 year of age with UTI is likely to have pyelonephritis and must be treated with intravenous antibiotics.

Choice of antibiotics

The choice of antibiotics is governed by the sensitivities of the urinary pathogen. The commonest causative organism is *Escherichia coli*. For this reason, Co-trimoxazole or Amoxycillin with clavuronic acid are suitable first-line oral antibiotics. Amoxycillin alone is not suitable because of the high numbers of resistant strains of *E. coli*. Nitrofurantoin and naladixic acid are poor antibiotics in the ill child as they do not give adequate tissue levels. Similarly, the new quinalones, although highly effective for treating adult UTI are unsuitable for children, as they may cause erosion of articular cartilage. Aminoglycosides are useful in serious upper UTI but need careful monitoring in the child with poor renal function, because of nephrotoxicity.

FURTHER READING

Brindle M. J. (1990) Children with urinary tract infection: a critical diagnostic pathway. *Clin. Radiol.* **41**: 95–97.

Hansson S., Hjalmas K., Jodal U. & Sixt R. (1990) Lower urinary tract dysfunction in girls with untreated asymptomatic or covert bacteriuria. *J. Urol.* **143**: 333–335.

Pyelonephritis: Pathogenesis and management update. *Dialogues in Pediatric Urology*, Vol. 13, No. 2 1990.

32

Vesicoureteric Reflux

Vesicoureteric reflux is the most common underlying anomaly in children with urinary tract infections (UTI). Reflux allows transfer of bacteria from the bladder into the kidney with the risk of pyelonephritis and renal scars.

PATHOGENESIS

The normal ureter runs between the bladder muscle and the bladder epithelium for some distance before opening into the bladder cavity. This part of the ureter, known as the submucosal tunnel, allows the increased pressure of bladder filling or micturition to compress the ureter against the bladder muscle and occlude its lumen. If the submucosal tunnel is short the ureter is not occluded by bladder filling and urine refluxes up the ureter into the kidney.

The urinary tract abnormalities seen in vesicoureteric reflux are due to two main causes:

(1) Congenital malformation: malformation of the ureteric bud will cause not only defects in the lower ureter with reflux but also poor formation of renal parenchyma. Thus many of the severe renal defects seen in association with reflux are congenital in origin

(2) Pyelonephritic scars: pyelonephritis may cause renal scars, and repeated episodes will cause progressive renal damage. Pyelonephritic scars mostly occur in infancy, while the kidney is growing rapidly.

In severe cases the combination of major renal parenchymal defects due to congenital malformation and subsequent damage from pyelonephritis may lead to renal failure. However, the spectrum of severity of vesicoureteric reflux is broad and most cases are mild and tend to resolve spontaneously with normal growth of the bladder muscle.

PRESENTATION

Urinary tract infection

Up to 40% of children with UTI have an underlying urinary tract abnormality of which vesicoureteric reflux is the most common. If a child has a urinary infection, proven by microscopy and culture of the urine, investigation should be undertaken to exclude urinary tract abnormalities, especially vesicoureteric reflux.

Antenatal diagnosis

Antenatal ultrasound is very sensitive in the detection of hydronephrosis and thus will detect reflux which causes pelvicalyceal dilatation. This early diagnosis enables prophylactic antibiotics to be commenced at birth and ensures that these children never have UTI.

Associated defects

Vesicoureteric reflux is associated with other urinary tract abnormalities such as: ureteric duplication and ureterocele; urethral valves; pelviureteric obstruction; vesicoureteric obstruction; and neuropathic bladder. A bladder diverticulum due to a muscular defect at the insertion of the ureter is particularly common with reflux. When one abnormality of the urinary tract is diagnosed it is important to investigate the whole of the urinary tract to exclude associated anomalies.

DIAGNOSIS

There are no clinical symptoms or signs specific to vesicoureteric reflux; it can be diagnosed only by special investigation.

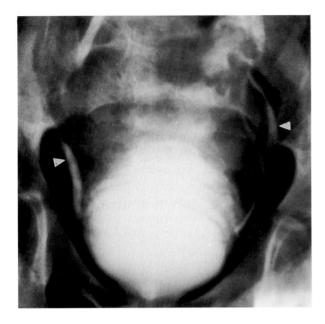

Fig. 32.1 Bilateral Grade I vesicoureteric reflux shown on MCU. The contrast in the lower ureters is arrowed. There is a good chance that reflux of this grade will resolve spontaneously.

Lower tract studies

The micturating cystourethrogram (MCU) is the key test for reflux. The bladder is filled with X-ray contrast or radionuclide and then emptied by voiding. The degree of reflux is assessed by the level to which urine refluxes up the ureter and the severity of ureteric dilatation (Figs 32.1, 32.2). On radionuclide studies, the presence of renal parenchymal damage can be documented as well. The MCU is an invasive, uncomfortable test because of the need for urethral catheterization. However, this test is the most reliable way to diagnose vesicoureteric reflux.

Upper tract studies

Renal ultrasound is the initial investigation to assess the status of the renal parenchyma. Loss of renal parenchyma occurs particularly at the upper and lower poles

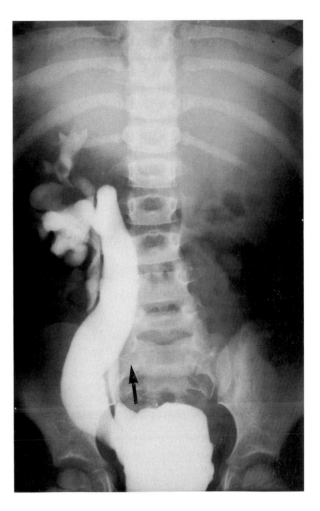

Fig. 32.2 MCU showing gross right-sided vesicoureteric reflux (arrow) up both ureters in a duplex system. There is no reflux on the left.

of the kidney. The other parenchymal defect seen in reflux is uniform thinning of the renal cortex over the whole kidney.

The renal isotope scan is an elegant way to image the renal parenchyma and is the most sensitive technique to identify renal scars. Intravenous pyelography seldom is used when there are good ultrasound and isotope facilities available.

The method of investigation of vesicoureteric reflux is controversial, but the combination of a renal ultrasound examination and an MCU is appropriate following a proven UTI. In children with repeated UTI MCU is mandatory, whereas in older children with a solitary minor UTI the MCU may be omitted in the initial investigation. However, if the child develops a further UTI the MCU must be performed.

NATURAL HISTORY

There is a strong tendency for vesicoureteric reflux to resolve spontaneously in the pre-school years with the normal growth and development of the bladder and ureter. While the child may well be born with congenital renal parenchymal defects in association with the reflux, further damage after birth only occurs with pyelonephritis.

MANAGEMENT

Medical management

The initial management of vesicoureteric reflux is medical. Infection is prevented by using long term low dose antibiotics given as a single night-time dose of one-half the daily therapeutic dosage level. The parents are instructed in the features of UTI in infants and children (e.g. malaise, vomiting, off feeds, pyrexia, irritability) and any breakthrough infections are detected quickly and treated promptly. In most cases of reflux, infection is controlled by prophylactic antibiotics and spontaneous resolution will occur. However, medical management requires close follow-up by the doctor and conscientious care by the parents. Anything short of these high standards leaves the child at risk of repeated episodes of pyelonephritis and subsequent renal parenchymal damage.

Surgical management

Surgery has an important role in the management of reflux:

Correction of structural defects

Vesicoureteric reflux associated with a para-ureteric diverticulum or a ureterocele will not resolve spontaneously and must be corrected surgically.

Failure of medical management

Medical management is not always successful. Breakthrough infections in the presence of reflux may cause pyelonephritis. If prophylactic antibiotics do not control UTI, reflux can be corrected surgically. Infection may still occur after surgical correction of reflux but these infections are usually due to cystitis and do not threaten the kidneys; they are thus less significant. The other problem seen with medical treatment is failure of spontaneous resolution of the reflux. This is often the case with the more severe degrees of reflux where there is gross dilatation of the ureter and pelvicalyceal systems.

The standard surgical technique for correction of vesicoureteric reflux is open reimplantation of the ureter. The ureter is dissected free from its short submucosal tunnel and a new long submucosal tunnel is fashioned. The success of open reimplantation of the ureter is high. Endoscopic techniques for the correction of vesicoureteric reflux (e.g. submucosal Teflon injection) are available also.

Whether vesicoureteric reflux is treated medically or surgically, a prolonged and careful follow-up of cases into adulthood is required. If there is renal parenchymal damage lifelong medical supervision is important because of the risk of hypertension.

FURTHER READING

Canning D. A. & Gearhart J. P. (1989) Limitations and alternatives to endoscopic correction of vesicoureteral reflux with Polytef paste. *Pediatr. Surg. Int.* **4**: 149–153.

Cass D. T. (1990) Surgical aspects of primary vesicoureteric reflux. *J. Paediatr. Child Health* **26**: 180–183.

Gonzales E. T. Jr, Decter R. M. & Roth D. R. (1989) Vesicoureteral reflux in boys. *Pediatr. Surg. Int.* **4**: 154–155.

Seruca H. (1989) Vesicoureteral reflux and voiding dysfunction: prospective study. *J. Urol.* **142**: 494–498.

Thomas D. F. M. (1989) Vesico-ureteric reflux: new perspectives. Editorial comments. *Pediatr. Surg. Int.* **4**: 147–148.

33

Obstructive Lesions of the Urinary Tract

Hydronephrosis is abnormal pelvicalyceal dilatation that results from obstruction of the urinary tract or from dilatation secondary to dysplastic growth of the urinary tract.

The patient with hydronephrosis presents an investigative challenge, because obstructive and non-obstructive lesions must be distinguished, and pathology in the ureter or bladder which may mimic pelvi-ureteric obstruction must be excluded.

AETIOLOGIC FACTORS

Pelviureteric obstruction

Partial obstruction of the pelviureteric junction is caused by stenosis or kinking of the ureter as it joins the renal pelvis. This leads to intermittent obstruction with good preservation of renal function in the early stages (Fig. 33.1). Infection and progressive renal obstruction lead to loss of renal function unless severe blockage is relieved surgically. Less severe degrees of obstruction in the newborn may resolve spontaneously.

Vesicoureteric obstruction

Stenosis or valve formation in the lower ureter causes partial ureteric obstruction with marked dilatation of the ureter (Fig. 33.2). Mild cases may resolve spontaneously leaving a persistently dilated ureter which is no longer obstructed. More severe cases require surgical correction.

Posterior urethral valves

In males, epithelial folds running down from the verumontanum in the posterior urethra impede the flow of urine with back pressure on the bladder, ureters and kidneys. When the obstruction is severe intrauterine renal failure occurs with fetal death *in utero* or death soon after birth from Potter's syndrome. Less severe valve obstruction allows a live birth but, if the problem is not detected early, septic complications from urinary tract infection (UTI) and metabolic abnormalities due to renal failure soon occur. The diagnosis can be made by detecting hydronephrosis on antenatal ultrasound. The postnatal features include a thick-walled, palpable bladder and a poor urinary stream in a newborn male infant; the diagnosis is confirmed on MCU (Fig. 33.3).

Vesicoureteric reflux

Massive reflux with associated hydroureter also can produce gross hydronephrosis when the upper tract distends with reflux.

Neurogenic (neuropathic) bladder

Neurogenic bladder causes hydronephrosis in a number of ways. Patients may have a functional bladder neck obstruction from sphincter dysfunction. Upper tract obstruction and dilatation may occur secondary to high intravesical pressure. Many patients with neurogenic bladder have reflux secondary to the neuropathy, and this also may lead to upper tract dilatation.

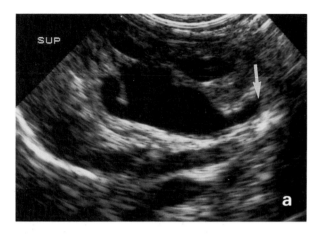

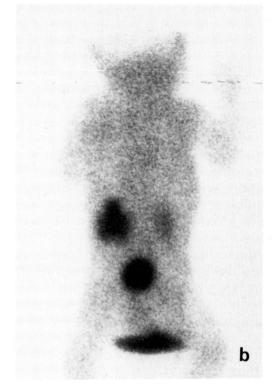

Fig. 33.1 Postnatal ultrasound examination in an infant in whom hydronephrosis had been recognized antenatally, showing pelviureteric junction obstruction (arrow) with pelvicalyceal dilatation, but good preservation of renal parenchyma (a); nuclear renal scan (DTPA scan) showing holdup at the pelviureteric junction at 45 min (b).

Double ureters and kidneys (duplex system)

Congenital duplex kidneys may cause hydronephrosis of either part of the duplex system. The upper moiety is usually the more abnormal (Fig. 33.4), and the dilatation is caused by dysplasia or distal obstruction (from uretero-cele; Fig. 33.5) or an ectopic position of the ureteric orifice (e.g. in the bladder neck). Ectopic ureteric insertion is often associated with dysplasia in a very poorly functioning subservient upper renal moiety. Dilatation of the more normal lower moiety may be caused by PUJ obstruction.

Stones (urolithiasis)

Rarely in children, a renal or ureteric calculus may cause an acute obstruction resulting in hydronephrosis.

CLINICAL PRESENTATION

The clinical presentations of urinary tract obstruction are shown in Table 33.1.

Pain is the most common presenting feature in the older child, and may be accompanied by infection or haematuria, especially after minor trauma. A distinguishing clinical feature is lateralization of the pain to

Table 33.1 Clinical presentation of urinary tract obstruction

Child	Infant/Neonate
Pain	Incidental finding
Infection	Infection
Haematuria	Loin mass
Loin mass	Haematuria
Incidental finding	Pain

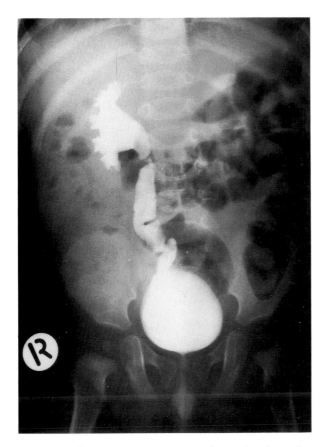

Fig. 33.2 Right vesicoureteric junction obstruction shown in intravenous pyelogram.

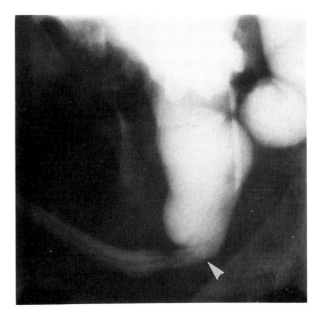

Fig. 33.3 Posterior urethral valves seen on a lateral view of the urethra on MCU (arrow). Note the reflux into a megaureter, bladder mucosal irregularity, massive dilatation of the posterior urethra, and a catheter in the urethra.

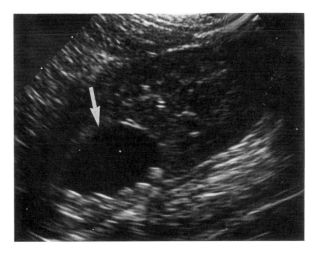

Fig. 33.4 Duplex kidney with a dilated upper moiety (arrow).

the loin, and accompanying nausea or vomiting. Symptoms are exacerbated by a fluid load and sometimes by position.

UTI is the most common presentation in infants and neonates. Hydronephrosis is often detected in the neonate as a palpable abdominal mass. Presentation as a loin mass is unusual except in a neonate, in whom 50% of all abdominal masses are renal in origin. Hydronephrosis is being detected frequently on antenatal ultrasonographic screening in centres where maternal ultrasound has become routine. The incidence of antenatal hydronephrosis detected in this way is about 1.5 : 1000 live births.

Another mode of presentation is where renal investigations are performed for suspected abnormalities in children with known multiple anomalies.

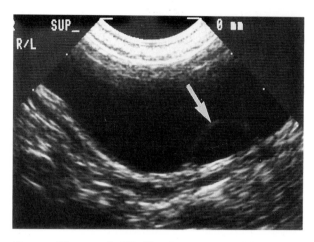

Fig. 33.5 Ultrasound of bladder showing ureterocele (arrow), in the same patient as Fig. 33.4.

INVESTIGATIONS

Investigation aims to:
(1) Prove obstruction
(2) Assess renal function (on both sides)
(3) Demonstrate the abnormal anatomy.

Ultrasound

Ultrasound is the first investigation performed on children with suspected obstruction. A good quality ultrasound will not only demonstrate any abnormal anatomy, but also may determine the likely cause of the problem. However, an ultrasound will not prove that a dilated system is obstructed; nor will it demonstrate function in the dilated system.

Micturating cystourethrogram

A micturating cystourethrogram (MCU) is essential in the investigation of children with dilated upper tracts, to exclude associated reflux, and distal obstruction, for example posterior urethral valves in boys.

Renal isotope scan

Renal isotope scans determine if there is obstruction and provide an estimate of the total function of the kidney. There are two kinds of renal scan: an excretory (DTPA) scan for demonstrating overall function and obstruction; and a parenchymal (DMSA) scan for demonstrating the amount of functional renal cortical tissue. The interpretation of renal scans is aided by computer analysis.

Intravenous pyelogram

Intravenous pyelography is used less commonly today for the demonstration of function, but is still an excellent investigation where it is essential to demonstrate the anatomy, particularly in duplex systems where both moieties are functioning.

Retrograde and antegrade pyelography

Both techniques are employed to demonstrate anatomy or obstruction where this is essential to the management of the patient. An antegrade pyelogram may be combined with a Whittaker test, where a set column of fluid is perfused through the system while the pressure is measured. This is a dynamic test aimed at demonstrating functional obstruction at high fluid loads.

Pitfalls of investigations

The immaturity of the neonatal kidney presents difficulties in interpretation of functional tests in the first month of life. As the concentrating ability and total renal function is low in the neonate, it is likely that functional studies will give misleading results. For this reason, it is best to defer any functional study for at least 6 weeks post-term.

MANAGEMENT OF OBSTRUCTIVE LESIONS

It is best to divide the investigation and management of hydronephrosis into two age-groups: those presenting in the neonatal period; and those presenting later.

Antenatal hydronephrosis

Not all hydronephroses on antenatal examination turn out to be significant. However, when hydronephrosis is detected, it is important to follow it throughout pregnancy. If other urinary tract abnormalities are detected on antenatal ultrasound this would suggest that the hydronephrosis is pathological. Increasing hydronephrosis with oligohydramnios is also pathological, suggestive of low urine output with posterior urethral valves.

It is important to commence all neonates with antenatally diagnosed hydronephrosis on antibiotics from birth while awaiting full evaluation, as there is significant risk of severe UTI developing in these children.

Preliminary investigations should include a careful clinical evaluation to exclude abdominal masses, and inspection of the perineum to detect clinically obvious abnormalities such as prolapsing ureteroceles.

All children with antenatally diagnosed hydronephrosis should undergo a postnatal ultrasound examination and a micturating cystogram within the first week. The ultrasound will confirm the degree of hydronephrosis (Fig. 33.1), and an MCU will exclude distal obstruction or vesicoureteric reflux, which accounts for 30% of hydronephroses in the antenatal period.

Functional evaluation is of limited value at birth because of the relative immaturity of the kidney and it is best to defer a renal DTPA scan or intravenous pyelogram until the baby is 6 weeks old. A DMSA nuclear scan, however, can be very useful in this period, as this shows up any functioning renal tissue.

Except for posterior urethral valves, definitive treatment can be deferred in most cases until full evaluation of the degree of obstruction is completed. A significant number of apparent neonatal pelviureteric junction obstructions improve spontaneously. However, severe obstruction in the neonatal period will require early surgery.

In posterior urethral valves the bladder is drained by a suprapubic catheter. The metabolic and septic complications are treated before endoscopic resection of the valves is performed.

Children with severe obstruction usually have gross hydronephrosis on postnatal ultrasound. The kidney is tense and usually palpable. A DTPA scan may show a non-functioning kidney, but if the DMSA scan shows an appreciable amount of renal cortical tissue, early repair will lead to significant recovery of renal function.

Management of older children with obstructive lesions

In the older child, the preliminary investigations should always include a renal ultrasound and MCU. These should be followed by a DTPA scan. Unless renal function is severely impaired (<10%) surgical relief of the obstruction should be undertaken. Where there is minimal function, the kidney should be removed (Fig. 33.6).

Percutaneous nephrostomy

This is a useful emergency measure to drain an obstructed kidney, particularly in the presence of infection. In a sick child with pyelonephritis it leads to rapid clinical improvement, as well as significant improvement in renal function. Percutaneous nephrostomy also allows evaluation of overall function and delineation of the anatomy by antegrade pyelography.

Open pyeloplasty

The standard operative procedure to relieve a pelviureteric obstruction is a Hynes-Anderson pyeloplasty. This requires excision of the narrowed segment and anastomosis of the spatulated ureter to the renal pelvis. The functional results of this operation are good, but these kidneys retain their dilated appearance permanently.

Percutaneous pyeloplasty

Endoscopic pyeloplasty is gaining popularity, but the long term results are not yet known. Through a small

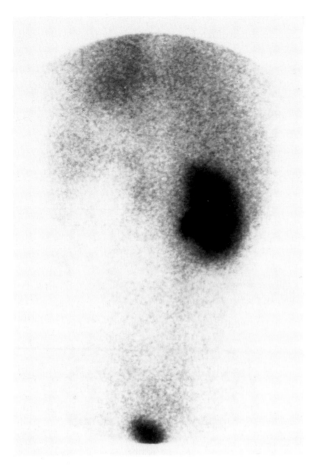

Fig. 33.6 Nuclear renal scan showing no function in the left kidney at 5 min (view taken from behind).

incision, a nephroscope is inserted into the kidney to divide the stricture, which is then stented for 6 weeks while healing occurs.

Total nephrectomy

Nephrectomy may be considered where the back pressure from the obstruction has destroyed the kidney. In such an instance, the dilated, poorly functioning kidney is a potential source of serious infection.

Partial nephrectomy

Duplex kidneys draining into an ectopic ureter or ureterocele (secondary to ureteric stenosis) are similarly likely to be very poorly functioning and a potential source of recurrent infections. These are treated by a partial nephrectomy and excision of the ectopic duplicated ureter.

Obstructed megaureters

Where the obstruction is at the ureterovesical junction, excision of the stenotic segment, and reimplantation of the ureter into the bladder is accepted treatment, and gives good results. Balloon disruption and dilatation of the segment has also been tried, but results are still to be evaluated.

FURTHER READING

Filmer R. B. & Spencer J. R. (1990) Malignancies in bladder augmentations and intestinal conduits. *J. Urol.* **143**: 671–678.

Jorgensen C. & Kullendorff C-M. (1989) Ultrasound diagnosis of fetal hydronephrosis: fetal renal pelvic size correlated to postnatal outcome. *Pediatr. Surg. Int.* **4**: 114–117.

Peters C. A., Bolkier M., Bauer S. B. *et al.* (1990) Urodynamic consequences of posterior urethral valves. *J. Urol.* **144**: 122–126.

Webb D. R., Tan H. L., Kelly J. H., Beasley S. W., Fowler R. & Woodward A. A. (1990) Management of urinary calculi using endourology and extracorporeal shockwave lithotripsy (ESWL). *Pediatr. Surg. Int.* **5**: 451–453.

— 34 —

The Child with Wetting

'Wetting' is one of the commonest symptoms in paediatrics. The symptoms are distressing, the cause may be obscure (Table 34.1) and the results of treatment are variable.

Table 34.1 Classification of wetting in children

(1) Wetting:
• Functional wetting
• Urinary tract infection, wetting, reflux syndrome
• Structural anomalies, for example ectopic ureter, urethral valves and phimosis
(2) Incontinence
• Hidden causes, for example sacral agenesis, spinal cord lipoma, dermal sinus and occult neuropathic bladder
• Overt neuropathic bladder, for example meningomyelocele

FUNCTIONAL WETTING

The detrusor muscle of the infant bladder contracts automatically to empty the full bladder. In older children voluntary control of bladder function involves continuous suppression of bladder activity until it is convenient to pass water. Functional wetting results from delay or imperfect development of this cerebral suppression of the bladder-emptying reflex.

Children with wetting can pass urine voluntarily but have accidents due to urge incontinence. The urge incontinence results from detrusor contractions in response to stimuli such as bladder filling, giggling or cold. This bladder dysfunction is known as bladder instability. A child with bladder instability may wet by day or night. Bedwetting alone usually has no underlying pathology as the child has demonstrated normal bladder function by day. Daytime wetting, however, may have an underlying cause in a few cases.

The assessment of functional wetting

The history is the most important diagnostic feature. Most of those affected are girls. There is good bladder sensation and the child can pass urine with voluntary control. The common presentation is urgency with involuntary passage of urine. The child develops unusual devices to try and control the wetting. For example, a girl may drop into a squat when she feels a detrusor contraction and jam her heel into the perineum to prevent the passage of urine until she can suppress the detrusor contraction. Physical examination reveals no abnormality. Particular attention is paid to palpation of the lower abdomen to exclude an enlarged bladder. The external genitalia and lower spine are examined for local anatomical abnormalities and spina bifida. Special investigations are indicated only if there are associated features, for example urinary tract infection or a strong family history of urinary tract malformation.

Treatment of functional wetting

Reassurance and support

Parents often need the assurance that there is no serious underlying abnormality. The child needs to empty her bladder frequently, especially before any vigorous activity which may bring on the wetting.

Medication

The main defect in daytime wetting is detrusor spasm and this can be treated with anticholinergic drugs (e.g. Oxybutinin), but these are helpful only in some children: they may be ineffective or their use limited by side effects such as mood change. Night wetting is treated with α-adrenergic drugs (e.g. Imipramine) which decrease detrusor tone to allow better bladder storage overnight and allow effective short term control of bed wetting. Other medications such as DDAVP are used occasionally to decrease urine output overnight.

Psychological behaviour therapy

The use of wetting charts, bell alarms and a system of rewards is a time-consuming but often remarkably effective way of treating wetting, particularly in school-age children. These methods are less effective in younger age-groups. Physiotherapy achieves the same ends with wetting charts and pelvic floor exercises.

URINARY INFECTION, WETTING, VESICOURETERIC REFLUX SYNDROME

Wetting may sometimes be associated with urinary tract infection and vesicoureteric reflux. Thus, if infection is diagnosed in conjunction with wetting, a micturating cystourethrogram and renal ultrasound should be performed. The reflux and infection are treated along usual lines. Control of infection with antibiotics often stops the wetting, but in a few, wetting may persist.

An underlying cause is found only occasionally in children with wetting.

STRUCTURAL DEFECTS

Ectopic ureter

A rare but important problem is the girl with constant low-grade incontinence from birth. An ectopic ureter does not cause wetting in boys because the ectopic ureter opens proximal to the external sphincter of the urethra. In the female the ectopic ureter opens outside the bladder neck or into the vestibule and causes constant minor wetting. The amount of urine which passes down the ectopic ureter is small because the ectopic ureter drains a poorly functioning upper part of a duplicated kidney. If the child is allowed to sit on a fresh sheet a small patch of urine may soon appear on the sheet—this is known as the 'patch test'. The diagnosis is confirmed by ultrasound which will show the upper renal moiety and its dilated ectopic ureter.

Excision of the upper pole renal segment and its subservient ureter will resolve the problem.

Phimosis

In boys, phimosis may be associated with a type of wetting with urine dripping away from the ballooned foreskin after micturition. Incomplete urethral valves or a urethral diverticulum may also be a hidden cause for wetting in males. Functional wetting is uncommon in males so further investigation is required more often.

TRUE URINARY INCONTINENCE

The difference between wetting and true incontinence is that in the latter there is no voluntary bladder control. Most children with urinary incontinence have spina bifida but some causes are hidden and may be treated as functional wetting for several years before the true diagnosis is made.

The history is critical. Children with incontinence secondary to a neuropathic bladder have poor bladder sensation and do not have urgency. Bladder emptying is abnormal and often is accomplished by abdominal straining. Overflow incontinence with continuous dribbling of urine is seen often. Frequent detrusor spasms are also seen in some patients. Physical signs include a palpable, non-tender bladder and occasionally there will be abnormalities of the lower spine, for example dermal sinus, dorsal midline naevi or hair and, in sacral agenesis, a shortened lower spine (Chapter 10). The physical signs are confirmed by X-ray. In some children with a neuropathic bladder there are no abnormal physical signs and no cause is found on special investigation. This rare group is known as 'occult neuropathic bladder'.

The management of neuropathic bladder depends upon the particular cause, but in general follows the line of treatment discussed in the chapter on spina bifida (Chapter 10).

FURTHER READING

Khoury A. E., Hendrik E. B., McLorie G. A., Kulkarni A. & Churchill B. M. (1990) Occult spinal dysraphism: clinical and urodynamic outcome after division of filum terminale. *J. Urol.* **144**: 426–429.

Yue P. C. K. (1974) Ectopic ureter in girls as a cause of wetting. *J. Pediatr. Surg.* **9**: 485–489.

35

The Child with Haematuria

Haematuria usually causes such alarm that the child is brought early for medical attention. Confirmation of the presence of macroscopic blood clots or microscopic red cells should be obtained, because haemoglobinuria, ingested dyes and plant pigments occasionally can be misleading.

Unfortunately, haematuria has often ceased by the time the child is examined, and the decision to investigate the child may be based solely on the observations of the parents or colleagues.

The causes are many, and in some the diagnosis is readily made (Table 35.1). In addition to generalized haemorrhagic disorders, haematuria can be due to inflammation, trauma, neoplasia or calculi in almost any part of the urinary tract.

It is not clear why, in the absence of infection, hydronephrosis and other malformations of the upper urinary tract so often should present with haematuria. It is seldom the sole presenting feature, and the clinical findings, examination of the urine and renal ultrasound or intravenous pyelography, usually make a diagnosis possible.

Table 35.1 Plan of investigation of a patient with haematuria

(1)	Cause obvious or readily determined	
	Renal mass	Overt glomerulonephritis
	Bleeding disorders	Urinary tract infection
	Hereditary haematuria	Meatal ulcer
(2)	Cause apparent on simple radiological investigation	
(a)	Plain film	Urinary calculi
(b)	Renal ultrasound	Hydronephrosis and hydroureter
		Cystic or malformed kidneys
(c)	MCU	Vesicoureteric reflux
		Vesical diverticulum
		Urethral polyp
(3)	Cause obscure without resort to more extensive investigation	
(a)	Endoscopy	Urethral membrane
		Vesical diverticulum
		Vascular anomalies
(b)	Retrograde pyelography	Small benign neoplasms of ureter or pelvis
(c)	Renal biopsy	Atypical nephritis
(d)	Selective renal arteriography	Vascular anomaly

HISTORY

A history of a recent streptococcal infection will be present in most of those with glomerulonephritis.

Frequency, dysuria, abdominal pains and fever point to an infection in the urinary tract; and injuries severe enough to damage the kidneys, ureter or lower urinary tract nearly always will present with an obvious history of trauma.

Haematuria sometimes has a familial background, and may be associated with familial deafness (Alport's disease) or related to exercise.

CLINICAL EXAMINATION

In boys who have been circumcised recently, the first thing to look for is a meatal ulcer. The typical story is of sharp pain at the meatus when voiding begins and of one or two drops of blood, which appear at the termination of voiding. In these boys, appropriate local measures will prevent unnecessary investigation. Occasionally it is seen in boys with phimosis after attempted forceful retraction of the foreskin.

Hypertension may point to chronic glomerulo-nephritis, and a palpable mass in the loin will focus attention on three conditions—hydronephrosis, Wilms' tumour and neuroblastoma—which are considered in greater detail in Chapter 25.

INVESTIGATIONS

Microscopy and culture of a mid-stream or catheter specimen of urine is the basis of diagnosis. Granular and cellular casts or persistent proteinuria in addition to 'glomerular' red cells, will lead to the diagnosis of glomerulonephritis, while pyuria and bacteriuria indicate infection as the cause of bleeding.

Phase contrast microscopy may show crenated and dysmorphic red cells to distinguish atypical focal glomerular lesions from lesions elsewhere in the urinary tract, which tend to give rise to more uniform red cell patterns.

Sterile pyuria accompanied by haematuria raises the possibility of a tuberculous infection.

Renal ultrasound

Except in children with meatal stenosis or readily demonstrable glomerulonephritis, a renal ultrasound is necessary in every case.

A non-functioning kidney accompanied by a palpable mass may be due to hydronephrosis or a tumour, and renal ultrasound will differentiate between the two.

Micturating cystourethrogram

A micturating cystourethrogram (MCU) will exclude vesical or urethral diverticula or urethral polyps. A plain X-ray prior to the MCU may show a calculus.

Endoscopy

In some patients with haematuria all investigations so far are normal. Cystoscopy may be undertaken next, preferably while haematuria is present, although this may be difficult in children, for bleeding is often of short duration. Occasionally cystoscopy reveals a vesical cause, for example a small haemangioma or a diverticulum not shown in an MCU or a urethral cause, for example urethral membrane.

Renal biopsy

Most children with 'idiopathic' or 'essential' haematuria have histological evidence of a focal type of glomerulonephritis in which haematuria is precipitated by physical effort or by an intercurrent infection. Biopsy is not required routinely, but does have a place when haematuria is persistent or severe.

Arteriography

When haematuria is too persistent and severe to be explained by atypical focal glomerulonephritis, and the renal ultrasound, MCU, cystoscopy and renal biopsy are all normal, renal arteriography may be needed occasionally to exclude the exceptionally rare vascular anomalies of the renal or ureteric vessels.

TREATMENT

Haematuria is a symptom which leads to a variety of diagnoses, and the treatment of these conditions depends on the diagnosis (see related chapters).

FURTHER READING

Boineau F. G. *et al.* (1989) Evaluation of hematuria in children and adolescents. *Pediatr. Rev.* **11**: 101–108.
Leading article (1970) Haematuria in childhood. *Br. Med. J.* **2**: 678.

36

Trauma in Childhood

Despite the majority of trauma being minor, it accounts for 50% of paediatric fatalities after the first year of life, and it is second only to acute infections as a cause of childhood morbidity. The causes of accidents in children are different from those of adults (Table 36.1).

Death from trauma occurs in three well-defined periods:

(1) Early (< 1 h post-injury): 50% of deaths occur and are secondary to disruption of the brain or major blood vessels

(2) 'Golden Hour' (1–2 h post-injury): 35% of deaths occur, mostly secondary to extradural haematomas, massive haemothorax or haemoperitoneum

(3) Late (> 2 days): 15% of deaths occur, from brain death, multi-organ failure and/or overwhelming sepsis.

Prevention of these injuries offers the best opportunity to reduce the mortality of childhood trauma.

INJURY PREVENTION

There are three ways to lessen or prevent childhood injury:

(1) Education of parents and children about potential accident situations

Table 36.1 The causes of accidents in children

Accident	%
Falls	62
Bicycles	12
Pedestrians	9
Motor vehicles	7
Others	10

(2) Minimization of injury in an actual accident, for example, use of car restraints or cycling helmets

(3) Limitation of injuries sustained after the accident, for example by first aid techniques. This requires an effective transport system which allows early, accurate assessment of injuries by trained personnel and rapid resuscitation prior to transport to an appropriate institution.

TRAUMA SCORES AND INJURY SEVERITY SCORES

Injury severity determination enables quantification of the magnitude of single or multiple injuries. Scores based on physiological data can be applied prospectively to determine triage destination and likely outcome, for example Champion Trauma Score and Paediatric Trauma Score. The Injury Severity Score (ISS) is based on the extent of tissue injury, which changes little following the initial insult. It is determined after physical examination, investigations, surgical intervention and/or post-mortem assessment. Thus, the ISS provides a retrospective assessment and cannot be used as a triage tool.

Glasgow Coma Scale

This was introduced to quantify central nervous system function. It documents three different brain functions: eye-opening, verbal response and best motor response, after different and graded stimuli (Table 36.2). The Glasgow Coma Scale (GCS) is used widely and enables rapid assessment of neurological injury.

Table 36.2 Glasgow Coma Scale

Score	Eye opening	Verbal response	Motor response
6	—	—	Obeys command
5	—	Oriented	Localizes pain
4	Spontaneous	Confused	Withdraws (to pain)
3	To voice	Inappropriate	Flexes (to pain)
2	To pain	Incomprehensible words	Extension (to pain)
1	None	None	None

Champion Trauma Score

To quantify the severity of trauma of different types a numerical value is assigned to five physiological parameters: systolic blood pressure, respiratory rate, respiratory effort, capillary refill and GCS. The sum of the assigned values is the trauma score. On a 0–16 range (where 16 is the least injured) (Table 36.3), a trauma score less than 13 is an indication for transfer to a major trauma centre.

Paediatric Trauma Score

This quantifies the severity of multiple injuries in children to enable speedy triage and despatch to an appropriate institution. It measures six different parameters: patient weight, patency of the airways, systolic blood pressure, neurological state, cutaneous wounds and the extent of bony injury. Each parameter is scored – 1, 1, or 2, with low scores indicating severe trauma (Table 36.4).

There are three categories of mortality risk: Paediatric Trauma Score (PTS) greater than 8 should have no mortality; PTS 8–0 has increasing mortality and PTS less than 0 has 100% mortality.

The Abbreviated Injury Scale and the Injury Severity Score

The Abbreviated Injury Scale (AIS) grades severity of injury from 1 (minor) to 6 (unsurvivable) in six different body regions: head and neck, face, chest, abdomen, extremities and external. The Injury Severity Score (ISS) calculates overall severity by determining the AIS value for each of the three most severely traumatized regions, squaring the scores derived from each and totalling the results. The ISS indicates increasing severity of injury on a scale from 0 to 75. Severe injury is defined by an ISS greater than 15.

Initial assessment and management

In assessing the injured child, many steps are accomplished simultaneously; for example, while conducting a rapid assessment of a patient's respiratory, circulatory and neurological status, the history and the events relating to the injury are obtained. There is often no adult witness to the accident present in the hospital, and it is the ambulance personnel who provide valuable information relating to the time and mechanism of the accident.

Table 36.3 Champion Trauma Score

Score	Respiratory rate (breaths/min)	Respiratory effort	Systolic BP (mmHg)	Capillary return (s)	Glasgow Coma Scale
5	—	—	—	—	14–15
4	10–24	—	>90	—	11–13
3	25–35	—	70–89	—	8–10
2	>35	—	50–69	<2	5–7
1	<10	Normal	<50	>2	3–4
0	None	Shallow/retraction	No pulse	Nil	—

Table 36.4 Paediatric Trauma Score

Score	Bodyweight (kg)	Airway	Systolic BP (mmHg)	CNS	Skeleton	Skin
+2	>20	Normal	>90	Awake	None	None
+1	10–20	Controlled	50–90	Obtunded/LOC	Closed fracture	Minor wound
−1	<10	Unmaintainable	<50	Coma/decerebrate	Open/multiple fracture	Major/penetrating

Mechanism of injury

The mechanism of injury may suggest that the severity of injury is greater than appears from the physiological state of the patient and the overt injuries. Factors which may indicate severe injury vary in different types of accidents and are discussed below:

(1) Motor vehicle accidents: important factors are high speed injury (> 60 km/h); ejection of the patient from the car; death of another person in the same accident; and the child being trapped in a fire

(2) Falls: important factors include the height of the fall (> 10 feet being significant); the part of the body which first struck the surface; and the type of surface, for example grass or pavement

(3) Vehicle and pedestrian/cyclist accidents: the speed of the vehicle and what happened to the child (for example thrown from vehicle or not) are important.

These factors predict that a child may have a major but as yet undetected injury, and this must be taken into account during assessment.

Establishing priorities

The Early Management of Severe Trauma course, (instituted by the Royal Australasian College of Surgeons) has developed a set of priorities which apply to both adults and children. It is important that patients are assessed and treated according to the nature of their injuries, the stability of the vital signs and the mechanism of injury. In general, patient management consists of a rapid primary evaluation, resuscitation of vital functions, followed by a more detailed secondary assessment; and when this has been done definitive care is initiated.

The primary survey: 'A, B, C's'

During the primary survey, life-threatening conditions are identified and management is begun simultaneously.

(1) A—Airways maintenance with cervical spine control

(2) B—Breathing and ventilation

(3) C—Circulation with haemorrhage control

(4) D—Disability: neurological status

Resuscitation phase

Shock management is initiated, patient oxygenation is re-assessed and haemorrhage control is re-evaluated. The life-threatening conditions identified in the primary survey are reviewed constantly as management continues. Tissue aerobic metabolism is assured by perfusion of all tissues with well-oxygenated blood. Replacement of lost blood volume with warmed crystalloid, colloid and blood is commenced, as are other modalities of shock therapy.

Secondary survey

The secondary survey begins after the primary survey (A, B, C) has been completed, and the resuscitation phase (management of other life-threatening conditions) has begun. Each region—head, neck, chest, abdomen, extremities—is examined individually and in detail. A careful neurological examination, including the GCS, is an integral part of the secondary survey. An assessment of the eyes, ears, nose, mouth, rectum and pelvis should not be neglected.

Definitive care phase

This phase involves the co-ordinated management of all the child's injuries including fracture stabilization and any necessary operative intervention. It may also involve stabilization of the child in preparation for transfer to a trauma referral centre.

Triage

Triage is the sorting of patients based on need for treatment. This is particularly important where the severity of injury may exceed the capability of the hospital and its personnel to treat, and is a reason for transfer to a more specialized institution.

SUPERFICIAL SOFT-TISSUE INJURIES

The extent and severity of soft-tissue injuries tends to be underestimated. It is ill-advised to attempt to explore and suture wounds under local anaesthesia. Most wounds require general anaesthesia for assessment of severity, debridement of contaminated and devitalized tissue, repair of important deep structures (e.g. tendons and nerves), and careful suturing of the skin. In small children it may be impossible to examine the external wound edges adequately without anaesthesia, let alone its deeper extensions. Lacerations through the deep fascia (where tendon or nerve damage cannot be excluded definitely) and those on the face (where a good cosmetic result is paramount) require surgical repair under anaesthesia, as do puncture wounds and those containing foreign bodies.

The only lacerations suitable for treatment in the emergency room or office are small lacerations that are not on the face, and where it is certain no deep structure is involved.

Debridement of wounds

The wound is explored aseptically to determine which structures are damaged and to remove foreign and devitalized tissue. Washing with soap and water, Savlon or chlorhexidine removes dirt and grass. Where gravel has been ground into the wound, a scrubbing-brush may be needed. Failure to remove dirt from an abrasion may leave the child with a 'tattoo'. Once the wound is clean and free of foreign material, the tissues are examined for capillary bleeding. If no bleeding occurs after cleansing, the tissue is likely to be avascular, and needs to be excised surgically. Non-viable tissue is removed until fresh bleeding occurs.

Special soft-tissue injuries

Some injuries and lacerations need special treatment because of their anatomical site.

The face

Facial lacerations rarely can be sutured under local anaesthesia because the child is often too frightened to lie still and the cosmetic result will be compromised. All except trivial lacerations should be referred to a paediatric or plastic surgeon.

The lip

Lacerations which cross the vermilion margin always need an experienced surgeon because failure to align the margin, even by a millimetre, will leave an ugly 'step'. Where the laceration is completely within the mucosa, exact apposition of the wound edges is unnecessary: here the more important feature is repair of the underlying orbicularis oris muscle to avoid a 'dent' in the lip.

The tongue

Despite initially vigorous bleeding and major deformity of the tongue contour, suture of the tongue is needed rarely. Most lacerations should be left to heal and remodel naturally. Infection of intra-oral lacerations is rare.

The forearm, wrist, hand and foot

These are the sites where even a superficial laceration can sever subcutaneous tendons or nerves. These serious injuries should be presumed by the site and size of the laceration and not on the presence of clinical signs of nerve or tendon injury: in small children these are extremely difficult to elicit. All these regions need exploration by an experienced surgeon under general anaesthesia. Further details of tendon injuries in the hand and fingertip lacerations are provided in Chapter 48.

The straddle injury

A slip onto the edge of the bath, bicycle bars or a fence may cause injury to the perineum. In females, this causes a tear in the posterior fourchette, often with significant bleeding. Where adequate assessment is not possible in the emergency room, the girl should be admitted for examination under anaesthesia. Minor splits require no sutures. Injuries through the hymen need careful repair. Where a laceration penetrates into the rectum, a colostomy for faecal diversion is required. Straddle injuries need careful assessment to exclude any possibility of sexual abuse (see below).

In boys, a straddle injury may tear the bulbous urethra and cause extravasation of urine into the scrotum and lower abdominal wall. A urethrogram demonstrates leakage of contrast and the need for catheter drainage of urine or primary urethral repair.

TETANUS AND GANGRENE

Successful prophylaxis against clostridial infections rests upon the triad of: (i) immunization; (ii) antibiotics; (iii) adequate surgical cleansing of wounds as described above.

Active immunization

Tetanus immunization should be part of routine childhood immunization. Primary immunization of infants is achieved with three doses of triple antigen (diphtheria, tetanus, pertussis) and a booster at 18 months. Primary immunization of children between 2 and 8 years involves three doses of CDT (diphtheria and tetanus) and beyond this age, with three doses of CDT at not less than 2 month intervals.

Booster doses

Although immunity following complete vaccination is long-lasting, it is considered reasonable to maintain immunity with booster doses at 10 year intervals. With a tetanus-prone injury, a booster dose of tetanus toxoid should be given if 2 or more years have elapsed since the previous dose. Active immunization against clostridial gas-producing organisms is not available.

Passive immunization

Tetanus immunoglobulin is available for the passive protection of individuals who have sustained a tetanus-prone wound and who have either not been immunized actively against tetanus or whose immunization history is doubtful. It should also be given to the fully immunized patient with a tetanus-prone wound when more than 10 years have elapsed since the last dose of tetanus toxoid. In all the above instances, active immunization should be commenced at the same time. Although tetanus immunoglobulin and vaccine can be given at the same time, they should be administered in opposite limbs using separate syringes. The minimum routine prophylactic dose for adults and children is 250 IU given by intramuscular injection.

ANTIBIOTICS

Antibiotics should be used when wounds are contaminated, but antibiotics are ineffective in the presence of dead tissue or foreign matter, and should never be relied upon to prevent infection in contaminated wounds.

CHILD ABUSE AND NEGLECT (BATTERED BABY SYNDROME)

Certain clinical signs and other features may raise the index of suspicion of abuse and point to the need for a closer examination of the psychosocial climate of the patient and family. The social and psychiatric aspects are often more important than the trauma itself, but lie outside the scope of this book.

General features

The incidence of intentional injury is difficult to determine, but it is probably far higher than is generally realized, and has been estimated to be from 0.3 to 3.0% of all injuries in childhood. Infants and children less than 3 years of age are particularly vulnerable.

Clinical features

The history of the supposed accident is variable but may be quite reasonable and acceptable; on other occasions it is conflicting or inconsistent, and sometimes utterly implausible. Information about previous injuries may be denied, distorted or difficult to obtain because the injuries were treated by a different doctor on each occasion.

The modes of presentation are diverse, but include:

(1) Unexplained fractures of limbs, especially when multiple

(2) Multiple bruises, soft tissue swellings and/or lacerations

(3) Subdural haematomas, particularly when bilateral

(4) Failure to thrive, with spectacular gains in weight when admitted for investigation.

Other patients present with features which suggest an obscure, non-traumatic disease of the central nervous system: a blood dyscrasia with haemorrhages, anaemia and ecchymoses. Accompanying findings which should arouse suspicion are listed in Table 36.5.

Investigation

A full blood investigation and clotting studies will exclude a blood dyscrasia as the cause of spontaneous haemorrhages, ecchymoses or anaemia. A bone scan will identify 'hot spots' which may suggest underlying fractures. These 'hot spots' are X-rayed for evidence of old or new fractures. In children less than 1 year old, a skull X-ray should be taken because the bone scan may be unreliable in determining a skull fracture.

Table 36.5 Observations suggestive of child abuse

(1)	Bizarre scars, scabs, weals, circumferential abrasions on the limbs and hemispherical bite marks
(2)	Multiple retinal haemorrhages
(3)	Periosteal thickening of long bones detected by deep palpation
(4)	Symmetrical burns or scalds in unusual areas
(5)	Multiple insect bites and/or infestations, for example pediculosis
(6)	Abnormal behaviour of the child in hospital, for example withdrawal or stark terror alternating with effusive affection for the ward staff as the parents come and go
(7)	An abnormal attitude in the parents to the injury. This varies considerably: for example, lack of affect, indifference, panic, guilt or belligerence. Their reactions may conceal an appeal for help
(8)	An apparently unrelated developmental abnormality: handicaps, both physical and neurological, which make the child 'different' can be associated with them becoming objects of abuse

Social history

An inquiry into the family's circumstances, the parents' personalities and the health of the siblings may well provide the grounds for diagnosis. While poverty, hardship and social inadequacy are found commonly, they are not present invariably; and cases in well-to-do, sophisticated families are by no means unknown. There is a high incidence of psychiatric disturbance in the parents, as well as alcohol- and drug-dependence.

Diagnosis

This depends to a large degree on an awareness of the possibility that serious injuries in young children may not be accidental. Thus it is important that where there is some suspicion of non-accidental injury, the child is admitted to hospital for assessment by the Child Protection Unit.

Management

The treatment of injuries is almost the least of the problems and is conducted along the lines described elsewhere.

A plan of management for the individual patient and family is required urgently, bearing in mind that indignation and a punitive attitude towards the person inflicting the injuries, though natural, is unfruitful. The following measures should be instituted:

(1)   Immediate protection for the patient

(2)   The assistance of a co-ordinating team composed of a paediatrician (to provide general care and advice); psychiatrist (for assessment and treatment); and medical social worker to undertake an investigation of the home and family, to supply social assistance and to aid rehabilitation of the family as a whole. The members of the team should be notified as soon as possible, ideally before the patient reaches the ward. Psychiatric assistance is refused rarely.

Prognosis

The long term prognosis of children suffering from abuse and/or neglect is unknown, although there is some anecdotal concern that it is an inter-generational problem.

FURTHER READING

Beaver B. L., Moore V. L., Peclet M. H., Haller A. Jr, Smialek J. & Hill J. L. (1990) Characteristics of pediatric firearm fatalities. *J. Pediatr. Surg.* **36**: 97–100.

Johnson C. F. (1990) Inflicted injury versus accidental injury. In: Reece R. M. (ed.), Child Abuse. *Pediatr. Clin. North Am.,* 791–814.

Lafferty P. M., Lawson G. M., Orr J. D. & Scobie W. G. (1990) The role of the paediatric surgeon in alleged child abuse. *J. Pediatr. Surg.* **25**: 434–437.

O'Doherty N. (1982) *The Battered Child. Recognition in Primary Care.* Baillière Tindall, London.

Peclet M. H., Newman K. D., Eichelberger M. R. *et al.* (1990) Patterns of injury in children. *J. Pediatr. Surg.* **25**: 85–91.

Schetky D. H. & Green A. H. (1988) *Child Sexual Abuse. A Handbook for Health Care and Legal Professionals.* Brunner/ Mazel, New York.

Tepas J. J. III, Di Scala C., Ramenofsky M. L. & Barlow B. (1990) Mortality and head injury: the paediatric perspective. *J. Pediatr. Surg.* **25**: 92–96.

37

Head Injuries

Head injuries cause a large number of deaths in the first decade of life. Despite this, children show remarkable powers of survival, but too often there are residual changes in behaviour, impaired intellectual performance and post-traumatic epilepsy.

DETERMINANTS OF INJURY

The pattern of head injuries in childhood is similar to that in adults, but there are some important differences related to the nature of the injury and the physical characteristics of the child's skull and brain.

The nature of the injury

Falls cause a high proportion (40–50%) of injuries, with traffic accidents next in frequency. More children are struck while running across the road than are injured as passengers compared with adults.

The nature of children's play also causes some characteristic injuries, for example small, localized, depressed and compound fractures, which result from blows by stones, sticks and other weapons.

The physical characteristics of the skull

The vault of the skull is thin and elastic and capable of much greater deformation than in adults. The increased elasticity permits more energy to be absorbed by the skull. This dampens down the acceleration or deceleration of the head after impact, and reduces the concussive effects. Children can tolerate blows of considerable severity without immediate loss of consciousness, although the conscious state is subsequently depressed by swelling and haemorrhage.

The elasticity causes more local brain damage at the point of impact than in adults. In the child, local indentation is often severe enough to produce a significant haematoma of the underlying brain. A child's skull can sustain considerable distortion without fracture, but when the limit is reached, the fracture which results is often extensive and frequently of the 'bursting' type. The skull sutures do not close until the fourth year, so that marked diastasis of the sutures may follow bursting injuries.

At the moment of maximal distortion a fracture line may open widely, causing the underlying dura to tear and separate, pushing out brain tissue through the fracture. As the distortion decreases in the next few milliseconds, brain or arachnoid membrane may be nipped by the closing fracture line, so that brain or CSF may be found outside the skull beneath the scalp (Fig. 37.1).

The physical characteristics of the brain

A child's brain is softer than an adult's and probably more prone to local damage; general oedema adds to the extent of local cortical injury.

CHARACTERISTIC INJURIES IN CHILDHOOD

Depressed fractures

These are one of the commonest injuries in childhood, and follow a blow with a small object or a fall onto a stone or sharp object.

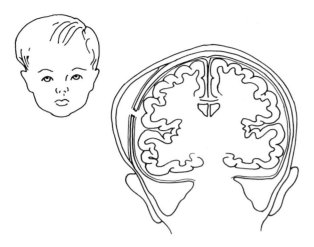

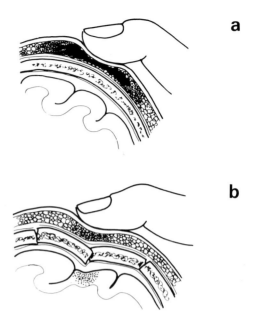

Fig. 37.1 Fractured skull. Cephalohydrocele, an accumulation of CSF beneath the scalp, following a laceration of the dura and arachnoid.

Fig. 37.2 Depressed fracture of the skull. Diagrams illustrating the similarity between (a) a haematoma with a peripheral clot, and (b) a depressed fracture.

Clinical findings simulating a depressed fracture (Fig. 37.2) can be caused by a scalp haematoma with a soft compressible centre. The fact that these findings are notoriously misleading may cause one mistakenly to dismiss the possibility of a depressed fracture. Radiography offers the only method of determining whether there is a depressed fracture, or a haematoma with or without a simple fracture (Fig. 37.3).

A compound fracture with penetration of brain and dura is not difficult to diagnose, but a small compound depressed fracture is often missed. The small superficial laceration is sutured or left to heal spontaneously, only to reveal an unsightly depression when the swelling subsides. When the story suggests a blow with a sharp object, skull X-rays with oblique views must be taken to determine whether or not there is an underlying depressed fracture.

Penetrating wounds

Small penetrating wounds caused by sharp objects, for example falls upon upturned nails, gardening tools, etc., are not uncommon. The point penetrates skull and brain with little general disturbance, and the incident may be

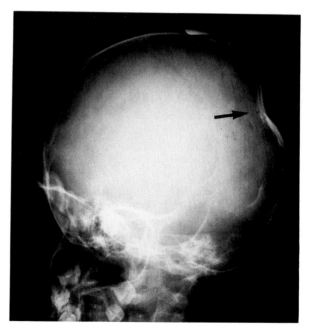

Fig. 37.3 Tangential skull X-ray is the best way to show a localized depressed fracture (arrow).

dismissed as trivial until infection or other complications ensue. Skull X-rays with oblique views must be obtained. Surgical debridement of the wound and exploration of the underlying fracture are necessary; computerized tomography (CT) scanning may indicate the degree of penetration.

Intracranial haemorrhage

Intracerebral haemorrhage

Intracerebral haemorrhage is common in childhood because the elastic skull is readily indented, thus causing oedema or haemorrhage which may extend deeply into the brain. This type of injury is most common where an indentation is most easily produced, that is in the posterior parietal region (Fig. 37.4), producing sensory and visual field defects on the opposite side.

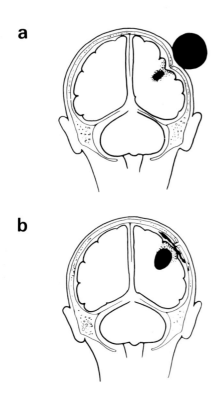

Fig. 37.4 Cortical laceration caused by (a) denting localized trauma and associated with (b) an intracortical haematoma.

Subarachnoid haemorrhage

A subarachnoid haemorrhage can occur in the child as a result of a minor head injury. The child falls, strikes his head and cries for a while; later headache, vomiting and drowsiness occur, often with fever and neck stiffness, all of which may suggest meningitis. A lumbar puncture excludes infection.

Sometimes deterioration of the conscious state is the main feature, and a subdural or extradural haemorrhage should be considered.

Subdural haemorrhage

After the first year of life this is uncommon. In the acute form which develops within hours of a fall, there are contralateral pyramidal signs and pupillary inequality (as seen in the adult), but there is also marked pallor from the blood lost into the subdural space, and the haemoglobin may fall to 5 g%.

The chronic form is rare in older children. In the infant it causes enlargement of the head (which may be asymmetric), mental retardation, irritability, and occasionally convulsions.

The acute form requires early and complete evacuation, but is often followed by a permanent neurological deficit or epilepsy.

Extradural haemorrhage

This is not as common in children as in young adults. The pattern is the same as in adults, but the volume of haematoma may amount for more than half the circulating blood volume in the infant. The resulting pallor and hypovolaemic shock can well be appreciated. CT scan allows diagnosis and treatment involves early evacuation of the haematoma.

Haemorrhagic diatheses

In some children, excessive haemorrhage following a mild injury may be the first sign of a blood disease such as acute leukaemia, thrombocytopenic purpura or haemophilia.

Intracranial birth injuries

Most birth injuries of the skull and brain come from excessive or rapid deformation of the skull as it passes through the birth canal or from compression by obstetrical forceps. Distortion may produce surface lacerations of the brain or tearing of superficial vessels, the large veins, or dural sinuses. The subsequent haemorrhage as well as cyanosis and anoxia from respiratory depression, may be catastrophic for the developing brain.

Depressed fractures of the skull during birth may occasionally be due to 'natural causes', but most result from incorrect placement of obstetrical forceps. The large 'pond-shaped' depression rarely produces neurological signs, but the fracture should be elevated without delay, because it is easiest and safest in the first 2 days of life.

Intracranial haematoma

Bleeding into the subdural space varies in rate, site and volume, and the clinical picture varies accordingly. Three varieties of the acute form are seen in infancy (Fig. 37.5).

Acute temporal haematoma

A clot surrounds the temporal lobe and spreads as a thin film over the parietal region. The fontanelle is bulging, there is a third nerve paresis on the affected side and weakness or lack of spontaneous movement of the contralateral limbs. The haemoglobin is below normal.

Craniotomy with early evacuation of the clot and irrigation of the subdural space is followed by rapid recovery.

Acute parasagittal haematoma

The clot can be reached with a needle inserted through the anterior fontanelle, and intermittent aspiration is often successful; if not, a craniotomy will be necessary.

Haematoma in the posterior fossa

This arises from a tear in or near the tentorium. Depres-

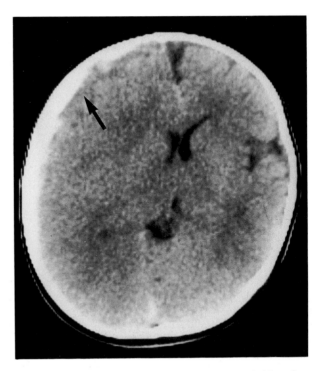

Fig. 37.5 Subdural haematoma on CT scan (arrow). Note the deviation of the midline in large part due to intracerebral swelling.

sion of respiration, opisthotonus, a tense fontanelle and no clot in the more usual anterior sites, provide clues to the diagnosis.

A suboccipital craniotomy is required, but the prognosis is poor in this fortunately uncommon type.

Chronic subdural haematoma

This type of haematoma may arise from birth trauma or a head injury during infancy. The collection develops slowly, giving the brain and skull time to adjust to the encroachment on the available space. If the lesion expands there is further compression of the brain and distension of the calvarium.

The clinical signs are an enlarging and sometimes asymmetrical head; delay in reaching the normal milestones; irritability; failure to thrive; and (occasionally) convulsions.

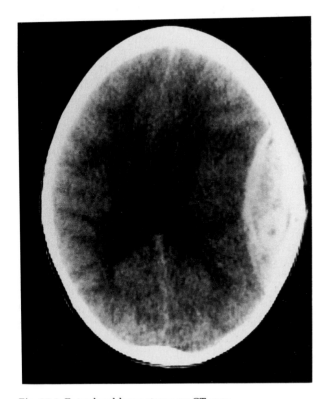

Fig. 37.6 Extradural haematoma on CT scan.

The diagnosis is confirmed by ultrasound or CT scanning or by needle aspiration of the fontanelle. Repeated aspiration may be sufficient, but persistent reaccumulation will require either open drainage, or internal drainage by means of a shunt (subdural, pleural or peritoneal).

SEQUELAE OF HEAD INJURIES IN CHILDREN

Although children show a surprising capacity for recovery after head injuries, they may suffer permanent disabilities as a result of the more severe injuries. A posterior parietal haematoma (see above) affecting the dominant hemisphere may cause a permanent defect in the contralateral visual field, and, perhaps more importantly defective visuomotor co-ordination, which

makes reading and writing difficult and results in reduced intellectual performance with all the psychopathological sequelae in its train.

The severe deceleration injury, so common in children involved in automobile accidents, affects the whole brain. This may result in disturbances of behaviour and intellect, but more obviously in spasticity, tremor and disturbances of speech from damage to the brain-stem, which is often the major manifestation of this injury.

Post-traumatic epilepsy is common after birth injuries, especially those which affect the temporal lobe. In older children it occurs after compound depressed fractures of the vault associated with a laceration of the cortex.

Internal compound fractures, for example a fracture of the base of the skull, may involve the frontal sinus, the nose, or the mastoid air cells and cause bleeding from the ear or escape of CSF when the dura beneath the fracture line is torn. The communication with the exterior through a mucosal space is a potential source of meningitis. Prophylaxis against such a complication begins with penicillin in the acute stage and continues with oral antibiotics for some weeks following injury.

If the communication persists meningitis may occur months or years later, and should be suspected when meningitis is recurrent. Leakage of CSF, or the demonstration of an old fracture line, will confirm the presence of a traumatic fistula and the need for repair with a fascial graft.

FURTHER READING

Amacher A. L. (1988) *Pediatric Head Injuries. A Handbook.* Waren Green, St Louis.

Caniano D. A., Nugent S. K. *et al.* (1980) Intracranial pressure monitoring in the management of the pediatric trauma patient. *J. Pediatr. Surg.* **15**: 537–542.

Hooper R. S. (1969) *Patterns of Acute Head Injury.* Edward Arnold, London.

Milhorat T. H. (1978) *Pediatric Neurosurgery.* F. A. Davis, Philadelphia.

Tepas J. J. III, DiScala C., Ramenofsky M. L. & Barlow B. (1990) Mortality and head injury: The pediatric perspective. *J. Pediatr. Surg.* **37**: 92–96.

38

Abdominal and Thoracic Injuries

INTRA-ABDOMINAL INJURIES

The majority of abdominal injuries in children are due to blunt trauma; penetrating trauma is rare. The commonest organs affected are the kidneys, spleen and liver. When the spleen and liver are injured, bleeding into the peritoneal cavity occurs. The injured kidney bleeds into the retroperitoneal space, and if the urothelium is disrupted urine may extravasate into the retroperitoneal tissues as well.

Haemoperitoneum

Haemoperitoneum, or blood in the peritoneal cavity, presents with signs of peritoneal irritation such as tenderness (often widespread) and a variable degree of reflex muscular rigidity (guarding). Abdominal distension results in part from the volume of blood in the peritoneal cavity, but mostly from swallowed air and the ileus which develops rapidly. The clinical evaluation of the abdomen is made easier and is more reliable if a nasogastric tube is inserted to decompress the stomach. There may be accompanying signs of blood loss and shock.

Knowledge of the mode of injury will often provide clues as to the likely organ(s) injured. For example, a bicycle handlebar injury to the left upper quadrant of the abdomen or to the lower chest is often associated with splenic trauma (Fig. 38.1).

Variations in posture and the time elapsed since injury result in wide variations in the distribution of the signs of haemoperitoneum and the site of maximum tenderness. When the spleen is ruptured the signs are usually maximal in the left upper quadrant, but it is not unusual for the signs, including pain at the shoulder tip,

to be more marked on the right side before the left, suggesting a ruptured liver. Of course, both the liver and spleen may be ruptured.

The recognition of haemoperitoneum is far more important initially than the diagnosis of damage to a particular organ.

Radiological investigation

Many children with minor blunt trauma to the abdomen require no specific radiological investigation. Computerized tomography (CT) with contrast is useful for unconscious patients with multiple injuries or where a specific organ injury is suspected (e.g. spleen, Fig. 38.2; liver, Fig. 38.3; or kidney). Nuclear scans for splenic or hepatic trauma and an intravenous pyelogram for renal injury are useful in some patients.

Recognition of hypovolaemic shock

Shock is recognized in the child by tachycardia, poor peripheral perfusion, cool extremities, and a systolic pressure less than 70 mmHg (although this is age-dependent). Familiarity with the age-dependent normal levels of pulse and blood pressure in children will lessen the chance of missing hypovolaemic shock, either initially, or if it develops after primary assessment.

The normal blood pressure in children is not only lower than in adults, but also it remains stable for longer with hypovolaemia, and then decompensation occurs quickly. Normotension, therefore does not exclude major blood loss in a child. The accurate measurement of blood pressure requires the correct-sized cuff. As a general rule, the cuff width ought to be two-thirds the length of the upper arm.

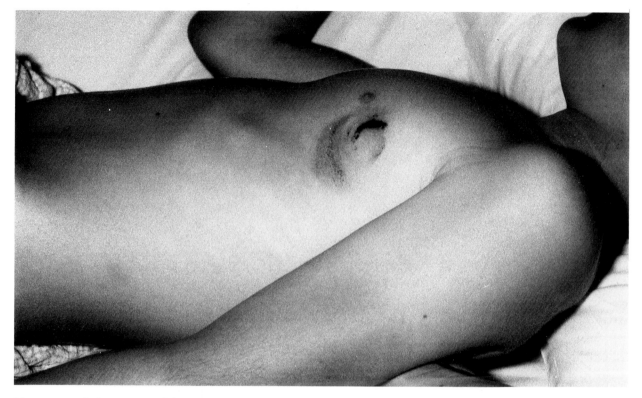

Fig. 38.1 Handle-bar injury with bruising over the lower ribs, which were so elastic the underlying spleen was torn without the ribs themselves being broken.

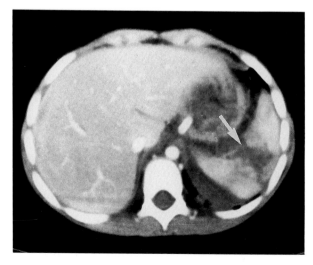

Fig. 38.2 CT scan of upper abdomen showing a ruptured spleen (arrow).

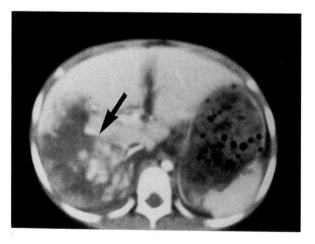

Fig. 38.3 CT scan of upper abdomen showing a ruptured liver (arrow).

Non-operative management

Non-operative management is appropriate for solid visceral injuries in children, provided they are kept under close supervision and are reassessed at frequent and regular intervals.

They are best managed in a facility with intensive care capabilities and an experienced paediatric surgeon. Intensive care must include continuous nursing staff coverage, monitoring of vital signs at frequent intervals, and immediate availability of surgical personnel and operating theatres, should they be required.

Indications for surgery

Indications for surgical intervention for blunt abdominal trauma, where injury to the spleen or liver is suspected, include:

(1)   Persistent or continued major bleeding, requiring more than 40 mL/kg of intravenous fluid resuscitation in the first 12 h to maintain cardiovascular stability

(2)   Persistent unstable circulation and hypotension despite appropriate resuscitation

(3)   A proven or suspected hollow visceral injury, that is gut perforation, on clinical examination or radiological investigation

(4)   Severe, concomitant head injury in which an unstable circulation cannot be tolerated, and where significant or ongoing intraperitoneal bleeding is suspected.

In splenic injuries requiring surgery, the spleen can be preserved by oversewing the tear ('splenorrhaphy') or partial splenectomy, avoiding the significant risk of post-splenectomy sepsis when the entire spleen is removed. If the spleen has to be removed completely, the child should be given Pneumovax vaccine and commenced on long term prophylactic antibiotics.

Peritoneal lavage

Diagnostic peritoneal lavage is not indicated in children because free blood in the peritoneal cavity *per se* is not an indication for surgery. Occasionally, peritoneal lavage is used in an unconscious child with a severe head injury where significant intra-abdominal injuries are suspected: in these children, continued hypovolaemia and an unstable circulation can exacerbate the secondary brain injury. Hartmann's solution is introduced at 10 mL/kg up to 1000 mL over a 10 min period. Remember that the child's abdominal wall is very much thinner than the adult's. Caution must be taken to avoid injury to the bowel during entry.

Haematuria

In all suspected intra-abdominal injuries, the presence or absence of blood in the urine must be established. Absence of haematuria virtually excludes a significant injury to the urinary tract, except in the rare instance of a transected ureter, which can be diagnosed when an intravenous pyelogram or CT scan show extravasation of contrast. Occasionally, there may be signs of extravasation in the flank or loin which prompt further investigation or exploration.

Urethral injury should be suspected in pelvic fractures and straddle injuries, from frank blood appearing at the external urethral meatus, from inability to void spontaneously (particularly in the presence of a palpable bladder) and from urine extravasation in the perineum. In these patients a urethral catheter must not be inserted blindly into the urethra, as this may convert a partial tear of the urethra into a complete transection. A carefully performed urethrogram must be obtained first, to delineate the injury. Depending on the type of urethral injury, either primary surgical repair of the urethra or temporary urinary diversion, for example suprapubic catheter, will be indicated.

Haematuria following relatively minor trauma suggests a predisposing factor such as hydronephrosis or Wilms' tumour. All children with haematuria, even after trivial injury, need a renal ultrasound or intravenous pyelogram to exclude these underlying lesions (Chapter 35).

Extraperitoneal extravasation

The signs of extravasation of blood or urine usually develop more slowly and less dramatically than those of intraperitoneal haemorrhage; they are also more consistently localized and less variable.

Renal injuries

Because the kidney is involved frequently, tenderness and muscular rigidity should be sought in the loin, but a perirenal haematoma may cause localized tenderness and sometimes a mass which is palpable through the anterior abdominal wall.

When haematuria accompanies tenderness and rigidity in the loin, an intravenous pyelogram or CT scan with contrast should be performed. This will distinguish between a contusion, which can be managed conservatively, and a rupture of the kidney with urine extravasation, which requires surgical exploration.

Early exploration, that is within 3 days of injury, rather than a non-operative approach to major renal injuries, is advocated. Delay in the recognition and management of injuries to the renal pelvis or parenchyma, which results in urine extravasation, is followed by severe inflammatory changes which prejudice attempts at conservation and later repair.

Bladder injuries

In extraperitoneal rupture of the bladder or membranous urethra, there are signs of extravasation of urine in the perineum, scrotum and suprapubic region.

When haematuria or urethral bleeding accompany signs of intraperitoneal or extraperitoneal haemorrhage or extravasation in the lower part of the abdomen, a cystogram will establish whether the bladder is intact. However, if blood, as opposed to blood-stained urine, is seen at the urethral meatus, the catheter should be passed only after a carefully performed urethrogram has demonstrated that the urethra is intact.

Ill-defined intra-abdominal injuries

Apart from those patients with intraperitoneal haemorrhage, extraperitoneal extravasation or haematuria, there is a difficult group with ill-defined symptoms and signs which may persist for several days after the injury.

Many probably have minor contusions of the abdominal wall or the intestine or its mesentery. Non-operative management usually is justified in these cases. Sometimes, lap belt deceleration injuries may cause severe trauma to the bowel wall when it is crushed against the sacral promontory. The injuries only become apparent after several days when the bowel perforates and peritonitis develops suddenly. The same type of trauma may also cause a periduodenal haematoma and pancreatic injuries, some of which may require surgical intervention.

Children who are comatose from concomitant head injuries are a specially worrisome group, requiring a high index of suspicion of intra-abdominal injuries. The indications for further investigation, which may involve laparotomy, include persistent or increasing pain; severe localized tenderness; the appearance of a localized abdominal mass; and generalized abdominal distension with vomiting.

Emergency diagnostic laparotomy may be required if there are signs of continued major concealed blood loss and cardiovascular instability despite appropriate resuscitation. In less urgent situations, the help of diagnostic imaging can be sought. Renal injuries show well on ultrasound, intravenous pyelogram and CT scan with contrast, but splenic and liver injuries show better on nuclear scanning. CT scanning is most helpful in complex multiple visceral injuries and in those where pancreatic injury is suspected, and should be performed using contrast in both the urinary and gastrointestinal tracts (Figs. 38.2, 38.3).

As abdominal injuries are frequently multiple rather than single, a systematic examination of all the viscera is mandatory at laparotomy.

THORACIC INJURIES

In contrast to their comparative frequency in adults, major thoracic injuries are not common in children. Most chest trauma in children is blunt; penetrating thoracic injuries are extremely rare. Blunt thoracic trauma tends to form part of a composite picture of multiple injuries which may include cerebral, abdominal and peripheral trauma, any of which may be the predominant threat to life.

The child's chest wall is very compliant and allows energy transfer to the intrathoracic structures, frequently without any external evidence of injury and without fractures to the ribs. The elastic chest wall increases the frequency of pulmonary contusions and direct intrapulmonary haemorrhage. Consequently, pulmonary contusion is the most common significant thoracic injury in children. Tension pneumothorax or haemopneumothorax are less common, but potentially lethal unless recognized and the tension relieved using intercostal drainage. Diaphragmatic rupture is extremely rare and may result from crushing of the torso and pelvis. Injury to the great vessels is less common than in adults and may reflect a lack of pre-existing vascular disease.

The diagnostic and therapeutic approach to chest trauma is the same for children as adults. Significant thoracic injuries rarely occur alone and are often a component of major multisystem trauma. Contusion of the lung and traumatic rupture of the diaphragm are unlikely to be recognized in the presence of these multiple injuries unless an X-ray of the thorax is taken as a routine. Pneumothorax, with or without haemothorax, may result from pulmonary contusion, and when of significant volume, should be relieved by an intercostal tube with an underwater seal.

Multiple fractures of the ribs are not common because of the elasticity of the thorax in children, and as a consequence, flail chest is rare. The small but vital respiratory excursion in childhood is not suitable for external compression or splinting, and when the flail area is large enough to cause respiratory embarrassment, internal splinting by positive pressure ventilation is preferable.

When penetrating injuries occur they may involve the heart or lungs, and the possibility of cardiac tamponade must be kept in mind.

Investigation and treatment

An X-ray of the chest should be taken in all cases of trauma with multiple injuries, in all thoracic injuries, and in all patients with respiratory insufficiency.

A penetrating injury should be assumed to have caused injury to underlying viscera until the contrary is proven. The possibility of combined thoraco-abdominal injury should always be kept in mind.

Respiratory symptoms demand investigation and treatment which may include intercostal drainage, thoracotomy or tracheostomy.

FURTHER READING

Bass D. H., Mann M. D., Cremin B. J. & Cywes S. (1990) A comparison between scintigraphy and computer abdominal tomography in blunt liver and spleen injuries in children. *Pediatr. Surg. Int.* **5**: 443–445.

Beasley S. W. & Auldist A. W. (1985) Management of splenic trauma in childhood. *Aust. NZ J. Surg.* **55**: 199–202.

Cosentino C. M., Luck S. R., Barthel M. J., Reynolds M. & Raffensperger J. G. (1990) Transfusion requirements in conservative nonoperative management of blunt splenic and hepatic injuries during childhood. *J. Pediatr. Surg.* **25**: 950–954.

Cywes S., Rode H. & Millar A. J. W. (1985) Blunt liver trauma in children: nonoperative management. *J. Pediatr. Surg.* **20**: 14–18.

Hardacre J. M. II, West K. W., Rescorla F. R., Vane D. W. & Grosfeld J. L. (1990) Delayed onset of intestinal obstruction in children after unrecognized seat belt injury. *J. Pediatr. Surg.* **25**: 967–969.

Hutson J. M. & Beasley S. W. (1988) Trauma. In: *The Surgical Examination of Children*, pp. 127–159. Heinemann Medical Publishers, London.

Ildstad S. T., Tollerud D. J., Weiss R. G., Cox J. A. & Martin L. W. (1990) Cardiac contusion in pediatric patients with blunt thoracic trauma. *J. Pediatr. Surg.* **25**: 287–289.

Lally K. P., Rosario V., Mahour G. H. *et al.* (1990) Evolution in the management of splenic injury in children. *Surg. Gynecol. Obstet.* **170**: 245–248.

Mandour W. A., Lai M. K. *et al.* (1981) Blunt renal trauma in the pediatric patient. *J. Pediatr. Surg.* **16**: 669–676.

Nakayama D. K., Ramenofsky M. L. & Rowe M. I. (1989) Chest injuries in childhood. *Ann. Surg.* **210**: 770–775.

Peclet M. H., Newman K. D., Eichelberger M. R., Gotschall C. S., Garcia V. F. & Bowman L. M. (1990) Thoracic trauma in children: an indicator of increased mortality. *J. Pediatr. Surg.* **25**: 961–966.

Touloukian R. J. (1983) Protocol for the nonoperative treatment of obstructing intramural duodenal hematoma during childhood. *Amer. J. Surg.* **145**: 330–334.

39

Fractures

Many fractures in children are misdiagnosed as sprains due to their proximity to joints. For practical purposes any child presenting following an injury with pain, swelling and loss of function must be assumed to have a fracture. The basic principles of fracture treatment are the same for all ages, but there are a number of important points pertinent to their treatment in childhood.

MAJOR DIFFERENCES IN CHILDHOOD FRACTURES

The flexibility of the paediatric bone (i.e. it is not brittle) and the presence of the growth plate produce a different spectrum of injuries from those seen in adults (Fig. 39.1).

Simple fractures

Complex and comminuted fractures rarely occur in the paediatric age group. Deformation producing a greenstick fracture is common and frequently missed unless high quality X-rays are obtained. (Fig. 39.1).

Speed of union

Delayed and non-union rarely occur in children and in fact most fractures unite rapidly and require quite short periods of immobilization. The younger the child the more rapid the union.

Reduction of fractures

In children reduction of fractures is usually by manipulation. With potential for remodelling anatomical reduction is not essential, provided alignment and restoration of length is obtained. Few fractures require open reduction or internal fixation.

Remodelling of fractures

Remodelling of fractures allows for correction of mild residual deformity. The remodelling capacity is best in the young and where the fracture is close to the growth plate. Overgrowth following fractures may occur and some overlap of fracture ends is acceptable. However, rotational deformities do not correct by remodelling.

Growth plate injuries

Growth plate injuries are a characteristic of the growing skeleton. It is essential to recognize those fractures which violate the germinal layer of the growth plate and thus have the potential for growth arrest. (Fig. 39.2). This may result either in shortening or deformity, depending on whether whole or part of the growth plate is involved. All fractures that may lead to growth plate arrest require anatomical reduction and commonly come to open reduction and internal fixation. It is recognized that with certain large growth plates even where the germinal layer is not violated, growth arrest may ensue (for example lower femoral epiphysis, fractures with a Salter Type 2 fracture).

Complications of fractures

The complications usually seen in adults rarely occur in children. For example, the skin in children is of such good quality that compound injury is not common. If a

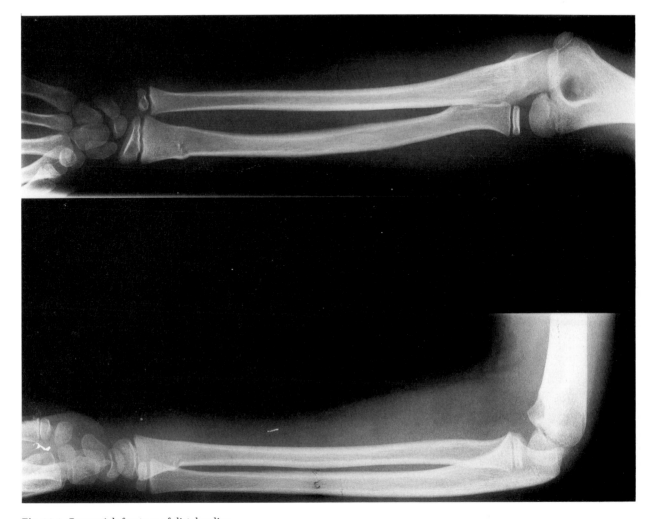

Fig. 39.1 Greenstick fracture of distal radius.

Table 39.1 Fractures in childhood

Feature	Implication	Example
Flexibility	Greenstick fracture	Shaft of radius and ulna
	Cortical kink	Shaft of radius and ulna
Presence of plate	Avulsion of epiphysis	Fracture of medial epicondyle and dislocation of elbow
	Compromised growth plate	Lower femoral epiphysis

child presents with a fracture and shock there is likely to be an internal organ injury, because shock from a bleeding fracture is rare.

Infection of a fracture site results from a compound wound or introduction of infection at the time of open reduction: neither of these circumstances is common in childhood fractures.

Fat embolism or shock lung is seen rarely in children with simple fractures.

Fractures in children unite rapidly and thus

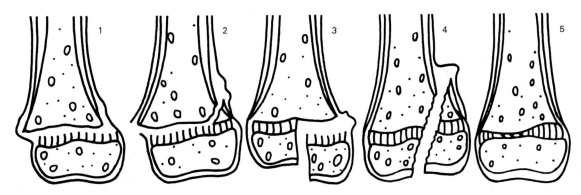

Fig. 39.2 Growth plate injuries as classified by Salter and Harris.

delayed union and non-union are exceedingly rare complications. Malunion likewise is not common because of the potential for remodelling.

PATHOLOGICAL FRACTURES

The common causes of pathological fracture are osteopenic conditions such as osteogenesis inperfecta and disuse osteoporosis in children with paralytic disorders. Other causes of pathological fractures include bony lesions such as simple bone cysts, fibrous dysplasia of bone and fibrous cortical defects (Chapter 47).

IMMOBILIZATION OF FRACTURES

Fractures in children always should be treated with a complete plaster which must be applied over a layer of plaster wool. If swelling is anticipated the plaster should be split to the skin from top to bottom. Following reduction of a fracture all patients should be given a list of instructions for plaster care. The patient should be reviewed 24 h following reduction to exclude complications from the plaster.

Complications of plaster immobilization

If pain is present the following should be excluded:

(1)   The plaster is too tight due to reactive swelling. The treatment is to split the plaster from top to bottom (including the plaster wool) and to elevate the limb

(2)   The plaster is causing local pressure. This can occur over bony prominences and if suspected a window in the plaster should be made to inspect the area

(3)   Arterial ischaemia is present. Arterial ischaemia can be caused by: (i) direct vascular injury; (ii) an over-tight plaster, or (iii) compartment syndrome. The features are summarized in Table 39.2.

If an excessively tight plaster is the likely cause the plaster should be removed, and if the circulation does not improve, fasciotomy is indicated as an urgent procedure to decompress the compartment.

If vessel injury is suspected, it should be diagnosed at presentation and treated by initial reduction and if there is no return of circulation, arterial exploration is indicated.

After-care

At the plaster check on day 1 following the injury, the following points should be checked:

Table 39.2 Features of arterial ischaemia in fractured limbs

(1)   Pain, severe and unremitting
(2)   Pallor of the digits with lack of capillary return
(3)   Paralysis with inability to move the digits. If full passive mobility produces pain, suspect ischaemia
(4)   Altered sensation

(1) Movement—pain free

(2) Circulation—capillary return or pulse felt

(3) Plaster adequate and intact.

All fractures requiring reduction should be reviewed at 1 week with a repeat X-ray to exclude displacement in the plaster. If displacement has occurred, re-manipulation under general anaesthesia or wedging of the plaster can be employed to regain an acceptable reduction of the fracture.

Rehabilitation

In children it is rarely, if ever, necessary to request physiotherapy assistance in mobilization.

SPECIFIC PROBLEM FRACTURES IN CHILDREN

Supracondylar fracture of the humerus

This is a common fracture after a fall onto the outstretched arm. The fracture line passes more or less transversely across the metaphysis close to the epiphyseal line. The shaft of the humerus may be driven forward into the cubital fossa (extension supracondylar), where it may involve the brachial artery or median nerve (Fig. 39.3). The periosteal hinge and the triceps muscle and tendon are intact on the posterior aspect of the fracture. Alternatively, the fragments may be driven forward and the humerus backward (flexion supracondylar).

Damage to the brachial artery with widespread arterial spasm is not common after supracondylar fractures. Vascular spasm leads to ischaemia of the forearm muscles, especially those in the flexor compartment, and of the nerves. If this is not relieved quickly, the muscles undergo ischaemic necrosis, which leads to muscle contracture and nerve degeneration. An immobile, clawed hand (Volkmann's contracture) results. The radial pulse and sensation should be monitored closely, and if compromised, treated by speedy reduction of the fracture or arterial exploration if reduction does not relieve the vascular spasm.

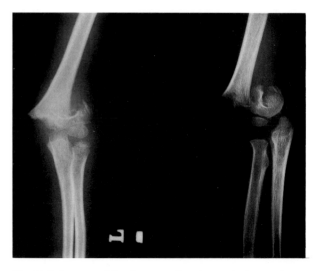

Fig. 39.3 Supracondylar fracture, showing typical posterior displacement of the lower fragment.

Reduction

In the extension type of supracondylar fracture, under general anaesthetic, the forearm is grasped and held with 20° of flexion at the elbow joint while an assistant provides counter-traction in the axilla; with firm traction the fracture is disengaged. Any rotational deformity is corrected and the elbow is flexed slowly. Medial or lateral displacement is corrected by direct pressure over the appropriate condyle. Finally, the posterior displacement is corrected by maintaining the traction and 'thumbing' the olecranon forward, flexing the fracture into an anatomical reduction.

When swelling is severe there may be considerable limitation of flexion at the elbow. A collar and cuff sling is applied with as much flexion as possible and the position checked on an X-ray. Failure to reduce the fracture may be caused by gross swelling or a delay in attempted reduction. If this occurs repeated attempts at reduction should not be attempted. The alternatives are either to manipulate the fracture into a reduced position under image intensifier control and pin with a percutaneous pin or alternatively, to return the patient to the ward and suspend the arm in Dunlop traction.

Unless the elbow is flexed beyond 90° usually the fracture will not be maintained in an anatomical position. Compromise to the circulation may prevent adequate flexion and if this occurs suspension in Dunlop traction is more appropriate with repeat manipulation at a later date when the swelling has settled, usually 4–5 days after injury.

Supracondylar fracture, flexion type

In this circumstance increased flexion of the elbow is likely to cause further displacement of the fracture and these patients are treated by immobilization in a cast in extension or alternatively by percutaneous pinning of the fracture, once reduced under image intensifier control.

After-care

The supracondylar fracture has great potential for vascular compromise and as a consequence it is advisable for all children to be admitted and kept under observation for 24 h to observe the circulation of the hand. X-ray at 1 week is essential to check that the position has been maintained and immobilization is required for approximately 3 weeks, after which the fracture can be mobilized. A full range of movement is not recovered until some 3–4 months after injury.

Fracture of the lateral condyle (capitellar fracture)

This fracture line extends obliquely from the lateral condyle of the humerus downwards and medially into the trochlea so that the lateral fragment consists of nearly half of the articular surface of the humerus (Fig. 39.4). This displacement of the fragment can be either very minor or quite significant.

Treatment

When the displacement is minimal treatment in a collar and cuff sling is all that is necessary. If there is dis-

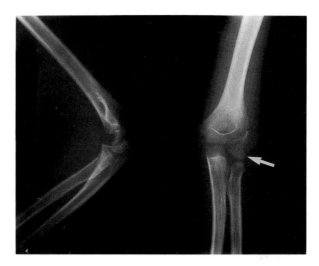

Fig. 39.4 Fracture of the capitellum showing displacement of the centre of ossification (arrow) by a fracture involving the articular surface of the elbow joint.

placement it should be recognized as a significant fracture involving the germinal layer of the growth plate and open reduction and internal fixation becomes mandatory.

Fracture of the neck of the radius

The small flat ossific centre of the radial head, together with the flake of the metaphysis, is broken off transversely, displaced and rotated.

Treatment

When there is only minimal angulation, reduction is unnecessary. When the fracture is still in contact and the angulation is less than 60° closed reduction is performed by extending the elbow while the forearm is firmly supinated, and exerting pressure over the head of the radius. If the angulation is over 90°, open reduction is preferable. The head of the radius must never be excised. Residual angulation of up to 30° after closed reduction is acceptable in children as remodelling will correct the remaining deformity. Immobilization of this fracture is only necessary for a period of 3–4 weeks.

Fractures of the forearm

A fall on the outstretched hand can result in fractures of the forearm region. The commonest of these fractures is a greenstick fracture of the radius (Fig. 39.1). This relatively innocuous fracture will not displace as it is a greenstick type and does not require prolonged immobilization. In most cases a period of 2 weeks in a below-elbow plaster or forearm slab is sufficient to give pain relief and allow resolution of the problem.

With more severe trauma a fracture of the distal radius with displacement or a fracture of the distal radius and ulna can occur. Many of these require reduction which can usually be effected by intravenous arm block analgesia followed by reduction and plaster, which should extend above the elbow. The period of immobilization varies with age from 3 weeks in the very young up to 6 weeks in the older child.

Fracture of the femur

A fracture of the femur occurs after major trauma and one must exclude other significant injuries, such as cranial, thoracic and abdominal injuries (see Chapter 36). A blood transfusion rarely is necessary for a fractured femur and if a child is hypovolaemic, internal haemorrhage should be suspected.

Treatment

Once the fracture has been diagnosed a femoral nerve block is very helpful in relieving pain in the emergency situation to facilitate handling and achieving immobilization. Children less than 2 years old are usually treated in 'gallows' (Bryant's traction) until early union is evident, when they are placed in a hip spica. In the 2–10 year age group an 'immediate' and carefully moulded hip spica is applied under general anaesthesia. Those over 10 years are usually treated in skin traction or Steinman-pin traction until union has occurred or on occasions for a shorter period followed by hip spica or a functional cast brace.

Where there is an accompanying head injury immediate external fixation is recommended to facilitate nursing and neurosurgical care. Alternatively, in the older age group an intramedullary nail can be employed to immobilize the fracture.

Fracture of the neck of the femur

The fracture of the neck of the femur in children is rare and is usually treated by immediate internal fixation as there is a high risk of avascular necrosis of the femoral head.

Spiral fracture of the tibia

In children, a twisting movement may cause a spiral fracture of the tibia alone. The toddler complains of pain in the lower leg but may be able to walk, sometimes leading to a delay in diagnosis and in which case may present later with a persistent limp. The fracture may be difficult to see on an anteroposterior film. The tibia is immobilized in an above-knee plaster for 6 weeks.

FURTHER READING

Rockwood C. A. Jr, Wilkins J. E. & King R. E. (eds) (1984) *Fractures in Children*, Vol. 3. J. B. Lippincott, Philadelphia.

Sharrad W. J. W. (1973) *Paediatric Orthopaedics and Fractures*. Blackwell Scientific Publications, Oxford.

Tachdjian M. D. (1990) *Pediatric Orthopaedics*, 2nd edn. W. B. Saunders, Philadelphia.

Williams P. F. & Cole W. G. (eds) (1991) *Orthopaedic Management in Childhood*, 2nd edn. Chapman & Hall, London.

40

Foreign Bodies

The infant's instinctive exploration of his environment and the spirit of experiment in the toddler and older child result in a wide variety of foreign bodies lodging in the oddest places. Most are found in the alimentary tract; others may enter the aural or nasal cavities, the bronchial tree or be accidentally driven into the soft tissues.

SWALLOWED FOREIGN BODIES

In infants, oral exploration of the environment may lead to accidental swallowing of a variety of objects. Older siblings may feed the 'new baby' inappropriate hardware. Accidental swallowing may be precipitated by a fall or a slap on the back. At any age, a bone hidden in food may be swallowed, for example a chop or fish bone. Ingestion of a foreign body occurs most commonly during the first year of life.

The vast majority of swallowed foreign bodies pass through the alimentary tract without a problem. If a foreign body becomes lodged in the oesophagus, however, it usually does so just below the cricopharyngeus muscle. With rare exceptions, objects which are first located below the diaphragm will pass naturally without hazard to the child.

The size of coins, the objects which are swallowed most often, determines whether they are likely to become impacted. When a coin or other foreign body becomes lodged in the oesophagus, it should be removed by endoscopy under general anaesthesia. Safety-pins may stick in the oesophagus, but if they enter the stomach they will almost always be excreted without difficulty, even if open.

Broken plastic toys are more dangerous, because they may be jagged or angular, and their radiolucency may lead to delay in diagnosis. Ulceration, mediastinitis, and even acquired tracheo-oesophageal fistulae may occur. A plastic bread-bag clip may cause bowel perforation. Bobby pins and 'Kirby grips' pass easily as far as the duodenojejunal flexure, but may be too long and rigid to negotiate this flexure in children less than 7 years of age, and require laparotomy for their removal. In children more than 6 or 7 years of age, observation for up to 1 week is justified, although impaction at the duodenojejunal flexure should not be allowed to continue for more than 10–12 days.

'Button' or 'disc' batteries used in micro-electronic toys, cameras and calculators, are particularly hazardous when swallowed by young children. Their small size ensures their passage into the stomach, and the great majority pass through the alimentary canal uneventfully. However, if any hold-up occurs, for example in the stomach, the nickel-cadmium shell can be eroded with release of strong alkali and cause local necrosis and perforation. Heavy metal poisoning (mercury, cadmium, nickel, zinc or magnesium) also has been reported. Complications from button batteries can occur in less than 36 h; when recently ingested in the absence of abdominal signs, a cathartic will ensure its rapid transit through the alimentary tract.

Clinical features

There may be no symptoms, and it is likely that innumerable small foreign bodies are passed uneventfully and unnoticed. In some cases an attack of gagging, coughing or retching is reported or the incident has been observed.

When the symptoms and history suggest lodgement in the mouth or throat, the oropharynx should be examined carefully. Oesophageal obstruction may present as excessive drooling and dysphagia.

If the accident has not been reported or observed, the first symptoms may be due to complications, for example progressive dysphagia or dyspnoea caused by pressure of the swollen oesophagus on the trachea.

Pain, swelling in the neck and fever are the signs of mediastinitis, and rarely a pneumothorax or pleuritic pain may be the first indication of perforation of the thoracic oesophagus by a foreign body.

Investigation

Radiographs of the head, neck, thorax and abdomen are required, because a radio-opaque object may be located anywhere from the base of the skull to the pelvic floor.

A radiograph will distinguish tracheal from oesophageal lodgement, for the maximum dimension of the trachea is in the sagittal plane, and that of the oesophagus in the coronal plane (Fig. 40.1).

Radiolucent foreign bodies are more difficult to detect radiologically, except on barium swallow.

Management

The vast majority of ingested foreign bodies do not need to be removed.

Endoscopic removal is required for all objects impacted in the oesophagus.

Foreign bodies first located beyond the oesophagus have a good chance of being excreted without incident

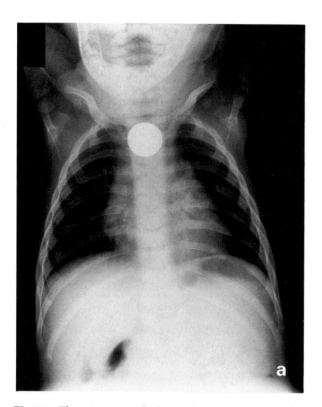
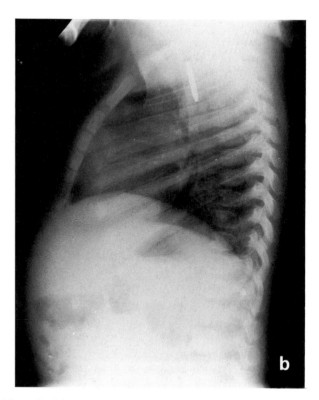

Fig. 40.1 The orientation of a foreign body (e.g. coin) will distinguish tracheal from oesophageal lodgement. Here a chest X-ray shows a coin in the coronal plane characteristic of the oesophagus. (a) AP view and (b) lateral view.

(Fig. 40.2). Blunt objects small enough to enter the stomach will almost all be passed; the patient should return only if abdominal pain or vomiting occurs. Further radiographs are not usually indicated, but will show that the object has been passed, often unrecognized.

In general, when a blunt foreign body has been impacted without progress for 6 weeks, removal at laparotomy should be considered even in the absence of symptoms.

Lead poisoning from objects which yield soluble lead salts is now very rare, particularly where legislation has banned lead fillers in paints. However, there have been instances of lead poisoning occurring within 10 days from the absorption of lead salts derived from thin lead foil retained in the stomach. Gastric lavage and analysis of the washings will indicate whether significant absorption is likely.

Multiple, minute, scattered opacities found in incidental X-rays of the abdomen, suggest bizarre appetites or oral habits (pica) and also raise the possibility of lead poisoning, such as from ingestion of flakes of paint gnawed from toys or other accessible articles. X-rays of the long bones showing a 'lead line' in the metaphysis, punctate basophilia in the erythrocytes, and a high content of lead salts in the blood or urine, will confirm this possibility.

Most sharp objects pass uneventfully and should be managed conservatively initially, although arrest and failure to progress through the bowel may raise concerns of impending impaction, ulceration and perforation.

A bezoar is a conglomeration of hair (trichobezoar) or vegetable material (phytobezoar) swallowed by emotionally disturbed or retarded children with bizarre appetites or habits (pica). The mass forms in the stomach or proximal gut and causes pain, vomiting or anorexia, malnutrition or unexplained anaemia. Less commonly, obstruction or perforation occurs. When X-ray studies indicate a mass of this kind, laparotomy and enterotomy are required.

Prevention

The area on which an infant crawls should be cleared of small objects, and articles should not be pinned to the clothing. Coins and buttons are unsuitable play materials for children less than 5 years of age.

FOREIGN BODIES IN THE TRACHEA AND BRONCHI

Sudden onset of coughing, spluttering and gagging with a residual wheeze are suggestive of inhalation of a foreign body. The exact clinical picture varies with the size of the object, the site of lodgement and the time elapsed since the object was inhaled. Large objects in the larynx or trachea produce obstruction which may be

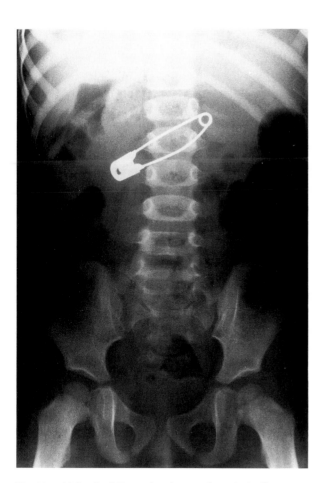

Fig. 40.2 Abdominal X-ray showing a safety pin in the stomach. This should pass spontaneously.

complete if they impact in the narrow glottis. Inspiratory stridor and retraction of the supraclavicular, substernal or intercostal areas indicate that the object is in the larynx or subglottic area.

Foreign bodies in the trachea or a bronchus cause a wheeze and clinical and radiographic evidence of a ball-valve type of obstruction during expiration resulting in emphysema. More distally impacted objects may present with symptoms of chronic chest infection from lobar or segmental consolidation.

X-rays may show an opaque object, or the segmental pulmonary collapse and lobar emphysema which occurs with small radiolucent objects. Films taken in expiration and inspiration show air trapping and assist in localizing the presence and size of small radiolucent objects in the lungs, for example a peanut.

In infants, respiratory symptoms can occur when the object is impacted in the oesophagus, for example acute dyspnoea or progressive stridor, a cough and wheeze. The orientation of the object by X-rays will identify the site of lodgement because the maximum diameter of the trachea is in the anteroposterior plane, compared with the transverse plane in the oesophagus (Fig. 40.1).

Removal at endoscopy under general anaesthesia is required. Mucosal abrasions and pulmonary changes, caused by the foreign body, its complications or manipulations during removal, are indications for a course of antibiotics. The earlier the diagnosis and treatment, the less the likelihood of residual pulmonary or mucosal damage.

FOREIGN BODIES IN THE EAR, NOSE AND PHARYNX

In the ear

Unless there is a definite history, children with a foreign body in the ear present with a blood-stained discharge, irritation or deafness. The requirements for the removal include sedation, local anaesthesia, good illumination and the correct instrument. The details of the technique are described in Chapter 14.

In the nose

The child, usually between 2 and 4 years of age, presents with nasal irritation and obstruction or a purulent discharge. The object often can be seen after the local application of an anaesthetic with adrenaline, but X-rays are sometimes necessary and the general principles of removal are the same as for those in the ear (Chapter 14). Suction is safe and effective for smooth, round objects, for example a bead or button.

In the pharynx

The commonest is a fish bone lodged in the tonsil, the piriform fossa or the back of the tongue. Subjective localization is poor and pain may be constant or felt only during swallowing.

After spraying the fauces and the pharynx with a local anaesthetic, the usual sites are examined with the aid of a spatula or a laryngeal mirror and proper illumination, and the object is removed with forceps.

FOREIGN BODIES IN THE URINARY TRACT

These are rare but most often involve the bladder, in girls in the pre-school age-group during play or in boys during puberty, when objects may be introduced in seeking erotic stimulation; or a fragment of a ureteric catheter may break off and remain after surgery to the urinary tract. Any of these objects may cause infection, haematuria or pain and may also act as a nidus for the formation of a calculus.

Foreign bodies in the urinary tract are removed by endoscopy. For foreign bodies in the vagina, see Chapter 27.

OTHER FOREIGN BODIES

In the hand

Apart from superficial splinters, a small fragment of metal or wood may be driven into the palm, and if it is unrecognized, a painless cystic swelling within a fibrous capsule may develop around the object. Exploration and removal under general anaesthesia are required, with tourniquet control. Unrecognized foreign bodies in the palm may cause deep web space infections similar to those seen in adult practice.

In the foot, knee, etc.

Nails, pins or needles driven into the foot or knee can be shown radiographically. When they are not visible through the skin, they are most easily and quickly removed under general anaesthetic by a pair of fine artery forceps inserted through a tiny incision and guided by an image intensifier.

FURTHER READING

Brown T. C. K. & Clark C. M. (1983) Inhaled foreign bodies in children. *Med. J. Aust.* **2**: 322.

Bundred N. J., Blackie R. A. S. *et al.* (1984) Hidden dangers in sliced bread. *Brit. Med. J.* **288**: 1723.

Groff D. B. (1986) Foreign bodies and bezoars. In: Welch K. J., Randolph J. G., Ravitch M. M., O'Neill J. A. & Rowe M. I. (eds), *Pediatric Surgery*, 4th edn, Vol. 2, p. 907. Year Book Medical, Chicago.

Jones P. G. (1963) Swallowed foreign bodies in childhood. *Med. J. Aust.* **1**: 236.

Kulig K., Rumack C. M., Rumack B. H. *et al.* (1983) Disk battery ingestion: elevated urine mercury levels and enema removal of battery fragments. *J. Am. Med. Assoc.* **249**: 2505.

Litovitz T. L. (1983) Button battery ingestions: a review of 56 cases. *J. Amer. Med. Assoc.* **249**: 2495.

Rivron R. P. & Jones D. R. B. (1983) A hazard of modern life. *Lancet* **ii**: 334.

Williams H. E. & Phelan P. D. (1969) The 'missed' inhaled foreign body in children. *Med. J. Aust.* **1**: 625.

41

The Ingestion of Corrosives

In children, swallowing corrosive fluids or solids nearly always is accidental, and the exploring toddler aged between 1 and 3 years is most often the victim.

PREVENTION

The most effective way to prevent such accidents is to keep all chemicals used in the home or garden out of reach of small children, and in their proper containers. They should not be stored under the kitchen sink or in unlabelled containers.

PATHOLOGY

The oesophagus is the most common organ seriously injured by corrosive ingestion. Extensive or circumferential oesophageal burns may lead to severe strictures which cause dysphagia within weeks of injury.

Burns of the buccal mucosa, soft palate or tongue suggest that the oesophagus has been damaged as well.

Mucosal injury and oedema of the larynx is rare, but can be life-threatening and lead to intubation or tracheostomy.

FIRST AID

(1)   If ingestion has just occurred, wash off any excess corrosive material from the lips and skin, using plenty of water

(2)   Immediately dilute any corrosive in the mouth, oesophagus or stomach by giving cold water or milk to drink. Do not attempt to use an 'antidote' acid or alkali because the corrosive may have been identified incorrectly, and the chemical antidotes themselves may cause mucosal damage

(3)   If ingestion of corrosive was not witnessed or confirmed by an adult, always assume it has occurred if the lips or mouth are blistered or if the toddler is drooling excessively and unable to swallow saliva

(4)   Where the nature or composition of the corrosive is uncertain, consult the Poisons Information Service by telephone. Induce vomiting with ipecac syrup only if directed by a Poisons Service. Large volumes of fluid alkali in the stomach may burn the gastric mucosa and may be best removed by vomiting, despite the 'double exposure' of the oesophageal and oral mucosae to the agent

(5)   Send a sample of the corrosive agent with the child when transferring to hospital if identification has not be made with certainty

(6)   All children should be sent to the nearest paediatric surgical centre as soon as possible after ingestion.

DEFINITIVE MANAGEMENT

An oesophagoscopy at 24 h is necessary in corrosive ingestion whenever injury to the oesophagus is suspected. This will determine the severity of oesophageal injury, and hence the need for prophylactic treatment to reduce the likelihood of subsequent formation of an oesophageal stricture. Where there is no damage to the oeosophageal mucosa on oesophagoscopy, no treatment is required.

Patchy oedema of the intact oesophageal mucosa is regarded as the minimal degree of burn and is not likely to cause a stricture. No treatment is required and the patient may leave hospital as soon as normal feeding is re-established. A white mucosal slough or circumferential ulceration is more serious and may lead to a stricture. In these patients, antibiotics are given to limit the effects of secondary infection. Steroids may diminish the extent of fibrosis, although their value is uncertain. Dilatation of the oesophagus is carried out daily by the passage of a mercury-filled Hurst bougie of appropriate size (e.g. no. 18, with a diameter of 1 cm, for a 2 year old). The unpleasant aspects are short-lived and the patient comes to tolerate the bouginage within a few days. Many older children can pass the bougie themselves.

This regimen is conducted initially in hospital, where the child's swallowing and the ease of bouginage can be assessed. Later the procedure can be performed at home. Oesophagoscopy is repeated 1–3 weeks after the injury, and if the mucosa has healed and there is no evidence of narrowing, treatment is discontinued. If there are abnormal findings at 3 weeks, treatment is continued for a further 6 weeks. Where there is worsening dysphagia and the stricture cannot be dilated effectively by bouginage, segmental resection and anastomosis may be required. Occasionally, an extensive resection and replacement of the oesophagus is inescapable; but in the long term, the best oesophagus is the patient's own, and prolonged bouginage is justified to avoid an extensive oesophagectomy.

FURTHER READING

Fyfe A. H. B. & Auldist A. W. (1984) Corrosive ingestion in children. *Z. Kinderchir.* **39**: 229–233.

Gillis D. A., Higgins A. & Kennedy R. (1985) Gastric damage from ingested acid in children. *J. Pediatr. Surg.* **20**: 494–496.

42

Burns

A burn causes partial or complete necrosis of the surface epithelium of the skin and, if more severe, of deeper tissues as well. It may be caused by heat (scald, contact with hot metal, flame), electricity, lightning, radiation (solar, atomic), chemical agents, or friction.

The care of a burned child requires the services of a multidisciplinary team and may extend over many years.

A burned child has a rapidly progressive illness: within a short time a healthy, alert, adventurous youngster may be in danger of losing his life. He will suffer pain and anxiety, and may develop lifelong physical and psychological scars.

PREVENTION

Most burns in children are due to scalds; are self-inflicted; involve boys (usually toddlers); and occur at home, mostly in the kitchen or bathroom. The child at greatest risk therefore is the male toddler, in the kitchen, while under the care of a parent preparing or drinking a hot beverage. Flame burns occur mainly in boys playing with fire, most commonly matches and flammable fluids.

Prevention of burns rests on three approaches:

(1)   Education, of both children and adults, concerning potential dangers, and the need for continual vigilance

(2)   Design, for example improvements in clothes, heating appliances, guards on stoves, temperature regulators in hot water systems

(3)   Legislation, for example government (legal) control of fireworks, nightwear materials and design regulations.

When visiting a home, the family doctor is in a unique position to prevent burning accidents by warn-ing the parents of specific hazards. These include: the ability of young children to reach table-tops and over-hanging saucepan handles on stoves; hot water in bath-rooms; old model radiators and unguarded fires; loose cotton nightwear; and access to flammable liquids.

TREATMENT

Early, competent assessment of the burn is essential. The child should be admitted to a burns unit when there is:

(1)   Full-thickness skin loss

(2)   More than 8% of the total body surface has been burned

(3)   Inhalation injury has been sustained

(4)   When important areas are involved, for example face, hands, buttocks and genitalia

(5)   Poor social circumstances and probable mal-treatment.

Treatment requires a team approach involving a surgeon, anaesthetist, social worker, school teacher, dietitian, physiotherapist and other paramedical thera-pists, all of whom confer and work together to ensure that the child is healed and back at home as soon as possible. The phases of treatment are summarized in Table 42.1.

First aid

First aid involves limiting the extent and severity of the burn. The child must be removed quickly from the source of injury; flames are smothered, by water if at hand; clothing should be removed immediately, es-pecially with a scald; the whole body or limb immersed in cold water for 10 min, and cold packs applied to the

Table 42.1 The management of burns in children

(1)	First aid
(2)	Transportation
(3)	Assessment
(4)	Resuscitation
(5)	Prevention and control of infection
(6)	Adequate nutrition
(7)	Care of the burn wound
(8)	Early excision of dead tissue and grafting
(9)	Minimizing scars and contractures. Pressure garments, splints etc.
(10)	Psychological support and rehabilitation
(11)	Reconstructive surgery to correct functional and cosmetic defects as necessary

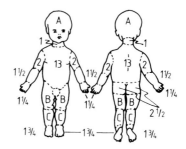

	Age 0	1 year	5 years	10 years	15 years	Adult
$A = \frac{1}{2}$ of head	$9\frac{1}{2}\%$	$8\frac{1}{2}\%$	$6\frac{1}{2}\%$	$5\frac{1}{2}\%$	$4\frac{1}{2}\%$	$3\frac{1}{2}\%$
$B = \frac{1}{2}$ of thigh	$2\frac{3}{4}\%$	$3\frac{1}{4}\%$	4%	$4\frac{1}{4}\%$	$4\frac{1}{2}\%$	$4\frac{3}{4}\%$
$C = \frac{1}{2}$ of leg	$2\frac{1}{2}\%$	$2\frac{1}{2}\%$	$2\frac{3}{4}\%$	3%	$3\frac{1}{4}\%$	$3\frac{1}{2}\%$

Fig. 42.1 Method of estimating the extent of burned surfaces, allowing for differences according to age (after Lund and Browder).

burned area(s). Iced water is dangerous because it may cause general hypothermia or local ischaemia, and thus is contra-indicated in children.

Transportation

In major burns, transport is arranged to a hospital, and intravenous fluids (e.g. Hartmann's solution) should be commenced early if delay in transportation is likely. If intravenous fluids are not available, a saline solution can be given orally, in small amounts at first, and later, in increased volume if tolerated. Intravenous morphine is administered and the child wrapped in a clean sheet and covered with a blanket to prevent hypothermia.

Assessment

The severity of a burn depends on the surface area and the depth of damage. The area burnt is more important than the depth, although deep burns cause more shock than superficial scalds of the same area. In children the area and depth of the burn are mapped on a figure chart (Fig. 42.1), which allows an accurate estimation of the area involved, according to age. Unless this estimate is charted carefully the area of the burn may be over-estimated and excessive fluids given.

A full-thickness skin burn (white, charred and painless) is usually obvious early, but partial skin loss may be superficial (erythematous, blistering, and painful white slough) or deep (mottled, red and painless). The depth of partial skin loss may not be evident for several days, even to the trained eye.

Resuscitation

If shock is present or the burn area exceeds 12% of the body surface (less in a young child), intravenous fluids are required, along with morphine (0.05–0.1 mg/kg), given slowly over 3–5 min.

Fluids required during the first 24 h after the burn include:

(1) Maintenance fluids (N/2 saline in 5% dextrose according to weight). One-third the estimated daily requirement is given every 8 h.

(2) Resuscitation fluids: 2–3 mL/kg bodyweight/1% burn surface are given, with one-quarter or one-half of the volume as colloid, for example stable plasma protein solution (SPPS), depending on the severity of the burn, and the remainder as Hartmann's solution. Half of the estimated volume is administered in the first 8 h and a quarter in each of the next two 8 h periods. The volume

required in the second 24 h is approximately half that of the first 24 h.

The rate of intravenous fluid administration depends on the general condition of the child and an expected urine flow of 0.75 mL/kg per h, obtained via a catheter in the bladder. If the expected urine flow is not reached, the intravenous fluid rate is increased, and later decreased once shock has been controlled and urine output established. After approximately 3 days, a diuresis will occur, and the serum electrolytes, urine osmolality and specific gravity will indicate the further requirements.

Blood transfusion rarely is required in the first few days after the burn, but is necessary when anaemia develops, and when the burn is to be excised surgically and grafted.

Milk and other oral fluids are introduced as soon as tolerated, and replace intravenous fluids.

The pH of the gastric juice is estimated regularly in severe burns, and antacids or sucralfate are prescribed to prevent the development of stress ulcers.

Infection

After shock, the next major cause of death is septicaemia, now less likely with modern regimens of antibiotic control.

On admission, swabs are taken from the nose, throat, faeces and the burned areas, but antibiotics are given only if there are specific indications, for example septicaemia, cellulitis or infected burns. Silver sulfadiazine (SSD) with chlorhexidine cream is applied topically to protect the burn from infection. Daily bathing, combined with aseptic techniques in burn dressing, are important factors in limiting infection. The control of *Pseudomonas pyocyaneus* has been dramatic, but multiple resistant staphylococcus can cause problems in serious burns.

Tetanus toxoid is given routinely.

Nutrition

Milk drinks in large volumes are given as early as possible in less severe burns, with added carbohydrate and protein in other drinks, to increase the joule intake. Extra vitamins and iron preparations are given routinely.

In severe burns, hypermetabolism occurs up to 2.5 times above normal and the rate of healing is dependent on the level of nutrition. Adequate nutrition is ensured by supplying maintenance requirements with additional carbohydrate and protein, according to the area burned: the greater the area, the higher the nutritional requirements. Sufficient nutrition, which may be given intravenously or via a gavage feeding tube, overcomes weight loss (the most important indicator of a balanced metabolism), prevents infection, and improves healing.

Wound care

After cleaning the wound with an antiseptic, loose skin is removed and gross blisters punctured, leaving removal of blistered skin to a later date. Very superficial burns, for example sunburn, can be left exposed or covered with a bland ointment, allowing a fine eschar to form; this lifts when the underlying epithelium has healed. Erythematous weeping burns do well with a closed dressing (tulle, or a plastic covering, e.g. Opsite) which is left undisturbed beneath gauze and a firm crepe bandage for 5 days. The inner dressing can be left to separate spontaneously, the outer dressings being changed as necessary.

When there is a burn slough, or a full thickness burn, the area is washed daily with a mild soap, and SSD applied, along with a non-adherent plastic dressing (e.g. Melolin) until healing has occurred or surgical intervention becomes necessary. Burns on the face or buttocks are left exposed, but other areas usually are treated by the closed method, which allows some freedom of movement and close contact with parents.

Surgical treatment

The aim of surgery is to excise dead skin and apply allografts as early as possible. Early skin coverage prevents many problems, including infection, long hospitalization, scar formation and psychological disturbances.

Full-thickness burns are treated as soon as the child has recovered from the shock phase. When a large area has been burned, the child is taken to the theatre twice a week for staged excision and grafting. If there is a lack of patient's skin, a homograft or a xenograft (pig) skin can be used as a 'biological dressing' while waiting to reharvest donor sites. Skin banks for this purpose are necessary.

Deep partial burns will heal in time from deeper cells remaining in the skin appendages but may form ugly hypertrophic scars. As soon as such a burn becomes evident (which may take up to 1 week), the area is submitted to 'tangential' excision, down to a living base of skin matrix, and then grafted.

Scars and contractures

Burn injuries, particularly deep dermal burns, are notorious for becoming hypertrophic and creating ugly scars. These will improve spontaneously but long term pressure garments will accelerate their resolution, and are very worthwhile. Application of silicon and Hypafix are valuable also.

Physiotherapy is employed from the time of admission, to assist movements of the chest, joints and muscles to achieve recovery of full function. Splints and pressure garments are tailored and may be needed for 6–12 months to prevent contractures and scars.

Psychological support and rehabilitation

Psychological support (ideally from parents, siblings and friends) is important during hospitalization and rehabilitation, and may be required for some years. Guilt feelings in the child and parents are common. Discussion groups for parents, and burn support groups should be available to help the child return to a normal life.

Reconstructive surgery

Contractures and scars can lead to functional disabilities and leave cosmetic blemishes. Surgical excision, inlay grafts, and corticosteroid injections may be required until adolescence is reached and active growth has ceased.

FURTHER READING

Carvajal H. F. & Parks D. H. (1988) *Burns in Children*. Year Book Medical, Chicago 106, 193.
Clarke A. M. (1975) Topical use of silver sulphadiazine and chlorhexidine in the prevention of infection in thermal injuries. *Med. J. Aust.* **1**: 413–415.
Solomon J. R. (1981) Care and needs in a children's burns unit. *Prog. Pediatr. Surg.* **14**: 19–32.
Solomon J. R. (1981) Nutrition in the severely burned child. *Prog. Pediatr. Surg.* **14**: 63–79.
Solomon J. R. (1985) Pediatric burns. *Crit. Care Clin.* **1**: 159–173.

— 43 —

Deformities

Deformities may be congenital or acquired, and fixed or mobile. To understand the nature of deformities it is necessary to know the meaning of some orthopaedic terms:

Fixed deformities are those which cannot be corrected by gentle pressure of the examining hand.

Varus and valgus are used according to whether the end of the extremity is displaced towards or away from the midline of the body: for example genu valgum (knock knee), genu varum (bowleg), pes valgus (everted heel).

Equinus is a deformity of the ankle joint in which the foot is plantar-flexed and the child walks with the heel off the ground.

Calcaneus is the opposite of equinus, and the weight is borne on the heel alone.

Cavus is a deformity of the midtarsal joint in which the longitudinal arch is abnormally high.

Planus is the opposite to cavus; the longitudinal arch is flattened.

Plantargrade is a term applied to the foot when no deformity is present and weight is born equally by the heel and the metatarsal heads.

Ankylosis means fixity of a joint: it may be fibrous (e.g. following rheumatoid arthritis) or bony (e.g. following septic arthritis).

METHODS AVAILABLE FOR CORRECTION OF DEFORMITIES OF THE LIMBS

Growth

Many deformities of childhood will correct themselves without treatment of any kind, for example knock knee.

Malunion in fractures often will disappear in the process of remoulding of the bone during growth. In some conditions, however, growth may aggravate the deformity, for example talipes equinus in cerebral palsy.

Manipulation or stretching

This may be carried out daily by a therapist or by the surgeon at less frequent intervals and usually without anaesthesia. In either case manipulation will be useless unless the correction obtained at the time is maintained by a splint or plaster cast; the aim is to obtain gradual correction, and the crushing of young bones and cartilage must be avoided. This form of treatment is common for talipes equinovarus.

Traction

This may be used in fractures to overcome shortening, or in joint diseases to correct a deformity. It may be applied via the skin by strapping or to a bone by a Kirschner wire or a Steinmann pin. In fractures in childhood skin traction is nearly always adequate. Pugh's traction is used commonly; the child lies flat in bed with skin traction on both legs, each attached to a weight over a pulley at the foot of the bed. Bryant's traction ('gallows') is used for femoral fractures in children less than 3 years of age. Russell's traction is the method of choice for fractures of the femur in children over the age of 3 years (Fig. 43.1).

Wedged plasters

These are most useful in correcting the alignment of fractures and deformities of joints. Two-thirds of the circumference of a complete plaster is cut through at the

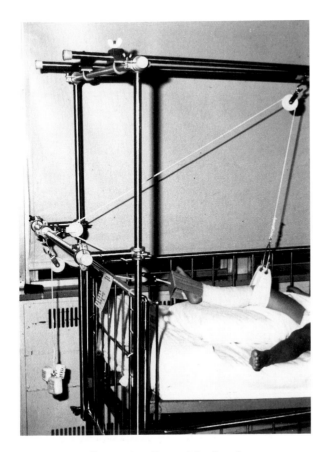

Fig. 43.1 Russell's traction. One weighted cord passes over four pulleys.

site of the deformity, and wedged open as far and as often as required.

Operations on soft tissues

These are used when conservative methods have failed or when experience has shown that surgery in the first instance is preferable. Tendons can be divided, elongated, or re-attached to reinforce or replace other tendons; and contracted fibrous fascial bands, in sheets or in muscles, can be divided or excised.

Bone operations

A long bone may be divided (osteotomy) to correct malunion or ankylosis in an undesirable position, and a joint can be fixed in a desirable position (arthrodesis), often after correction of the pre-existing deformity.

CONGENITAL DEFORMITIES

Very little is known about the causes of congenital deformities. In a few, there is a family history of the same condition, for example congenital dislocation of the hip and to a lesser extent talipes. Some drugs, for example Thalidomide, are well-known to produce fetal abnormalities, but in the majority the cause remains unknown.

Some defects which are present at birth are due to poor 'packaging' *in utero*, for example metatarsus adductus and talipes calcaneus, and these usually recover without treatment. Others are due to defects of 'manufacture' (e.g. talipes equinovarus), and these always require correction.

TORTICOLLIS

The common causes of torticollis in infants and children are, in order of frequency:

(1) Fibrosis in the sternomastoid muscle (Fig. 43.2)

(2) Postural torticollis (a legacy of the position *in utero*)

(3) Cervical hemivertebrae; and

(4) Imbalance of the ocular muscles.

Postural torticollis is present from birth and disappears in a few months. Likewise, the associated plagiocephaly (Chapter 12) and scoliosis do not require treatment, for they are caused by intrauterine moulding.

Cervical hemivertebrae produce a mild angulation of the head and neck. The cause is readily seen in X-rays, which should be taken in all cases of torticollis where the sternomastoid muscle is not tight. No treatment is necessary, for the degree of torticollis is mild and the course is not progressive.

Ocular torticollis is not detectable until the age of 6 months and usually is not noticed until the child is at least 1 or 2 years old. Strabismus suggests that this is the cause, but it is not always obvious and may be latent or intermittent. An ocular imbalance is the most likely cause of torticollis in a child without hemivertebrae, with normal sternomastoid muscles and a full normal range of passive rotation (i.e. the chin can be made to touch each acromion). Treatment is the correction of the imbalance by adjusting the attachment of the eye muscles to the globe.

STERNOMASTOID FIBROSIS

This is found in two groups of patients:

(1) Infants 2–3 weeks old present with a localized swelling in one sternomastoid muscle, that is a sterno-mastoid 'tumour' (Fig. 43.2)

(2) Older children present with torticollis and a tight, short fibrous sternomastoid muscle. Rotation of the head towards the affected side is limited, growth of the face on the side of the affected muscle is reduced (hemihypoplasia of the face; Fig. 43.3) and the ipsilateral trapezius muscle is wasted.

The aetiology is unknown, but prenatal or peri-natal trauma is suspected in some cases. On histology there is endomysial fibrosis around individual muscle fibres, which undergo atrophy.

Clinical features

The 'tumour' is so characteristic that it is diagnostic: a hard, painless spindle-shaped swelling 2–3 cm long in the substance of the sternomastoid muscle. Sometimes the fibrosis may affect the whole length of the muscle.

Angulation of the head is not always present, and the infant can turn the head towards the opposite side without angulation. Plagiocephaly (Chapter 12) is evident in the first 3 months of life as a result of this preferred position, and can be limited by putting the infant down to sleep on each side in turn.

Hemihypoplasia of the face (Fig. 43.3) describes the decreased growth of one side which may occur as a

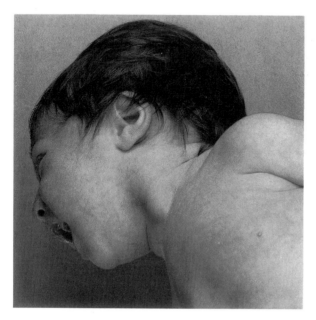

Fig. 43.2 Sternomastoid 'tumour' in an infant.

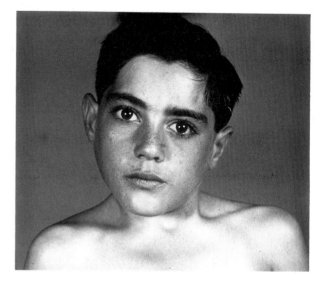

Fig. 43.3 Sternomastoid torticollis. Hypoplasia of the left side of the face and a tight left sternomastoid muscle is apparent.

non-specific result of any type of immobilization and not directly attributable to fibrosis in the sternomastoid.

Treatment

Babies with a sternomastoid 'tumour' should be managed non-operatively, because in 90% it will subside completely in 9–12 months.

In the remaining few the fibrosis causes permanent muscle shortening and persistent torticollis. Division of the sternomastoid muscle is indicated if there is persistent torticollis after the age of 12 months or hemi-hypoplasia of the face. The symmetry of the face improves after operation, but may take several years, and probably never recovers completely.

SCOLIOSIS

The causes of scoliosis are summarized in Table 43.1.

In postural scoliosis, the curvature disappears entirely when the child touches his toes; there is no bony, muscle or nerve abnormality, and the prognosis is excellent. Treatment is the same as for other postural conditions (see below), because a postural curve never develops into a structural curve. In compensatory scoliosis, the legs are unequal in length and the pelvis tilts downwards on the side of the shorter leg, producing the scoliosis. Treatment is directed towards the cause, for example by raising the level of the shoe or by surgical shortening or lengthening of one leg. In structural scoliosis, there is an abnormality in or around the vertebral column (Fig. 43.4).

Clinical features

The first step is to establish that the legs are of equal length by palpating both anterior iliac spines while the child is standing. The next step is to exclude postural scoliosis. The child is asked to touch his toes; if the curve disappears, the scoliosis is postural and no further inquiry is necessary. If it does not disappear, the neurological examination and X-rays of the whole spine will usually indicate which type of scoliosis is present.

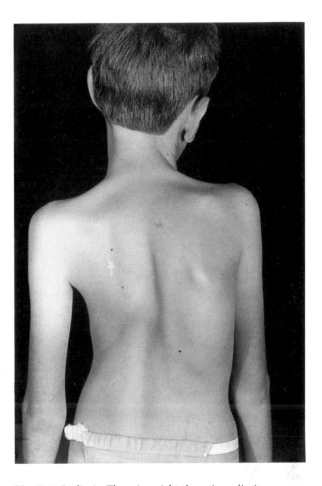

Fig. 43.4 Scoliosis. There is a right thoracic scoliosis producing prominence of the right scapula and ribs due to rotation of the vertebral bodies. The left shoulder is lowered and the left waist is increased. The deformity of the spine and chest is more apparent on forward bending.

Table 43.1 Causes of scoliosis

(1) Postural
(2) Compensatory
(3) Structural:
 —congenital, for example hemivertebrae
 —neuropathic, for example poliomyelitis, neurofibromatosis
 —myopathic, for example muscular dystrophy
 —idiopathic

Treatment

All structural curves tend to worsen with growth. Minor curves should be observed only, and an X-ray taken every 6–12 months. Once the curve becomes decompensated, or measures more than about 40°, active treatment may be indicated with either a brace or surgical fusion of the spine.

'DISCITIS'

This is an unusual inflammatory disease of the intervertebral discs in childhood (Fig. 43.5). The aetiology is not fully understood, although some may be bacterial in origin, that is a form of osteomyelitis.

The lumbar spine is the usual site, and children present with pain in the back and down the legs, refusal to walk or sit, abdominal pain or general irritability and malaise. There is stiffness and reduced mobility in the spine, and X-rays show narrowing of a disc space without any abnormality in the vertebrae (Fig. 43.5).

Osteomyelitis should be suspected in those with pyrexia, severe pain and acute signs, and in this type the treatment is the same as for osteomyelitis in other sites (Chapter 46). All non-suppurative cases are treated by rest. The prognosis is excellent.

KYPHOSIS IN ADOLESCENCE (SCHEUERMANN'S DISEASE)

This is more common in boys and presents in early adolescence. There is irregular growth of the vertebral epiphyseal plates, probably caused by gravity and poor muscular development. The resulting disability is both cosmetic and functional, and pain in the back may develop in later life.

Clinical features

The upper thoracic spine has a kyphotic curve (Fig. 43.6) and greatly limited flexion and extension. X-rays show wedging of the vertebral bodies and irregular ossification in the epiphyseal plates (Fig. 43.7).

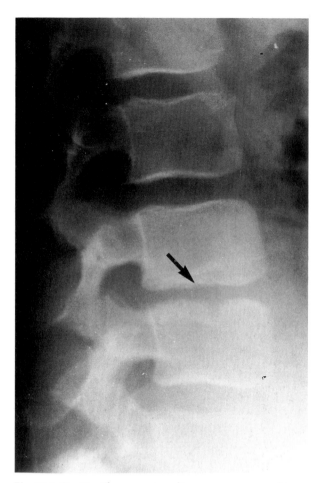

Fig. 43.5 Discitis. The upper two disc spaces are normal in height and shape. The next lower disc space is narrow with irregular margins typical of discitis (arrow).

Treatment

Preventive measures are begun in early adolescence, for example sleeping on a firm flat mattress, extension exercises and active participation in sports. In severe cases a brace is indicated and capable of producing complete correction of the deformity.

CONGENITAL DISLOCATION OF THE HIP

This occurs in 1.5 : 1000 births in Australia. Girls are affected four times more frequently than boys, and in

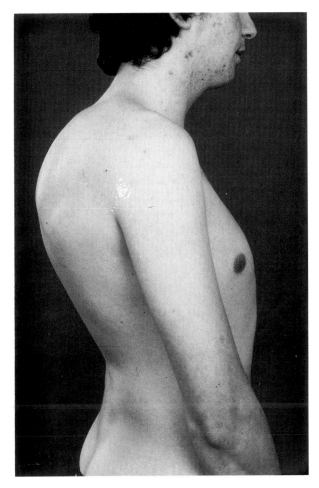

Fig. 43.6 Scheuermann's disease. Severe thoracic kyphosis and increased lumbar lordosis.

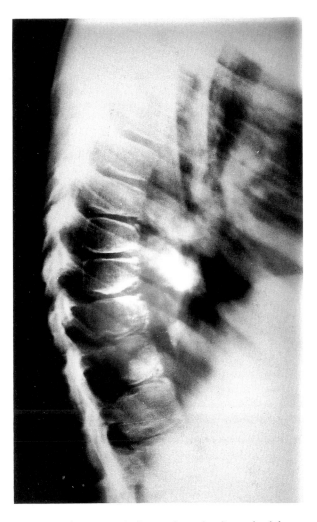

Fig. 43.7 Scheuermann's disease. Lateral radiograph of the thoracic spine showing wedging of the mid-thoracic vertebral bodies with irregularities of the epiphyseal plates.

one of every four cases both hips are dislocated. Heredity undoubtedly plays a part, and there is a higher incidence in the daughters of affected mothers. Capsular laxity at birth (due to hormonal factors), breech delivery, or sudden extension of the hip after birth may be contributory factors.

Early diagnosis

The diagnosis should be made in the first few days of life, because when treatment is commenced at this age, nearly every affected hip will develop normally. The older the patient at the time of diagnosis the less favourable the prognosis.

Diagnosis in infancy is only possible if every newborn is systematically examined for Ortolani's sign (Fig. 43.8). The baby is undressed, placed on a firm bench and given a feed, for the muscles must be completely relaxed and the examination should be gentle. The knees are flexed, each hand grasping a leg so

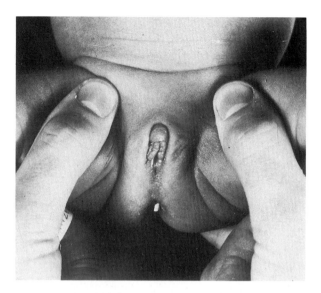

Fig. 43.8 Congenital dislocation of the hips. Ortolani's test: the thumbs are placed over the front of the hip joints as both are fully abducted with the knees and hips flexed.

that the thumb is over the front of the hip and the fingers grasp the trochanter behind; the hips are flexed to a right angle and then abducted as far as possible.

Laxity in the hip joint is detectable without any jerk during abduction of the hips in many babies during the first few days of life, especially if premature or shocked; it usually disappears within a week. Persisting laxity beyond this period is significant and should be treated as a congenital dislocation.

In congenital dislocation of the hip, there is a palpable, visible forward jerk of the head of the femur as it slips over the posterior lip of the acetabulum and becomes reduced at the end of abduction: this is Ortolani's sign.

If a faint click is palpable in the joint, but is not associated with any abnormal movement of the femur on the pelvis it is of no significance.

X-rays in the neonatal period are of no value in diagnosis because the femoral epiphysis does not appear until about 4 months of age. Dynamic ultrasound examination of the hips is undertaken if the clinical signs are equivocal or when the clinical signs are absent in 'at risk' children, that is those with a breech birth and a family history of congenital dislocation of the hip.

Late diagnosis

If the diagnosis is missed at birth, these children do not present until there is delay in walking or an abnormal gait is noted. If the dislocation is unilateral, the gait is typical of an unstable hip, and if bilateral there is a characteristic waddle. The clinical and radiological signs of congenital dislocation of the hip in older children are summarized in Table 43.2 and illustrated in Fig. 43.9.

Treatment

The basic principle is to achieve and maintain reduction.

At birth and in infancy, reduction occurs spontaneously during Ortolani's test, and treatment consists of holding this position in some form of suitable retention (Fig. 43.10) for approximately 3 months. Ultrasound examinations are required to monitor the reduction and development of the acetabulum during harness treatment. An X-ray is taken at 4 months and periodically afterwards. The child is reviewed regularly until growth is completed.

Table 43.2 Signs of congenital dislocation of the hip in older children

Clinical	Radiological (Fig. 43.9)
The leg on the affected side is short	The capital nucleus is smaller on the affected side
The trochanter is high and wide	The acetabulum is shallow and shelved, more like a saucer than a cup
The abductor creases are asymmetrical	The femoral head is displaced outwards and upwards
Abduction of the hip, especially in flexion, is restricted	
Trendelenburg's sign is positive	

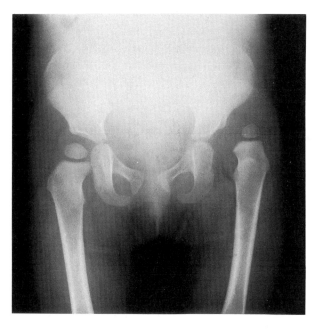

Fig. 43.9 Congenital dislocation of the hip. X-ray showing permanently dislocated hip and poor acetabular development in an infant where the diagnosis was missed at birth.

THE KNEE

Injuries to the knee in childhood are uncommon compared with the high incidence in young adult life, but three traumatic conditions occur: dislocation of the patella, foreign bodies in the knee joint and chondromalacia patellae.

Dislocation of the patella

This is more common in girls and is usually the result of a sudden strain while playing sport. The patella dislocates laterally and the knee is painful and held flexed. The dislocation can be reduced by extending the knee, and a plaster cylinder should be worn for 3 weeks followed by a limited-motion knee orthosis and physiotherapy. Failure to treat the initial episode properly can lead to recurrent dislocations.

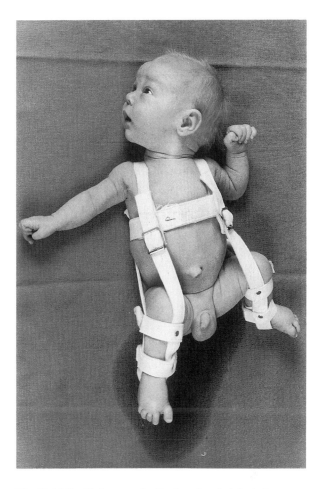

Fig. 43.10 Pavlik harness. In the flexed and abducted position the dislocated hip is held in the reduced position.

Foreign bodies in the knee joint

The knee joint is subcutaneous and prone to penetrating injury by needles or splinters of glass and wood. The possibility of a foreign body in the joint should be borne in mind when a child presents after the supposedly total removal of a foreign body from this region. If part of the foreign body has been retained, the wound must be thoroughly explored and the joint cavity opened; but this must be done under general anaesthesia and using a tourniquet.

Chondromalacia patellae

This is common in adolescents and presents with pain in the knee, which is reproduced when the patella is pressed against the femur. Occasionally, there is a history of locking. The condition always resolves with time and healing is not influenced by any form of treatment, conservative or operative. Other rare causes of internal derangements, for example a loose body or an injury to the meniscus, should be excluded.

SWELLINGS AROUND THE KNEE JOINT

Three types of swelling occur in this area: Osgood-Schlatter's disease (Chapter 45), semimembranosus bursa and cysts of the lateral meniscus.

Semimembranosus bursa

This bursa becomes distended with fluid and forms a cystic swelling on the back of the leg just below the joint line and towards the medial side. It may cause a little discomfort, but treatment is unnecessary and the condition almost always resolves, although it may take many months or years.

Cyst of the lateral meniscus

On the lateral portion of the joint line there is a swelling which disappears when the knee is flexed. It is due to cystic degeneration of the meniscus, and if pain (usually most troublesome at night) persists, arthroscopy and partial meniscectomy is necessary.

OSTEOCHONDRITIS DISSECANS

This can occur in various sites, but is most common in the lateral aspect of the medial femoral condyle or the lateral femoral condyle. There is a localized area of aseptic necrosis in the subchondral bone, and the overlying cartilage is involved secondarily. The cause is obscure, but is probably traumatic.

Clinical features

There is intermittent swelling, aching, and a small effusion of the knee, as well as some wasting of the quadriceps femoris. When the fragment has separated, there is a click on movement and/or episodes of locking. X-rays using standard views of the knee may not show the lesion, which can be seen clearly in special projections (Fig. 43.11).

Treatment

In children under 10 years of age with the fragment still *in situ*, healing is the rule and only some restriction of sport is needed. X-rays are taken every 3 months to follow its progress, and reincorporation may take up to 12 months.

After the age of 10 years, separation of the fragment is likely (and in adults is the rule). Treatment is withheld until full separation occurs and then the loose body is removed at arthroscopy.

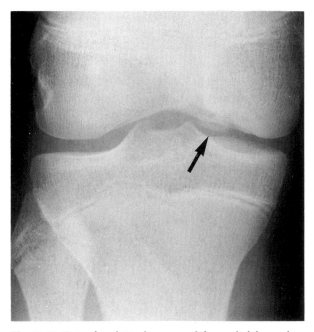

Fig. 43.11 Osteochondritis dissecans of the medial femoral condyle, the usual site. The fragment is partially detached.

THE FOOT

Feet vary so much in size, shape and posture that it is difficult to define 'normal'. However, they are regarded as normal if they function normally in standard footwear without subsequently deforming it.

The height of the longitudinal arch is not important, but if it is too high (pes cavus) it is difficult to fit a shoe and prone to metatarsalgia in later life; if too low (pes planus) it is liable to strain.

The final shape of the foot is probably determined more by genes than by treatment.

Talipes

This is a general term for any foot which is not plantargrade; the deformity may be congenital or acquired (paralytic, spastic, ischaemic, etc.). Congenital talipes occurs in two forms: equinovarus and calcaneovalgus.

Talipes calcaneovalgus

This is a defect in which the foot has been folded back against the front of the tibia (Fig. 43.12). The deformity produced is mobile and easily corrected, and treatment is not required unless there are secondary contractures in front of the ankle, in which case a short period of splinting in equinus is desirable.

Talipes equinovarus

This occurs in 1 : 1000 births and is nearly twice as common in males as in females. The diagnosis is made at birth: the foot is held rigidly in equinus and varus, and passive correction is not possible (Fig. 43.13). The calf muscles are poorly developed, and the foot and leg are slightly shorter on the affected side.

In the normal newborn the feet are often held inverted so that the soles face each other, but the feet can be moved easily into calcaneovalgus. Talipes may be associated with other abnormalities, for example congenital dislocation of the hip, or a more general defect such as arthrogryposis (see below).

The aim of treatment is to correct, and then overcorrect, the deformity as soon as possible after birth and to retain correction until skeletal maturity. There is a persistent tendency to relapse and constant supervision is required. Correction must never be forcible, especially in the newborn, for it is more likely to crush the fragile tarsal bones and destroy articular cartilage than to stretch contracted ligaments and muscles.

Denis Browne splints are used in the initial correction in which the feet are secured to the sole plates by adhesive strapping and connected by a metal bar which holds them in eversion. The splints should be renewed

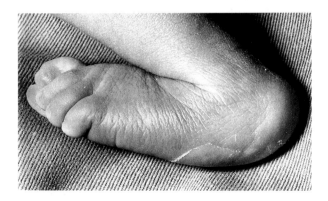

Fig. 43.12 Congenital talipes calcaneovalgus. The foot has been folded back against the front of the tibia, but there is no fixed deformity.

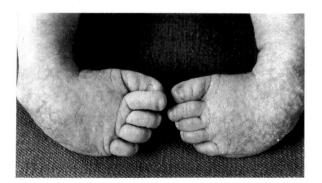

Fig. 43.13 Congenital talipes equinovarus. The foot lies in a typical position and is rigid.

at intervals of 2–3 weeks and full correction should be obtained within 6 weeks of birth. However, the splint must be retained for 4–6 months, by which time the feet are large enough to control in a calcaneus night-splint.

If correction proves difficult, or if relapse occurs quickly, surgical release of the contracted structures in the calf and ankle may be required in the first 12 months. A series of plaster casts may be used as an alternative, but whichever method is chosen, a high degree of skill is required and these infants should be treated by a paediatric orthopaedic surgeon.

Flat feet

When a child first stands, the feet always appear flat, because the longitudinal arch is filled with a pad of fat and incomplete control causes the foot to roll over into valgus. Hypotonic children may develop extremely flat feet, and require arch supports.

The common form of postural flat foot persists, in diminishing degrees, until the age of 3 years, at which time the feet begin to assume their final form. It is very doubtful that wedges on the inner edges of the heels do any good and their use is not recommended. Similarly, arch supports have little value in the otherwise normal child except perhaps to prevent distortion of the shoes.

Extreme pes valgus in early adolescence may require surgery.

Pes cavus

The longitudinal arch is high, the toes are clawed, and the heel may be turned into varus (Fig. 43.14). The deformity may be familial or may occur in neurological conditions such as Friedreich's ataxia, poliomyelitis and sciatic palsy, or in anomalies of the lumbar spine.

Children with pes cavus usually present after the age of 7 years with the complaint that shoes are difficult to fit and rapidly lose their shape.

Careful neurological assessment is required before treatment is commenced. In severe cases the plantar fascia is divided and the foot moulded into a better shape and held in plaster.

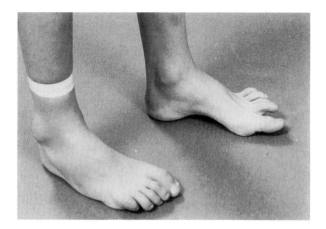

Fig. 43.14 Pes cavus. Both feet have high arches and claw toes.

Metatarsus adductus

In most newborn babies, the feet tend to curve medially with the forefoot adducted on the hindfoot so that the inner border is concave (Fig. 43.15). When this is marked it is called metatarsus adductus; it has a natural tendency to disappear during growth.

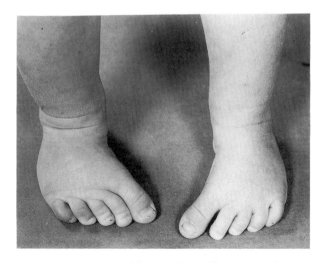

Fig. 43.15 Metatarsus adductus. The midfoot and forefoot are adducted, but the heel is normal.

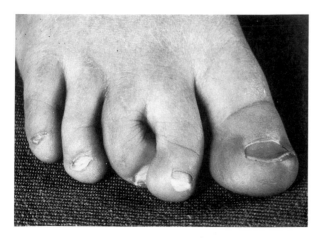

Fig. 43.16 Curly third toe due to contracture of the flexor tendon.

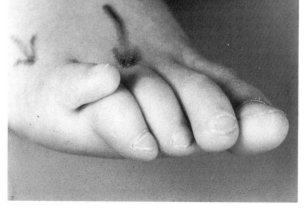

Fig. 43.17 Over-riding fifth toe.

In a few children this posture persists beyond the age of 18 months and treatment is necessary. The most simple form of treatment is wearing shoes both day and night. Sometimes serial plasters are required for correction.

Hammer toes

One or more toes are held in flexion by a congenital contracture of the flexor tendon (Fig. 43.16). Contracture of the long flexor produces a C-shaped toe, and of the short flexor tendon, a Z shape. Splinting and strapping are ineffective, and in most cases the flexor tendons will require division. This should be delayed until 3 years of age, for spontaneous improvement occasionally occurs in the early years.

Overlapping little toe

This is usually bilateral and often familial. The little toe is directed medially and overlies the base of the fourth toe, being held there by a tight skin fold and a contracted extensor tendon (Fig. 43.17). The position of the toe is not compatible with normal footwear and should be corrected surgically after the age of 5 years.

Painful heels

Two conditions cause pain at the back of the heel in children between 10 and 15 years of age.

An enlarged posterolateral angle of the os calcis rubs on the counter of the shoe and the skin becomes reddened or, later, bruised. Most of these children can be helped by softening the counter of the shoe, although in few the 'exostosis' must be removed.

Pain in the heel may occur after playing sport and is probably due to a strain of the insertion of the tendo-Achilles or to minor trauma to the apophyseal plate. The symptoms always disappear as the child becomes more mature, and can be relieved by raising the heel half an inch. Restriction of activity is not necessary.

ARTHROGRYPOSIS MULTIPLEX CONGENITA

This is an uncommon clinical syndrome in which contractures or absence of muscles cause rigidity or, dislocation of joints (especially the hip), and absence of skin creases, producing a 'featureless' cylindrical limb.

The aetiology is unknown, but the basic lesion appears to be muscular rather than neural, and is sometimes confined to one limb. More often all joints in all four limbs are involved to a variable degree, and the spine and jaw may also be affected. Intelligence is not impaired.

Correction is difficult and there is a liability to relapse. Serial plasters and splints are useful in some situations, but surgical release and lengthening of contracted muscles are often required, especially in the knees and feet.

FURTHER READING

Williams P. F. & Cole W. G. (eds) (1991) *Orthopaedic Management in Childhood*, 2nd edn. Chapman & Hall, London.

Tachdjian M. O. (1990) *Pediatric Orthopedics*, 2nd edn. W. B. Saunders, Philadelphia.

Morrissy R. T. (1990) *Lovell and Winter's Pediatric Orthopedics*, 3rd edn. J. B. Lippincott, Philadelphia.

Dandy D. J. (1989) *Essential Orthopaedics and Trauma*. Churchill Livingstone, Edinburgh.

44

Posture and Gait

Children change in shape and proportion as they grow. At a given age, the posture may be quite different from that of the adult, and it is essential that these 'normal' variants are recognized so that unnecessary treatment can be avoided.

Sometimes there is an accentuation of a normal component of posture, which must be considered abnormal and is unlikely to correct spontaneously during further growth. Some form of simple treatment or restriction of certain activities, is usually all that is required to help normal growth work effectively.

Importantly, posture at any age may be influenced by organic disease, for example chronic respiratory infection, and emotional disorders.

THE SPINE

In the erect position the spine should be straight when viewed from behind, but in profile there is a series of curves which change with growth, and individuals differ widely in the curves they exhibit when growth is completed.

After birth the infant lies on the side with the spine curved like a banana from occiput to sacrum. At about 2 months of age head control is achieved and the cervical spine develops its characteristic curve, concave posteriorly. When the infant can sit up at 6–8 months the lordotic lumbar curve develops and the thoracic spine becomes much straighter. When walking starts, the lumbar lordosis is exaggerated, the child is pot-bellied and walks on a broad base with steps of varying length and direction.

In later childhood the same curvatures are maintained, but the exaggerated lumbar lordosis should decrease. If it does not, the posture is poor. Similarly, the dorsal curve may increase and, together with collapse of tone in the scapular and cervical muscles, produce the round-shouldered child.

All these postural abnormalities can be corrected by voluntary effort, so if any treatment is required, the effort must be supplied by the child, not the therapist.

THE LEGS

The legs of normal children are not straight. Nevertheless, the phases of normal growth may cause parents great anxiety, and are common reasons for referral.

Treatment rarely is required, but effective reassurance must include an explanation of the facts.

Bow legs

In the first 2 years of life the tibia has an outward curve and an inward twist (internal torsion), which is often unnoticed until the child first stands and appears to be bandy and pigeon-toed. The outer border of the foot is presented to the floor so that the ankle rolls over into valgus and accentuates the normal 'flat' appearance of the feet at this age (Fig. 44.1).

Bow legs usually are more pronounced in very sturdy children, and may increase for the first 6 months after walking begins. Later, spontaneous improvement occurs and by the age of 2 years the appearance of the tibia has returned to normal.

A careful explanation is the mainstay of treatment. Orthoses are ineffective and osteotomies rarely are required.

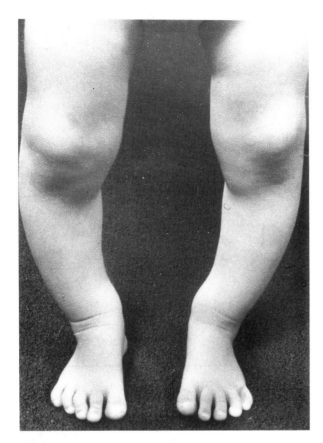

Fig. 44.1 Bow legs: the tibia has an outward curve and an inward twist (internal torsion), both of which accentuate the normal 'flat' appearance of the feet.

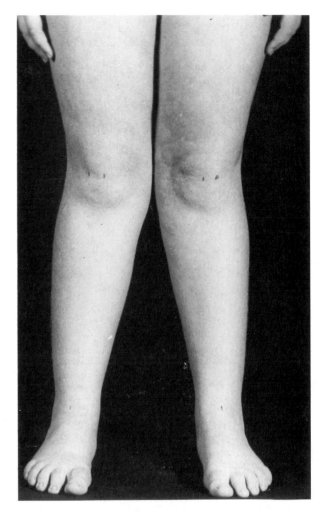

Fig. 44.2 Knock knees, 'genu valgum'.

Knock knees

Shortly after the age of 2 years, the legs may develop a knock-knee posture (genu valgum, Fig. 44.2) which increases to a maximum at the age of $3\frac{1}{2}$ years, at which stage gradual improvement begins, continuing until the legs are finally 'straight' at 6–7 years.

The deformity is caused by unequal growth in the femoral condyles so that the plane of the knee joint becomes oblique. It is not due to laxity of the ligaments of the knee joint.

Treatment is not required, except in children who are excessively overweight, and then it is directed to their diet; the legs will look after themselves. The traditional wedged heels have no proven value, are expensive to maintain, and merely make the child more awkward on his feet. Surgery is rarely required.

'In-toeing'

This is a common presenting complaint, and has three different causes:

Metatarsus adductus

The foot itself may be incurved (metatarsus adductus, Chapter 43), a posture often seen at birth and which has a natural tendency to correct in the first few years. The shoes may be worn on the opposite feet, both day and night, for several months if the condition is marked. Very occasionally, correction in plaster casts or splints may be necessary.

Tibial intorsion

In children under 2 years of age, tibial intorsion (usually accompanied by bowing) causes the child to walk 'in-toed'. Spontaneous correction of the torsion often lags behind that of the bowing, but is usually complete by $2\frac{1}{2}$ years.

The 'inset' hip

In the adult, the ranges of external and internal rotation of the hip are equal and in walking the feet point straight ahead. In many children, however, there are 90° of internal rotation and only 10° of external rotation, so that the walking position corresponds to 40° of internal rotation and the hip is said to be 'inset'.

These children can:

(1) Sit on the floor with their thighs together and the medial surface of both knees in contact with the floor (Fig. 44.3)

(2) Walk with both the knees and feet turned inwards

(3) Run in an ugly fashion, throwing their feet out sideways

(4) Appear bandy, because the legs when viewed from the side are slightly curved, and the plane of the curve changes as the legs are internally and externally rotated

(5) Develop secondary flat feet as they roll out into valgus in an attempt to overcome the in-toeing.

The 'inset' hip may present in a variety of ways, and its recognition is important in understanding many of the problems of posture and gait.

Treatment is unnecessary, for the arc of rotation is adjusted slowly during growth and, in most cases,

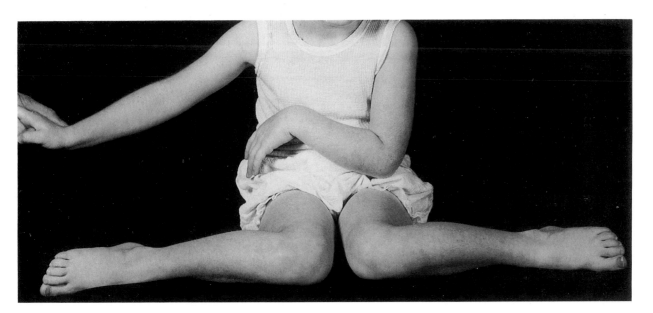

Fig. 44.3 The inset hip: the child can sit on the floor with her thighs together and the medial surface of both knees in contact with the floor.

normality is reached at maturity. Occasionally, a small degree persists into adult life. At worst, this is only a minor cosmetic problem.

THE TREATMENT OF POSTURAL DEFECTS

Many defects of posture correct themselves in the course of normal growth; treatment is not indicated but careful explanation of the natural history is essential. However, in some children with poor spinal posture, active measures are advisable. It is necessary to make a distinction between 'exercise' and 'exercises'. Formal programmes of exercises are of limited value, whether supervised by a therapist or a parent. Instead, emphasis should be placed on sports such as swimming, gymnastic activities and all forms of group sport. The child is encouraged to be 'normal' rather than 'abnormal', and the emphasis is on play rather than medical treatment.

FURTHER READING

Williams P. F. & Cole W. G. (eds) (1991) *Orthopaedic Management in Childhood*, 2nd edn. Chapman & Hall, London.

45

The Child with a Limp

'Gait' is the term applied to the rhythmic movements of the whole body in walking, and a limp is an abnormality of gait. It is one of the commonest presenting symptoms in childhood, and is frequently painless. The causes (Table 45.1) range from a plantar papilloma (wart) or unsuitable footwear to a cerebral tumour, and considerable clinical acumen may be required to identify the cause.

INVESTIGATIONS

A careful history includes the duration of the limp, its progression and associated symptoms. A prolonged labour, prematurity, neonatal anoxia or jaundice, or delay in reaching the developmental milestones, suggest cerebral damage.

Physical examination begins by observing the child walking in underpants, in an attempt to recognize the pattern of the limp. With experience it is possible to reach a working diagnosis by observation alone. Hopping on one leg at a time is a valuable test, for if this can be done normally, it is unlikely that the cause of the limp is of much importance. While the patient is on his feet, spinal movements are tested and the anterior iliac spines are palpated to determine whether the legs are of equal length.

Finally, each hip is tested for Trendelenburg's sign. When a normal child stands on one leg, the buttock on the opposite side rises slightly; if it falls, the test is

Table 45.1 The child with a limp: Causes

Age (years)	Common conditions	Uncommon conditions

1–2	Spiral fracture of the tibia
	Cerebral palsy
	Congenital dislocation of the hip
		Congenital abnormalities causing short leg, for example
		  Coxa vara
		  Hemiatrophy
		  Short femur

2–5	Mono-articular synovitis Mild spastic hemiplegia Perthes' disease	Muscular dystrophies
5–10	'Irritable hip' Perthes' disease Kohler's disease	
10–15	Slipped upper femoral epiphysis Osgood-Schlatter's disease	Hysteria
All age groups	Trauma Osteomyelitis Suppurative arthritis	Spinal infections Tumours

positive and indicates that there is instability of the weight-bearing hip joint. A soft flat buttock on the affected side is evidence of a lesion in the hip joint which has caused wasting in the gluteal muscles.

The child then is placed supine on the examination couch. Attention is directed first to the area under suspicion, for example a complete neurological examination is performed when cerebral palsy is suspected.

The real and apparent lengths of the legs are measured, and fixed flexion in the hip joint is sought by Thomas's test. This involves flexing the normal hip up onto the abdomen to remove the lumbar lordosis; a flexion deformity is present if the other hip cannot be extended to lie flat on the couch.

Each joint in the lower extremities is examined for swelling, tenderness and restricted movements. The soles of the feet are examined, as are the shoes, for evidence of abnormal wear on the outside and projections on the inside.

TYPES OF ABNORMAL GAIT

Spastic gait

A child with a spastic hemiplegia holds the arm flexed at the elbow and tends to walk on the toes of the affected leg; the diplegic is recognized by a tendency to 'scissoring', that is crossing the legs in full adduction when trying to walk.

Ataxic gait

An ataxic gait is characterized by a lack of balance and co-ordination with a tendency to trip and fall, and difficulty in negotiating corners or doorways.

'Antalgic' gait

When there is a painful lesion in the lower extremity the weight is transferred to the good leg as quickly as possible, and when walking is very painful, a hopping gait is the result.

Trendelenburg's gait

In an unstable hip, active abduction while weight-bearing is impossible so that the affected hip is pushed into passive abduction by the muscles in the opposite leg. The shoulder on the affected side drops sharply, and when both hips are affected the gait becomes a waddle.

Short-leg gait

This can be recognized easily, for the pelvis tilts when the patient stands up, and during walking the opposite knee remains slightly bent.

Hysterical gait

When the gait is bizarre and no obvious cause can be found, hysteria should be suspected. It is not unknown in older children, but the diagnosis must be made only after all other causes have been eliminated. With the information obtained from clinical examination, a tentative diagnosis usually can be made.

COMMON ABNORMALITIES OF GAIT

The commonest orthopaedic causes of a limp in childhood are:
(1) 'Irritable hip'
(2) Perthes' disease
(3) Slipped upper femoral epiphysis (less common than the other two).

Tuberculosis is exceptionally rare in Australia, but should be considered in areas where the incidence is still significant.

The 'irritable hip'

The commonest disease of the hip joint in childhood is a synovitis of uncertain origin and short duration which is relieved by rest. Trauma, viruses and even allergy may play a part.

Clinical features

The child, usually between 2 and 5 years of age, presents with a painless limp of short duration, and on examination there may be no evidence of general illness or toxaemia. There may be a slight fever at the onset, but the white cell count usually is normal, and as a rule the only abnormal findings on examination are protective spasm and some limitation of all movements in the hip joint, particularly abduction. X-rays show nothing unusual, or only slight regional osteoporosis.

Differential diagnosis

Although most patients quickly respond to rest, it may be difficult to be sure that it is not an early stage of a more serious condition. Rheumatic fever and rheumatoid arthritis may present in this way, but the subsequent course will distinguish them.

Suppurative arthritis, either primary, or secondary to osteomyelitis of the upper end of the femur, must be identified or excluded as soon as possible (Chapter 46). When the signs are more severe, with fever and toxaemia, the hip joint should be aspirated with a wide-bore needle under general anaesthesia, and blood for culture obtained at the same time. X-rays are normal initially and fail to show any evidence of changes in the bone for 7–14 days. The white cell count is raised, for example, above 10 000/mm, and polymorphs predominate (Chapter 46).

Treatment of the irritable hip

Bed rest with both legs in skin traction is continued for 1–2 weeks or until there is a full range of painless movement. When traction is removed, active movements in bed are permitted, and if there is no recurrence of signs, the patient is allowed to bear weight on the leg 1 week later. A further examination, including X-rays, should be carried out 1–2 months later.

Perthes' disease (Legge-Calvé-Perthes; pseudocoxalgia)

This is a form of osteochondritis juvenilis which affects the head of the femur, mainly in boys (80%) between 3 and 10 years of age. In 10% of children both hips are affected.

The cause is unknown, though trauma is believed to be at least partly responsible.

Clinical features

There is an intermittent painless limp, but sometimes pain and disability are more severe. On examination the typical findings are slight limitation of some (but not all) movements of the hip joint, especially abduction in flexion. Wasting of the gluteal muscles produces a flat soft buttock on the affected side. Trendelenburg's sign is present in established cases.

Radiology

The typical X-ray sign in the early stages (Fig. 45.1) is 'widening' of the joint space, decalcification in the metaphysis and the femoral head becomes more dense

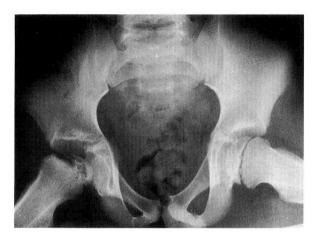

Fig. 45.1 Typical X-ray appearance of Perthes' disease.

and slightly flattened. Later still, the head becomes fragmented and vacuolated as osteoid tissue gradually replaces the nucleus.

Finally, the uniform texture of the normal femoral head is restored, but the femoral neck may remain both wider and shorter than on the unaffected side.

Natural history and prognosis

Most affected children have a painless intermittent limp for approximately 2 years and during this period can live a relatively normal life. A few develop stiffness in the hip and a severe limp. Some develop deformity of the femoral head, which may lead to pain or osteo-arthritis of the hip in later life. Various factors influence the prognosis in Perthes' disease (Table 45.2).

Treatment

For the patient with a good prognosis, the parents are reassured and told that the child may be normally active without damaging the hip. The child should not do prolonged walking or exercise. Vigorous con-tact sports are avoided but swimming is encouraged. The child may need admission to hospital for a short period to rest the leg in Pugh's traction or slings.

Table 45.2 Factors influencing prognosis in Perthes' disease

Factor	Good prognosis	Poor prognosis
Age of onset	Under 6 years of age	Over 8 years of age
Amount of femoral head involved	The anterior portion	The whole head
Extension of the head outside the limits of the acetabulum	Little or none	Marked extension
Movement present in the affected joint	Little restriction	Gross restriction

Progress is assessed by 4 monthly clinical and radio-logical examinations.

For the patient with a poor prognosis, it is neces-sary to contain the head of the femur within the acetabulum so that the acetabulum will act as a mould for the soft head, leading to maintenance of the normal spherical shape of the femoral head. Containment can be achieved by:

(1) A plaster cast, or orthosis (splint), which holds the legs apart while allowing flexion and extension at the hip

(2) Osteotomy of the pelvis to turn the acetabulum forward and laterally over the femoral head

(3) Osteotomy of the femur, with varus angulation at the osteotomy site, to turn the head under the acetabulum.

Slipped upper femoral epiphysis

This is most common in tall, fat boys between 10 and 15 years of age who have relatively small external genitalia; in 20% both hips are involved. The cause is uncertain, although an endocrine basis is suggested by the general facies, the age and sex incidence, and the number of bilateral cases.

The epiphysis may slip suddenly ('acute' slip) or gradually ('chronic' slip), and it slides backwards and downwards so that the leg rolls out into external rota-tion; there is an associated synovitis in the hip.

Clinical features

The boy with an acute slip has all the features of a fracture of the neck of the femur. He cannot walk, the leg lies in full external rotation, and attempts to move the leg cause pain.

In a chronic slip there is a history of ache in the hip, thigh or knee for several months, and an 'antalgic' limp has developed. On examination there is a slightly 'irri-table' hip and a variable degree of fixed external rotation depending on the degree of slip. These symptoms and signs may be passed off as a 'sprained hip', but there is no such condition.

Radiology

The earliest X-ray evidence is widening and irregularity of the epiphyseal plate. A line drawn on the X-ray film along the upper border of the neck of the femur normally passes through the lateral aspect of the head; when it misses the head, slipping has occurred (Fig. 45.2). A lateral view is essential, for it shows that the axis of the femoral neck and that of the epiphysis no longer coincide.

Treatment

In an acute slip, avascular necrosis of the femoral head is a common outcome. To reduce the incidence of this complication the haematoma in the hip is aspirated urgently under general anaesthesia. The femoral head is reduced over several days with skeletal traction and then secured with one or more threaded pins. Weight bearing is deferred until fusion of the epiphyseal plate is complete.

In a chronic slip, the femoral head is pinned without attempting to improve the position. Avascular necrosis occurs rarely in a chronic slip.

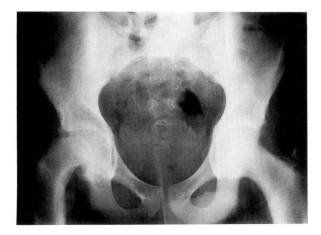

Fig. 45.2 Anteroposterior view of hip in slipped upper femoral epiphysis.

Osteochondritis juvenilis

This is the name given to several conditions with a similar natural history and which involve the epiphyses of growing bones. In general they are troublesome rather than serious and have a self-limiting course over about 2 years, during which there is a cycle of radiographic changes terminating in the restoration of normal texture, though not always normal shape.

The clinical symptoms are a mild ache and (in some cases) a variable degree of reflex muscular spasm. Each site of osteochondritis has an eponymous name, and each is a distinct clinical entity with a slightly different age incidence (Table 45.3).

Osgood-Schlatter's disease

This affects the tibial tuberosity at the insertion of the ligamentum patellae, predominantly in boys between 8 and 14 years of age.

The presenting symptoms are swelling, an ache after strenuous activities and pain on kneeling. The tibial tuberosity is enlarged and tender. X-rays show fragmentation of the tibial tuberosity.

The symptoms are more a nuisance than incapacitating, and management is based on a full explanation of the condition to the patient and his parents, including the information that it is self-limiting and that although it may last months, there will be no permanent

Table 45.3 Osteochondritis

	Peak age range (years)
Tarsal navicular (Köhler's disease)	5
The head of a metatarsal (Frieberg disease)	14–18
The patella (Larsen-Johansson disease)	
The vertebral epiphyseal plates (Scheuermann's disease)	13–16
The capitellum of the radius (Panner's disease)	
The carpal scaphoid (Kienböck's disease)	
Perthes' disease	3–10
Osgood-Schlatter's disease	8–14

disability. It is one of the 'over-use syndromes' in which the load applied to the tendon attachment is excessive.

The amount of discomfort is variable; when severe, it can be alleviated by wearing a plaster cylinder for a month.

In general, this condition does not prevent a boy from doing what he wants to do. He may continue playing sport if he wishes; his knee will hurt, but it will come to no additional harm.

FURTHER READING

Williams P. F. & Cole W. G. (eds) (1991) *Orthopaedic Management in Childhood*, 2nd edn. Chapman & Hall, London.

46

Bone and Joint Infections

OSTEOMYELITIS

Osteomyelitis usually is due to a *Staphylococcus aureus* infection of the metaphysis of the lower femur or upper tibia (Table 46.1).

In early-acute osteomyelitis, the child is unwell and febrile for less than 24 h and refuses to use the involved limb. Careful examination reveals reduced or absent spontaneous motion of the limb, and swelling and tenderness over a metaphysis. At this early stage there are no signs of a subperiosteal abscess. The adjoining joint is non-tender and X-rays are normal.

In late-acute osteomyelitis there is a severe systemic illness and marked local signs including the features of a subperiosteal abscess. The X-rays are abnormal after 10 days, but the radiological abnormalities appear a few days earlier in neonates. Late-acute osteomyelitis usually occurs because of delay in diagnosis, particularly in neonates and infants, but is sometimes seen in children over the age of 10 years.

Neonatal osteomyelitis

There are two clinical forms:

(1) A severe and life-threatening septicaemia culminating in inflammation in a long bone, typically the upper end of the femur or around the knee joint. Multiple sites are often involved

(2) In the more common form there is a misleadingly benign course, with virtually no general systemic symptoms and minimal local signs which are easily overlooked despite advanced destruction of the bone. Typically the infant is 5 or 6 weeks of age and afebrile, feeding and sleeping normally, but cries when the napkins are changed. Movement of the hip causes pain and there is a mass from an underlying abscess. X-rays

taken on the day of diagnosis commonly show extensive bone damage.

Smith's arthritis of the hip is primarily osteomyelitis of the upper end of the femur which has already involved the hip joint. Pathological dislocation of the hip and necrosis of the head of the femur are common and may be already present at the time of diagnosis.

Osteomyelitis in older children

Delay in the diagnosis of acute osteomyelitis is common in children over the age of 10 years, when it may be confused with other causes of acute limb pain such as sprains or sporting injuries, and when it involves the pelvis or spine.

Treatment

Early diagnosis and treatment is vital because early-acute cases can be cured. Late-acute cases have more

Table 46.1 Sites of acute osteomyelitis in 61 consecutive admissions

Site	No.
Femur	17
Tibia	15
Fibula	5
Radius	4
Ulna	3
Humerus, ileum, metatarsal, phalanx, maxilla	2 each
Neonates (multiple sites)	3
Cervical, os calcis, skull, mandible	1 each
Total	61

extensive bone destruction and occasionally irreversible damage to adjoining growth plates.

(1) Blood is collected for culture. *Staphylococcus aureus* is the commonest organism. There is no need to aspirate the periosteal region

(2) Intravenous flucloxacillin (100–200 mg/kg per day in four doses) is used to combat *Staphylococcus aureus*. Alternative antibiotics may be required according to the organism responsible and its sensitivities. Gentamicin is added in neonates

(3) The limb is immobilized in a plaster slab designed to allow repeated examination of the area affected

(4) Open drainage of subperiosteal pus is required in approximately 20% of cases of acute osteomyelitis. The underlying bone is not drilled.

Patients with early-acute osteomyelitis respond to treatment rapidly, with resolution of the systemic and local signs in a few days; at which stage oral antibiotics are commenced. A single antibiotic is used if an organism has been cultured, but if cultures are negative flucloxacillin (100 mg/kg per day in four doses) orally is continued for a total of 3 weeks in early-acute osteomyelitis, and for a minimum of 6 weeks in late-acute osteomyelitis. Cure is expected in the early-acute cases, while late-acute cases may require further treatment because of damage to the growth plate in young children or sequestra in older children.

SUPPURATIVE ARTHRITIS

Suppurative arthritis results from blood-borne infection of the synovial membrane. *Staphylococcus aureus* is common while *Haemophilus influenzae* is found in 25% of children between 4 months and 4 years of age. Suppurative arthritis also presents as an early-acute or late-acute illness.

In the early-acute case there is a systemic illness with fever and local signs of acute synovitis. The joint is swollen, tender and there is restriction of movement in all directions. Tenderness is maximal over the joint line, with no tenderness over the metaphysis. It may be difficult to distinguish from osteomyelitis when the infection involves the shoulder or hip joints, but in many neonates and infants both the bone and joint are involved.

Late diagnosis of suppurative arthritis is common in neonates, infants and in children over 10 years of age. In neonates and infants, this is usually due to failure to recognize that there is an abnormality in the limb, whereas in the older child, delay results from confusion with other diseases, for example rheumatoid arthritis.

Treatment

(1) Blood is collected for culture

(2) Under general anaesthesia, the affected joint is aspirated and the joint fluid cultured. If the pus aspirated is thin, a joint such as the knee and elbow can be washed out with normal saline. In the hip and shoulder, which are difficult to aspirate, an arthrotomy is preferable. If aspiration of the hip yields clear fluid, it is likely that the child has the 'irritable hip syndrome' (Chapter 45), not a suppurative infection.

(3) Intravenous antibiotics (flucloxacillin and amoxycillin 75 mg/kg per day in three doses) are commenced after samples have been obtained for culture. Antibiotics may need to be changed according to the organisms cultured and their sensitivities

(4) The limb is immobilized in a suitable plaster slab designed to permit repeated examination of the area affected.

Oral antibiotics are commenced after acute symptoms and signs have settled; cefaclor is used if the cultures are negative, but a suitable single antibiotic is continued for a total of 3 weeks in early-acute cases, and 6 weeks in late-acute cases. Cure is to be expected in early-acute cases of suppurative arthritis, but in late-acute cases the end result depends upon whether there is damage to the articular cartilage.

DIFFERENTIAL DIAGNOSIS OF THE CHILD WITH AN ACUTE LIMB

A variety of clinical conditions causing similar symptoms may prove difficult to distinguish and tend to delay diagnosis and treatment of bone and joint infections

(Table 46.2). Careful clinical and radiological assessment is required.

Osteomyelitis is characterized by acute tenderness over a metaphysis.

Cellulitis may be confused with osteomyelitis, but the initial treatment is the same. X-rays taken at least 10 days after the onset of the illness will distinguish cellulitis from osteomyelitis. A nuclide bone scan also may distinguish these conditions.

Suppurative arthritis causes inflammatory changes that are maximal over the joint with limitation of all movements.

Other causes of acute arthritis may be confused with suppurative arthritis: rheumatic fever, viral arthritis, and Henoch-Schönlein purpura.

An undisplaced spiral fracture of the tibia is a common cause of an acute limp in a toddler (toddler's fracture). Tenderness over the mid-shaft of the tibia and a fine crack on the X-ray are noted. The child lacks the systemic features of acute infection.

Pain in a limb may be due to a malignant condition (Chapter 47). In leukaemia, neuroblastoma and Ewing's sarcoma, the child may have a systemic illness as well as local signs of tenderness and refuses to use the limb

Table 46.2 Differential diagnosis of the 'acute limb'

(1) Osteomyelitis
(2) Cellulitis
(3) Suppurative arthritis
(4) Other causes of acute arthritis
  —rheumatic fever
  —viral arthritis
  —Henoch-Schönlein purpura
(5) Undisplaced spiral fracture of tibia
(6) Malignancy:
  —leukaemia
  —neuroblastoma
  —Ewing's sarcoma
  —osteosarcoma

normally. Other malignant tumours, such as osteosarcoma, also produce acute pain. The X-rays point to the diagnosis.

FURTHER READING

Williams P. F. & Cole W. G. (eds) (1991) *Orthopaedic Management in Childhood*, 2nd edn. Chapman & Hall, London.

47

Bone Cysts and Tumours

BENIGN BONE TUMOURS

Benign tumours are much more common than malignant lesions and many of the benign conditions are seen only in children.

Solitary bone cyst

This usually presents as a pathological fracture, less often as an incidental finding on an X-ray. It occurs in the long bones, particularly at the proximal end of the humerus and femur.

On X-ray the cyst appears as a rounded translucent area with thinning of the cortex but without expansion, and there is no reaction around the margin (Fig. 47.1).

At operation the cyst may contain yellow fluid and a lining is difficult to find. Section of this lining shows a few giant cells in a fibrous stroma, appearances not to be confused with a 'giant-cell tumour' (osteoclastoma), which does not occur in childhood.

Treatment

If a fracture is present, this should be allowed to unite. Treatment may be required if repeated fractures occur or if the lesion is at a likely fracture site, for example in the neck of the femur. Aspiration of the fluid and installation of a depot form of corticosteroid gives comparable or better results than curettage and bone grafting.

Recurrence of the cyst is fairly common when treatment is performed under the age of 10 years.

Osteochondromas

These occur singly or in large numbers (hereditary multiple exostoses, diaphysial aclasis) although the

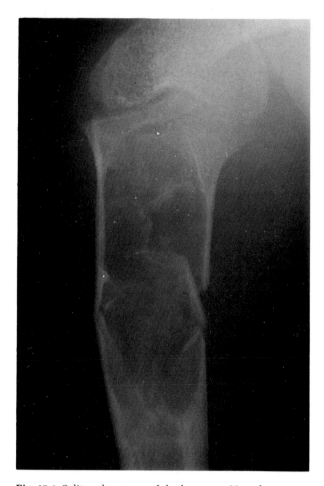

Fig. 47.1 Solitary bone cyst of the humerus. Note the fractures of the thinned cortex.

pathology is the same in both conditions. Most arise near one end of a long bone as a cap of cartilage on a bony outgrowth from the cortical surface (Fig. 47.2). The

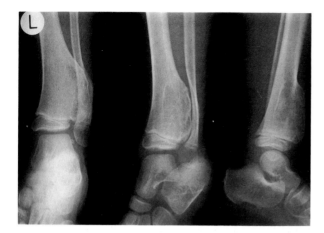

Fig. 47.2 Osteochondroma of the metaphysis of the distal tibia. The exostosis is protruding anterolaterally. The central radiograph is an oblique X-ray showing the distortion of the fibula that has resulted from the growth of the osteochondroma.

child may present with a visible lump on a subcutaneous bone or with pain on movement caused by the exostosis catching on an adjacent tendon or nerve. Very rarely the cartilaginous cap may give rise to a chondrosarcoma.

Excision may be indicated for cosmetic reasons or because of pain and discomfort.

Aneurysmal bone cyst

This is an uncommon lesion occurring in the vertebrae and flat bones as well as in the long bones. It is caused by a local circulatory disturbance resulting in the formation of numerous vascular spaces so that the area is transformed into an expanded blood-filled sponge.

The patient presents with a swelling or a fracture and an X-ray shows an expanded cyst of honeycomb texture. The tumour is progressive and destructive, so that treatment is always necessary. Cure is achieved by saucerization or excision of the cyst.

Osteoid osteoma

This curious 'tumour' occurs in practically every bone except the skull. It never grows to more than about 1 cm

in diameter, but causes very typical symptoms: characteristically it produces localized pain which increases in severity, especially at night, and is relieved specifically by aspirin. In cortical bone it provokes widespread cortical thickening with increased density (Fig. 47.3), while in spongy bone there is only a thin rim of reactive sclerosis surrounding the tumour nidus.

Treatment consists of surgical excision of the nidus of osteoid tissue; relief of pain is immediate and permanent.

Eosinophilic granuloma

This represents one variant of a generalized condition now designated 'histiocytosis X'. There are three clinical types:

(1)   A solitary eosinophilic granuloma of bone

(2)   Multiple bone lesions and visceral involvement (Letterer-Siwe's disease, a fatal disease of infancy)

(3)   A chronic illness with multiple lesions, visceral involvement, multiple cranial lesions, and diabetes insipidis (Hand-Schüller-Christian disease).

The solitary granuloma arises most commonly in the skull, but may be found in any of the long bones as a reddish-yellow gelatinous tumour. The radiographic appearance is a punched-out area without any surrounding reaction. The cortex is not expanded but may be destroyed, and a firm palpable swelling results, for example in the scalp.

The child presents because of pain or a swelling at the site of the lesions.

Treatment

An isotope bone scan is required to determine whether there are other lesions. Open biopsy is undertaken and the lesion is curetted or injected with corticosteroid at the same time. Chemotherapy is effective for recurrent or multiple granulomas.

MALIGNANT BONE TUMOURS

Primary malignant tumours of bone are classified according to the cell of origin (Table 47.1). The average 5-year survival with treatment is 60%.

Table 47.1 Malignant bone tumours

Ewing's sarcoma
Osteosarcoma
Chondrosarcoma
Fibrosarcoma
Reticulum cell sarcoma

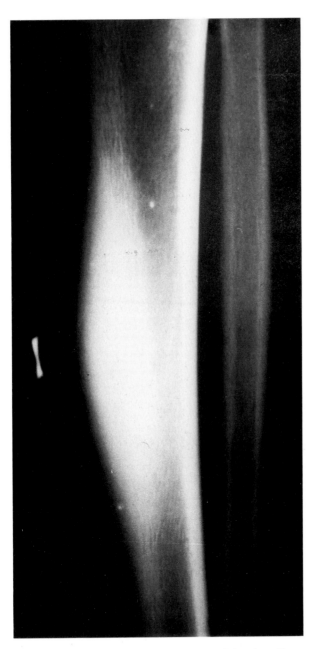

Fig. 47.3 Osteoid osteoma in the diaphysis of the tibia. This lateral radiograph shows dense ossification of the anterior cortex of the tibia. Tomography revealed a central radiolucent nidus typical of an osteoid osteoma.

Ewing's sarcoma

Ewing's tumour is a highly malignant neoplasm, more common than osteosarcoma in childhood. It can arise in either long bones (Fig. 47.4) or in the short flat bones, and may mimic osteomyelitis in causing fever, leucocytosis and material which resembles pus. Although very radiosensitive, results of treatment were poor until the introduction of chemotherapy.

High doses of combination chemotherapy usually result in rapid shrinkage of the primary tumour. The tumour is then resected and when this is not possible, an amputation is carried out. Ewing's sarcoma is sensitive to radiotherapy, but the large doses required interfere with joint function and growth, and there is a high incidence of local recurrence of the tumour.

Osteosarcoma

Oestosarcoma arises during puberty in the metaphysis of a long bone. The lower end of the femur and the upper end of the tibia together account for 75% of cases. The tumour is either osteoblastic or osteolytic, causing much variation in the histological and radiographic findings.

Clinical features

Pain and swelling are common, and examination shows a firm to hard spindle-shaped swelling of the metaphysis with distended veins in the overlying skin. In advanced disease there is invasion of the soft tissues and pathological fractures occur. Dissemination by the bloodstream to the lungs occurs early.

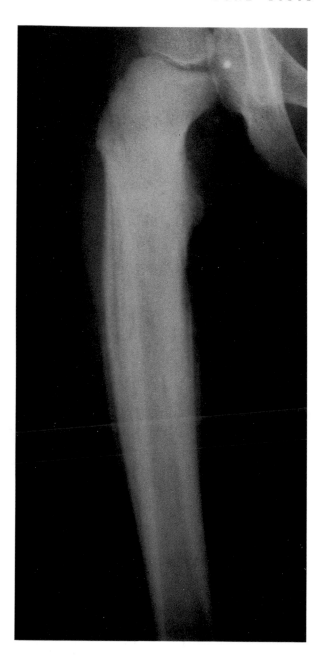

Fig. 47.4 Ewing's sarcoma involving the proximal half of the diaphysis of the femur, with layers of new bone and fusiform swelling of the soft tissue.

Diagnosis

Pain and swelling in a long bone always should arouse suspicion of osteosarcoma and an X-ray is the most helpful investigation: it may show irregular destruction of bone, soft-tissue shadows or the formation of new bone, sometimes in radiating spicules ('sun-ray' sign).

Plain X-rays and computerized tomograms of the lungs are taken to detect pulmonary metastases. Isotope bone scans reveal skeletal metastases and the extent of the primary tumour. Computerized tomography and magnetic resonance imaging are also used to determine the extent of the primary tumour.

Treatment

Pre-operative intensive combination chemotherapy is used to shrink the primary tumour and to assess its responsiveness to these agents. A good prognosis can be expected when the tumour responds well: in these patients the same chemotherapy drugs are continued postoperatively for approximately 6 months. The cytotoxic regimen is changed when there is a poor response to preoperative chemotherapy. After several cycles of chemotherapy the initial investigations are repeated and wherever possible the primary lesion is resected and replaced by an artificial joint or vascularized bone graft. If the tumour is not resectable an amputation, commonly transfemoral, is required. Pulmonary metastases are resected.

Secondary malignant metastases in bone

Practically the only tumour in childhood which metastasizes to bone is neuroblastoma. Most arise in the adrenal gland in the first 2 years of life. Secondary deposits in the skull, orbits and long bones are characteristic, and in the orbits they are sometimes bilateral.

Treatment is directed to the primary tumour, though irradiation and cytotoxic agents may be effective in treating metastases, at least initially (Chapter 25). The overall results are poor.

FURTHER READING

Dandy D. J. (1989) *Essential Orthopaedics and Trauma.* Churchill Livingstone, Edinburgh.

Jones P. G. & Campbell P. E. (1976) *Tumours of Infancy and Childhood.* Blackwell Scientific Publications, Oxford.

Morrissy R. T. (1990) *Lovell & Winter's Pediatric Orthopedics,* 3rd edn. J. B. Lippincott, Philadelphia.

Tachdjian M. O. (1990) *Pediatric Orthopedics,* 2nd edn. W. B. Saunders, Philadelphia.

Taylor W. F., Ivins J. C., Pritchard D. J., Dahlin D. C., Gilchrist G. S. & Edmonson J. H. (1985) Trends and variability in survival among patients with osteosarcoma: a 7-year update. *Mayo Clin. Proc.* **60**: 91.

Williams P. F. & Cole W. G. (eds) (1991) *Orthopaedic Management in Childhood,* 2nd edn. Chapman & Hall, London.

48

The Hand

The hand of a child is one area where the results of reconstructive surgery are much better than for similar conditions in adults.

Injuries should be repaired immediately, while correction of malformations should be deferred until a proper evaluation of the abnormality has been made or, rarely, until bone growth is complete.

DEVELOPMENTAL ABNORMALITIES

These are common and varied. A classification based on embryological failures is useful in describing and recording malformations (Table 48.1).

Deformities may be localized to the hand or be a local manifestation of a generalized condition, such as arthrogryposis multiplex congenita. Some deformities, for example certain forms of syndactyly, are strongly familial; others are sporadic with no known cause. Association with other congenital malformations is common, and some are sufficiently clear-cut to be recognized as syndromes, for example Apert's syndrome.

Table 48.1 Classification of developmental abnormalities of the hand

(1) Failure of formation of parts (amelia, phocomelia etc.)
(2) Failure of differentiation of parts (syndactyly)
(3) Duplication (polydactyly)
(4) Overgrowth (gigantism, macrodactyly)
(5) Undergrowth (hypoplasia and brachydactyly)
(6) Congenital constrictive bands (congenital amputations)
(7) Generalized skeletal abnormalities (achondroplasia)

TREATMENT

A child with a deformed hand has two problems: (i) a functional handicap; (ii) a cosmetic disability, which often is the more important. A child born with a malformed hand knows no other, and will learn to use it with dexterity provided certain basic anatomical elements are present.

In the first year of life, treatment simply consists of observation and splinting when joint deformities are the major feature.

In polydactyly one or more digits usually need to be removed for aesthetic reasons and to restore the balance of the hand. This can be done at any time after the neonatal period, provided that the surgery will not interfere with any growth centres.

All other forms of surgery are deferred until functional capacity can be estimated, which is not possible until the child develops purposeful, co-ordinated movements. However, reconstructive procedures should be completed as early as possible, to take advantage of the extraordinary capacity for adjustment and re-education that exists in the early years.

Correction of syndactyly, transposition of digits, and tendon transplants are performed at 1–3 years of age. More complicated procedures involving micro-neurovascular transfer of other digits, for example toes, may be required to provide useful apposition in children with missing fingers.

When the hand is absent reconstructive surgery has nothing to offer and prosthetic substitutes should be provided at about 6 months of age, when the child has achieved sitting balance.

TRIGGER FINGER

A 'trigger finger' or 'trigger thumb' is a common and frequently bilateral abnormality which is sometimes identified at birth, but usually found in children 1–5 years of age. The primary lesion is a fusiform thickening in the long flexor of the thumb, less commonly in one of the fingers. There is an associated narrowing of the tendon sheath in the region of the thickening, and once the affected finger is flexed, extension may be hindered or prevented by lodgement of the nodule proximal to the narrowing.

The terminal phalanx or phalanges are 'held' flexed, and can only be extended with assistance from the other hand or a parent. Frequently, even passive extension is impossible.

Clinically, the nodule in the tendon can be palpated at the level of the head of the metacarpal in the palm. A similar nodule can sometimes be palpated in the identical position in the opposite hand, and may or may not give rise to symptoms.

Treatment involves a small skin incision and a longitudinal incision in the tendon sheath, to allow full excursion of the swollen tendon through the area of narrowing.

INJURIES TO THE HAND

In children of more than 7 or 8 years of age, the repair of injuries to the hand differs little from that in adults, except that the results generally are better. Restoration of function is more rapid and more complete; prolonged physiotherapy is rarely necessary and re-education takes days or weeks instead of months or years.

The major problems in young children with an injured hand arise from failure to diagnose the extent of the injury when the child is first seen. Subjective tests for nerve injuries are of little value, and co-operation during a detailed examination is unlikely. Injuries to tendons and nerves may be overlooked until loss of function is noted by the parents, weeks or months later. Awareness of the likelihood of these injuries in lacerations of the hand is essential; the possibility of nerve injuries at an age when no reliable confirmatory clinical tests can be applied is particularly important.

Postural changes in the fingers with the hand at rest suggest possible tendon injuries. When no fracture is present, any disturbance of the normal posture of a finger in relation to the other finger indicates a tendon injury.

In young children, soft tissue damage rarely is severe; most injuries are cuts and tissue viability is not usually a problem. Restoration of function is so rapid and complete that in most cases primary repair is indicated, after adequate cleansing of the wound, provided this is undertaken within a reasonable time after the injury.

Exploration of a wound under local anaesthesia purely for the purpose of establishing the diagnosis is strongly contra-indicated. Any wound in a child which cannot be adequately examined, and which overlies an important structure, must be explored under general anaesthesia, so that any damage to tendons and nerves can be repaired primarily, under ideal conditions.

Deferred repair of nerves or tendons, frequently advocated in certain types of adult injury, is indicated only rarely in young children. The only possible exception to this rule arises when both flexor tendons are cut in the tendon sheath of the finger, in which situation primary repair will depend on the age of the patient, the site of the tendon division and the extent of damage to the tendon sheath. In some cases, secondary tendon grafting may be preferable to direct suture.

The greatest difficulty in small children is immobilization of the hand and fingers during healing; plaster and bandage technique is of great importance if immobilization is required.

INJURIES TO FINGERTIPS

Crushing and slicing injuries, with loss of part of the fingertip, are common in childhood.

In most crush injuries the tissue remaining after judicious debridement is viable, even though the soft tissue pedicle may be very narrow. Careful alignment of the small flaps will give a satisfactory result. If possible, a portion of the tip of the finger should be left exposed, so that the circulation can be observed in the early postoperative period.

In slicing injuries with skin loss, some form of primary closure with a free graft or a local flap is desirable, to speed healing and prevent the hypersensitivity associated with slow healing and a thin scar over exposed nerve ends. In children less than 4 years of age, the cross-sectional area of the fingertip is small, and after trimming any protruding bone, healing is rapid and the subsequent disability is minimal. No graft is required unless the line of section is very oblique.

GANGLION

A ganglion is a cystic dilatation of a tendon sheath and contains synovial fluid. They occur most frequently on extensor tendons with the back of the hand being the commonest site. Ganglia rarely enlarge more than 1–2 cm. When the ganglion causes discomfort it can be removed, although recurrence after excision occurs occasionally.

FURTHER READING

Lyndsay W. K. (1986) Congenital defects of the hand. In Welch K. J., Randolph J. G., Ravitch M. M., O'Neill J. A. & Rowe M. I. (eds), *Pediatric Surgery*, 4th edn. Vol. 2, p. 1405. Year Book Medical, Chicago.

Rayner L. R. W. (1987) The hand. In: Muir I. R. K. (ed.) *Plastic Surgery in Paediatrics*. Lloyd-Luke (Medical Books), London.

49

The Breast

In the paediatric age group, there are no serious conditions involving the breast in either sex, but there are a number of minor conditions which may give rise to anxiety or inconvenience.

ABSENT BREASTS AND MULTIPLE NIPPLES

Absence of the breast is a rare anomaly in which the breast and nipple are absent on one side; this is frequently part of a regional dysplasia which also affects the pectoral muscles and subjacent ribs (Chapter 50).

Multiple nipples, which can occur anywhere along a curved line in front of the anterior fold of the axilla, are also rare. It is even rarer to have a supernumerary breast, which is usually in the axilla. These can be removed simply by surgery.

NEONATAL ENLARGEMENT

The transplacental passage of lactogenic hormones may lead to hyperplasia and the secretion of breast milk in newborn babies of either sex. The enlargement usually lasts a week if left alone, but any attempts to empty the breast by massage will prolong and increase milk production. Unusually overactive secretion can be stopped within 24 h by oral oestrogens, but this is rarely necessary. The engorgement predisposes to infection, but this is not particularly common.

If an abscess forms, it should be drained by a small incision placed peripherally in girls to minimize disruption of the canaliculi beneath the nipple. Since the entire breast is no larger than the areola, extreme care is required to avoid unintentional mastectomy or physical damage to the breast bud.

PRECOCIOUS PUBERTY

This is very uncommon but may occur in girls as early as 12–18 months of age. Menstruation and bilateral hyperplasia of the breasts should always raise the possibility of an underlying cause, for example an ovarian tumour or an intracranial lesion, but in the constitutional type no cause is found and the possibility of dwarfism from excess production of oestrogens should be investigated.

PREMATURE HYPERPLASIA

This is probably the commonest minor physiological aberration, and when unilateral presents a diagnostic problem. The usual finding is the development of one breast in girls, sometimes as young as 5 years, though more commonly 7–9 years of age.

The presenting feature is a firm discoid lump 1–2 cm in diameter, situated symmetrically and concentrically beneath the nipple. It is initially symptomless and found accidentally, although it may become tender, possibly due to repeated palpation and to anxiety. There are no other signs of puberty, which develops at the normal time. The danger is that a biopsy will be performed, for it is tantamount to a total mastectomy.

The clinical signs are so diagnostic that no confirmation by other means is required. This is not precocious puberty, for the menarche occurs at the normal age. The affected breast may return to normal, but the swelling commonly remains static and the same changes usually appear in the opposite breast within 3–12 months; both then remain static without further increase in size until puberty. Reassurance and explanation are all that are required. Biopsy is an avoidable disaster.

PUBERTAL 'MASTITIS'

This occurs in boys as well as girls. In girls there is some tenderness, discomfort, a granular texture on palpation and serous fluid can be expressed from the nipple; one breast is often affected more than the other. It is a temporary phase and no treatment is required.

In boys the discoid, subareolar lesion as described in premature hyperplasia occurs in one or both breasts at about 12–14 years. No treatment is necessary.

GYNAECOMASTIA

This occurs in several conditions, perhaps most commonly in a spurious form in obese pre-adolescents, when it is formed of fat alone.

In thin boys, the possibility of ambiguous sexual development requires elucidation by a close examination of the genitalia, chromosomal studies, the estimation of ketosteroids in the urine, urethroscopy, biopsy of the gonads, or even laparotomy (Chapter 11).

It may arise as a side effect of oestrogen therapy for some other condition.

In most cases no cause can be found, and if the enlargement is of sufficient magnitude to cause embarrassment, simple mastectomy is justified. The standard curved submammary incisions should not be used, for the scar may simulate the contour of a breast even after it has been removed. A straight transverse incision is preferable, or a half-circle peri-areolar incision if the breast is not too large.

FURTHER READING

La Franchi S. H., Parlow A. F. *et al.* (1975) Pubertal gynecomastia and transient elevation of serum estradiol level. *Am. J. Child.* **129**: 927.

50

Chest Wall Deformities

Deformities of the chest wall are almost all congenital and are classified as follows:

(1) Primary depression deformities of the sternum (funnel chest: pectus excavatum)

(2) Primary protrusion deformities of the sternum (pigeon chest: pectus carinatum)

(3) Deficiency deformities of the chest wall

(4) Failure of midline sternal fusion.

AETIOLOGY

The deformity is a primary condition, except in a few of the protrusion deformities, where it may be secondary to chronic asthma, congenital heart disease, a massive lung cyst, diaphragmatic hernia or hydatid cysts of the liver. Extremely rarely, depression deformities may be seen in Marfan's syndrome, homocystinuria and congenital laryngeal stridor with inspiratory retraction.

A hereditary factor can generally be established, but is recessive and consequently may slip one or more generations. The fact that the deformity may be so mild as to pass unrecognized, and the frequent paucity of available information, may account for the apparent lack of a pertinent family history in some cases.

Abnormal action of the diaphragm may influence the nature of the anomaly whether there is protrusion or depression. It is important to realize that the type of deformity is not always the same in successive generations or even among siblings.

DEPRESSION DEFORMITIES (FUNNEL CHEST)

Clinical features

These are four times as common as pigeon chest, appreciably more frequent in males and may be symmetrical or asymmetrical. These children are usually thin; muscular and ligamentous laxity is marked and posture tends to be poor. The sternal depression is always maximal at the sterno-xiphisternal junction, but may extend up the sternum to any level.

When most of the sternum is affected, the depression is shallow and the deformity may be described as the 'saucer' type. A localized depression is compatible with a well-developed upper chest and the very localized 'funnel' may be referred to as the 'cup' type.

In asymmetrical lesions the sternum is rotated, usually from right to left around its longitudinal axis, producing prominence of the costal cartilages on one side and recession of those on the other.

A shallow sulcus may extend laterally on each side from the sterno-xiphisternal junction, a sulcus which corresponds to the attachment of the diaphragm to the lower costal cartilages, that is Harrison's sulcus. The costal margin on each side may become generally everted or protrude as a boss. Postural kyphosis is common and scoliosis not infrequent.

The deformity may be of any degree of severity, from being barely detectable to one in which the lower sternum almost touches the front of the vertebral column (Fig. 50.1).

A funnel chest may be present at birth or become apparent at any age up to 16 years. There is a group of males in which it develops rapidly at about 15 years of age, when rapid growth in height is occurring.

When the deformity is severe at birth, there is paradoxical reaction of the sternum on inspiration. This ceases at about the age of 4 years and is replaced by orthodox respiratory movement of subnormal amplitude. In the great majority of cases there is a tendency for the deformity to progress until growth ceases, but in others it becomes less severe.

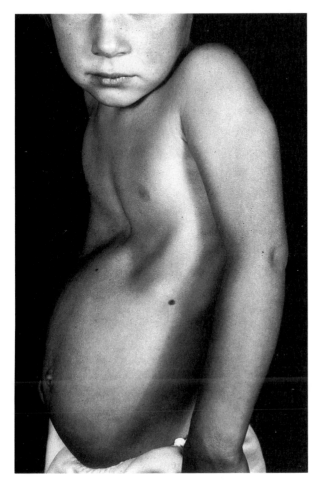

Fig. 50.1 Depression deformity. An extensive deep depression centred on the xiphisternal junction. Note the lateral sulcus, in profile, on the right side.

Symptoms

These are largely related to psychological effects and to cardiac function.

Psychological features may become apparent from an early age. The child resents being 'different' and when undressed for examination, brings the arms together to try to conceal the shape of the chest. Older children may refuse to go swimming for fear of becoming an object of attention. Comments from schoolmates may be frequent and unkind. The psychological effects can completely alter the child's personality and his reaction to his environment.

Diminished exercise tolerance is uncommon and confined to those with severe deformity. Pain may be mentioned, but has no organic basis. The deformity is not responsible for any supposedly increased tendency to respiratory infections.

The progression and severity of the condition, and its significance to the patient and his parents, can best be assessed by several examinations at yearly intervals, with photographs recording the deformity at each visit.

An X-ray of the chest may be taken to demonstrate the position of the heart and to establish the distance of the sternum from the vertebral column.

Treatment

The deformity cannot be improved by any form of exercises or retaining apparatus. Encouragement of participation in physical activity helps some children to become less self-conscious about lesser degrees of depression deformity. In selecting patients for surgical correction of the deformity, it is important that the patient wants to have the deformity corrected. Only in very severe cases is surgery indicated in the first decade of life.

At operation, which is usually performed at puberty, the chest cage is exposed through a transverse incision, with elevation of muscle flaps. The sternum is mobilized and the costal cartilages divided to correct the deformity. The corrected position of the sternum is maintained by struts (usually of steel) placed transversely behind the sternum.

PROTRUSION DEFORMITIES (PIGEON CHEST)

A high protrusion

This may be associated with a deficiency deformity and is never an acquired lesion. The sternum is angulated forwards at the level of the third sternochondral junction, and below this point it recedes as a depression. There may be 'pinching-in' of the lower costal cartilages.

The radiographic findings are unique, for there is osseous fusion of all the synchondroses of the sternum, which probably occurs before the age of 1 year.

The symptoms produced are purely the result of the cosmetic defect. The deformity tends to increase with age, and never regresses spontaneously.

Surgical treatment is for cosmetic reasons and achieves excellent results. In less severe cases in girls, the decision to operate may be deferred until after puberty, for breast development may help to mask the deformity.

Low protrusion

These may be secondary, particularly to chronic asthma. In a few of those in whom it is a primary condition, there is a tendency to spontaneous improvement, which is usually apparent by the age of 8 years; otherwise, there is a general tendency for the deformity to increase until growth ceases.

The maximal protrusion is at the sterno-xiphisternal junction or a little higher, and there is usually some pinching-in of the lower costal cartilages (Fig. 50.2). Prominence of the costal cartilages on each side near their junction with the sternum may be present, forming a median trough which, though locally depressed, is still part of the sternal protrusion. Rotation of the sternum producing an asymmetrical deformity is not uncommon.

Radiography is necessary to confirm the degree of protrusion and to exclude the presence of any intra-thoracic condition which might be contributory. The symptoms are related entirely to the cosmetic defect.

Treatment

Secondary deformities usually resolve spontaneously after elimination of the underlying cause.

Primary lesions may also show a tendency to spontaneous improvement. In the first decade of life, repeated observation will indicate the trend. Many patients present for the first time after puberty.

Operation is indicated in the patient with severe and/or progressive cosmetic deformity.

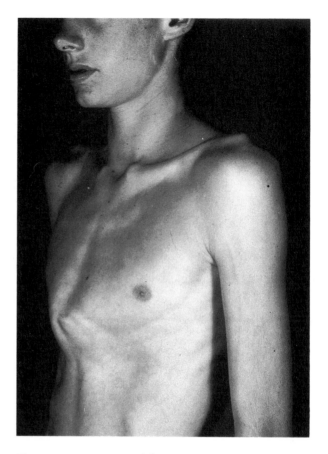

Fig. 50.2 Low protrusion deformity maximal just above the sterno-xiphisternal junction.

DEFICIENCY DEFORMITIES

In the usual type, the pectoral muscles are absent on one side and there is a variable degree of hypoplasia of the underlying ribs and costal cartilages.

The third and fourth cartilages may be deficient anteriorly, with some paradoxical respiratory movement visible through the chest wall. (This is rarely of any clinical significance.) All elements of the breast may be absent, but usually the nipple and areola are present. Hypoplasia of the upper limb on the affected side and syndactyly may occur (Poland's syndrome;

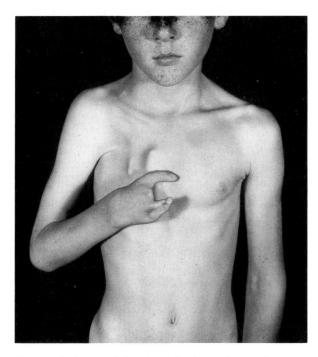

Fig. 50.3 Deficiency deformity. Poland's syndrome; absent nipple, areola and pectoral muscles with hypoplasia of the chest wall and syndactyly.

Fig. 50.3). The sternum in these patients may show a high protrusion deformity of cosmetic significance. The dominant problem, however, is the soft tissue deficiency.

Treatment

Surgery is only rarely indicated for filling in the bony chest wall deficiency or for correction of sternal protrusion. Muscular flaps, utilizing the latissimus dorsi, can be used to provide soft tissue bulk, to be followed in girls by augmentation mammoplasty. It is more difficult to replace absent tissues than it is to reorganize disordered tissues; despite this, much can be done to improve the appearance in these children.

FURTHER READING

Bax N. M. A., Ottenschot T., Gil D. & Vosmeer H. (1990) Does early subperichondral removal of several costal cartilages interfere with chest wall growth? An experimental study in kittens. *Pediatr. Surg. Int.* **5**: 165–169.

Chetcuti P., Dickens D. R. V. & Phelan P. D. (1989) Spinal deformity in patients with oesophageal atresia and tracheo-oesophageal fistula. *Arch. Dis. Child.* **64**: 1427–1430.

Howard R. N. (1958) Pigeon breast (protrusion deformity of the sternum). *Med. J. Aust.* **2**: 664–666.

Ireland D. C. R., Takayama N. & Flatt A. E. (1976) Poland's syndrome: a review of 43 cases. *J. Bone Joint Surg.* **58A**: 52–58.

Martinez D., Juame J., Stein T. & Pena A. (1990) The effect of costal cartilage resection on chest wall development. *Pediatr. Surg. Int.* **5**: 170–173.

Ravitch M. M. (1986) The chest wall. In: Welch K. J., Randolph J. G., Ravitch M. M., O'Neill J. A., Rowe M. I. (eds), *Pediatric Surgery*, 4th edn, pp. 563–589. Year Book Medical, Chicago.

Shamberger R. C. & Welch K. J. (1990) Sternal defects. *Pediatr. Surg. Int.* **5**: 156–164.

von der Oelsnitz G. (1990) Operative correction of pectus excavatum. Experience at the Children's Hospital of Bremen. *Pediatr. Surg. Int.* **5**: 150–155.

51

Lungs, Pleura and Mediastinum

While the principles of diagnosis and treatment of pulmonary disease in children are similar to those of adults, there are, in addition, some aspects which need to be considered:

(1) The respiratory passages are small and any encroachment upon the lumen by exudate or oedema from inflammation or trauma is more likely to cause obstruction of the airways

(2) The cough reflex is relatively ineffectual in infancy and retention of secretions may have serious consequences

(3) Obstruction may cause both superimposed infection and patchy or lobar collapse

(4) Hypoxia develops rapidly in neonates and increased respiratory effort increases the consumption of oxygen; the vicious circle may culminate in respiratory failure

(5) Disturbances of intrathoracic pressure relationships are tolerated poorly, and if a tension pneumothorax remains unrecognized, there is a danger of irreversible cardiorespiratory failure, particularly if there is pre-existing lung disease.

With few exceptions, for example hydatid disease, operations on the lungs and pleura in childhood are of two kinds: the resection of pulmonary tissue and the provision of pleural drainage. Resection, usually lobectomy, is required for a variety of developmental anomalies, for example lobar emphysema, hamartoma, sequestrated lobe and for carefully selected cases of bronchiectasis. Metastatic tumours, for example osteosarcoma or Wilms' tumour, may also warrant resection.

Inhaled foreign bodies are important in childhood, but may produce few symptoms. The final diagnosis of an intrabronchial foreign body is occasionally made only after resection of a diseased segment of lung.

Pleural drainage may be necessary in three conditions:

(1) Pneumothorax, for example neonatal pneumothorax (Chapter 4); traumatic pneumothorax (Chapter 38)

(2) Empyema (see below)

(3) Haemothorax, an unusual condition because of the rarity of major thoracic injuries in childhood.

Aspiration of the pleural cavity may be used diagnostically to obtain pleural fluid for microscopy and culture or as a preliminary step in providing immediate continuous drainage of an empyema by means of an intercostal catheter.

STAPHYLOCOCCAL PNEUMONIA

This occurs usually as a complication of a viral infection of the upper respiratory tract (Fig. 51.1).

Diagnosis

Although X-rays make the diagnosis with a high degree of certainty, identification of the organism responsible is the absolute criterion. When *Staphylococcus aureus* is isolated from a throat swab or sputum and typical changes are present in lung radiographs, the diagnosis is at least presumptive. The development of a pleural complication and culture of staphylococcus from a specimen of pus from the pleural cavity confirm the diagnosis.

The diagnosis may be delayed at presentation because the clinical signs suggest upper respiratory tract infection, and the pathological changes initially are confined to this area. When the condition progresses to

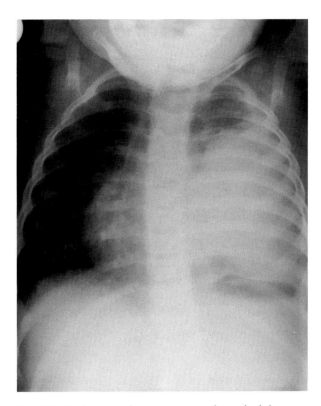

Fig. 51.1 Staphylococcal pneumonia involving the left hemithorax.

pneumonia, this may not be recognized immediately. The baby or young child become worse rapidly because of the following factors:

(1)   Toxaemia, with or without septicaemia, and a shock-like state of collapse

(2)   An air leak under tension at one or more of three sites: (i) intrapleural—pneumothorax; (ii) intrapulmonary—pneumatocele; (iii) in the mediastinum—pneumomediastinum

(3)   A collection of pus: (i) intrapleural—empyema, or a pyopneumothorax when, as is common, both pus and air are present; (ii) intrapulmonary—single or multiple lung abscesses

(4)   Obstruction of the airways.

Treatment

Antibiotics are given, and until the results of culture and sensitivity tests are known, an effective combination is flucloxacillin and gentamicin. X-rays are repeated at short intervals because of the rapid evolution of the pathological changes on radiology.

Complications and sequelae

Suppurative pericarditis, meningitis, septicaemia and osteomyelitis may complicate staphylococcal pneumonia, but are uncommon when appropriate antibiotics are given early and in adequate dosage.

Surgery may be required for an empyema, a lung abscess or a pneumatocele.

Lung abscesses in staphylococcal pneumonia are usually small and rarely require drainage. Pneumatoceles are mostly small and resolve spontaneously, though this may occur slowly, over a course of 6–12 months. Surgery should not be considered unless resolution does not occur.

EMPYEMA

Spread of infection from the lower respiratory tract may cause a fibrinous or serofibrinous pleurisy, a pyopneumothorax or an empyema.

An empyema may be unilateral or bilateral, generalized or loculated, and the rate of resolution is variable. These factors determine the clinical course and the type of treatment required.

The incidence of empyema, the causal organisms and their sensitivities, reflect the antibiotics used in the community and the bacteria currently prevalent.

Staphylococcus aureus predominates and 80% are resistant to penicillin. Other Gram-positive cocci, for example pneumococci and streptococci, and Gram-negative bacilli, for example *Escherichia coli*, are encountered less commonly. In 75% of patients, an acute respiratory infection, apparently viral, is the precipitating factor. The exanthems (particularly measles), focal staphylococcal infections or an underlying pulmonary disease are responsible in the other 25%.

Those with an underlying disease form a heterogeneous group which includes developmental anomalies, prematurity, birth injury, degenerative diseases of the CNS, anaemia, skin diseases, and malabsorption syndromes.

Clinical features

The onset of staphylococcal pneumonia is marked by acute toxaemia associated with cough, dyspnoea and grunting respirations, but usually without localizing signs in the chest. As toxic signs become less severe, the clinical features of an empyema can be recognized: diminution in the movement of the chest, dullness to percussion and diminished air entry. In others, the illness remains static or progresses more slowly; but in either type, the clinical picture may become suddenly worse with the occurrence of an 'air leak' caused by a bronchopleural fistula and leading to a pneumothorax or pyopneumothorax. These may occur in any type of infection, but they are particularly typical of staphylococcal pneumonia (Fig. 51.1).

In staphylococcal empyema, cyanosis is a variable feature, and peripheral circulatory failure may develop; but the interpretation of the clinical signs is virtually impossible without concomitant X-rays, for the same clinical signs can be caused by a pneumothorax with tension, which demands urgent relief.

The symptoms and signs of an empyema, other than staphylococcal, vary widely according to the underlying disease, the duration of illness and the age of the patient. As in other infections, the picture in the neonatal period is frequently quite different, and there may be a minimal fever or toxaemia, even when there is extensive intrathoracic suppuration.

Investigation

Bacteriological investigation will determine the organisms present in the nasopharynx, in focal areas of sepsis, and in the empyema.

The radiographic findings are a composite of those in the underlying lung and in the pleura. The course of the disease and the response to treatment are closely followed by means of serial X-rays.

Treatment

Treatment is directed to the underlying condition and drainage of the empyema. Intermittent paracentesis has a limited place and in most cases continuous drainage is required. Open thoracotomy and drainage is the method of choice when paracentesis has failed, the pus is thick, or there is evidence for loculation.

Drainage is needed in most cases, and an early surgical consultation is desirable in a child with an empyema. The surgeon should observe the early stages of a disease, so he can advise whether and when thoracotomy is appropriate. Chronic empyemas are very rare in childhood and decortication is practically never required.

In previously healthy children, the mortality is minimal and most deaths occur early when the infection is fulminant and the child is septicaemic. The highest mortality is in the newborn, in bilateral empyemas and in those with serious pre-existing pulmonary disease.

PNEUMOTHORAX

Clinical features

The clinical picture is determined by the age of the patient, the size of the pneumothorax, the presence or absence of tension and the nature of underlying pulmonary disease, if present (Table 51.1). The symptoms include pain in the chest, dyspnoea, and in some, those of the underlying disease.

The signs arise from displacement of the mediastinum, that is displacement of the trachea and the apex beat, diminished movement of the chest wall, a hyperresonant percussion note and diminished air entry.

X-rays are virtually diagnostic (Fig. 51.2), but there are other conditions with similar findings, for example a huge lung cyst or unusual types of diaphragmatic hernia.

Table 51.1 Causes of pneumothorax

(1) Rupture of a subpleural abscess in staphylococcal pneumonia (see earlier)
(2) Neonatal pulmonary disease
(3) Rupture of subpleural emphysematous bulla, for example in asthma or cystic fibrosis
(4) Traumatic, following injuries to the chest wall (Chapter 39)
(5) Perforation of the oesophagus by an ingested foreign body or during oesophagoscopy
(6) Iatrogenic, for example after paracentesis of the pleura
(7) Rupture of a hydatid cyst, spontaneously or following misdiagnosis and needling
(8) Complication of tracheostomy (very rare)
(9) Postoperative—after thoracotomy

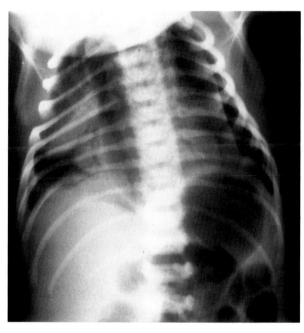

Fig. 51.2 Neonatal pneumothorax. The tension pneumothorax has caused displacement of the mediastinum to the right with collapse of the right lung.

Treatment

Urgent relief of tension is required, by needling or intercostal drainage with an intercostal chest tube, and the underlying cause may require investigation and appropriate treatment.

Table 51.2 Causes of pleural effusions

(1) Pulmonary infections, either acute (e.g. staphylococcal pneumonia) or chronic (e.g. tuberculosis)
(2) Disturbed haemodynamics (e.g. in congestive cardiac failure or hypoproteinaemia)
(3) Malignant disease of the lung, pleura or mediastinum
(4) Chylothorax—damage to or obstruction of the thoracic duct

PLEURAL EFFUSION

The accumulation of fluid (pus, serofibrinous exudate, blood, chyle or transudate) in the pleural cavity occurs in a variety of conditions (Table 51.2).

The physical signs are usually unmistakable, but radiographs are necessary and may require careful interpretation to distinguish a pleural 'collection' from such conditions as hydatid cyst or neuroblastoma.

Paracentesis provides information on the nature of the fluid and material for cytological and bacteriologic examination, and indicates the necessity for further drainage.

Chylothorax occasionally occurs spontaneously, but more usually after thoracic operations; some cases require aspiration or even thoracotomy. Replacing the fat content of the diet with medium-chain triglycerides which are absorbed via the portal vascular system may control, or even cure, the condition; long-chain fats enter the lacteals and travel via the thoracic duct.

BRONCHIECTASIS

Recurrent or chronic bronchitis is the most common precursor of bronchiectasis. This type of bronchiectasis tends to be widespread, although the disease is usually most marked in one particular area. Bronchiectasis may complicate an exanthem.

Infection associated with permanent collapse of one or more lobes of one lung may be the cause, but the bronchiectasis may remain 'dry', that is structural changes can be demonstrated by bronchography but symptoms and signs are minimal or absent if the affected area remains free of infection.

Other causes include pulmonary tuberculosis, hydatid disease, congenital weakness of the bronchial wall (bronchomalacia), cystic fibrosis and the inhalation of a foreign body. In healed tuberculosis, the bronchiectasis is usually 'dry', while in bronchomalacia and cystic fibrosis, dilatation of the bronchi is usually widespread and associated with copious sputum.

Clinical features

A careful history is the first requirement. Physical signs may be diffuse, localized or even absent, according to the aetiology and the extent of the disease. Clinical assessment of the nature and amount of sputum, any interference with normal life and school attendance, and the frequency of acute toxic episodes of pneumonitis, should precede any investigations.

Bronchoscopy and bronchography aim to confirm the diagnosis and determine the distribution and severity. Culture of the sputum is a useful guide to chemotherapy, particularly during exacerbations of infection.

Treatment

Conservative treatment, with physiotherapy, postural drainage and antibiotics, is usually effective. The co-operation of fully informed parents is all-important in the success of this programme.

Lobectomy and/or segmental resection is required occasionally, and, in localized disease, is curative. As a general rule, resection should be deferred until late childhood in case progressive disease in the remaining lobes of the lungs develops. When the bronchiectasis is more widespread, resection of a particularly diseased area may considerably improve the patient's well-being and reduce the amount of sputum produced, although some coughing may persist.

CONGENITAL MALFORMATIONS

Congenital lobar emphysema and congenital cystic lung (Chapter 4) may present in older children, and there is no typical clinical pattern. Often recurrent respiratory infections lead to an X-ray examination of the chest and the diagnosis.

Bronchography may provide additional information, and fluoroscopy may demonstrate 'trapped air' in the lobe concerned, that is movement of the mediastinum towards the affected side during inspiration, and aways from it during expiration.

Treatment involves removal of the affected portion of the lung.

PULMONARY SEQUESTRATION

A sequestrated lobe is pulmonary tissue which has no connection with the bronchial tree and an arterial supply from a systemic vessel, usually the aorta. It does not participate in the normal function of the lung and is particularly prone to infection. Two types are recognized: extralobar and intralobar.

In extralobar sequestration, there is complete anatomical and physiological separation from the relevant lung and the sequestrated portion may be above or below the diaphragm. This is sometimes seen in association with congenital diaphragmatic hernia.

In intralobar sequestration, the more important type, the abnormal tissue is contiguous with the related lung which partially surrounds it. This type is practically always in the posteromedial portion of the right or left lower lobe, but cases are recorded in which the whole of one lung, or both lungs, are affected.

The sequestrated lobe may consist of a large cyst, multiple cysts, branching bronchi without cysts, or all three of these. The ectopic arterial supply is usually derived from the aorta or one of its immediate branches, above or below the diaphragm. The blood vessels, one to four in number, are large, thin-walled and prone to atheroma. They may supply sequestrated tissue only, or both sequestrated and normal tissue, and the venous blood usually enters the pulmonary veins and occasionally the inferior vena cava.

Clinical features

The usual history is of repeated episodes of pulmonary infection with signs confined to one area. Although the infection commonly subsides, acute suppuration may supervene. Subsidence of the acute phase leaves in its wake chronic suppuration with poor health, a persistent cough and sometimes low grade pleural pain. Haemoptysis occasionally occurs.

Chest X-rays show an opacity in the posteromedial part of one of the lower lobes or cystic spaces with or without fluid levels in a lower lobe. In the acute phase, the opacity increases in size and may produce mediastinal displacement. Bronchograms typically show no filling in the posterior part of one lower lobe and anterolateral displacement of the adjacent bronchi. Occasionally, the contrast material enters the abnormal lobe and outlines the dilated bronchi or cystic spaces.

Aortography demonstrates the anomalous arterial supply, confirms the diagnosis, and is useful in planning the surgical approach (see Fig. 4.3).

Treatment

Resection is indicated because of the susceptibility to infection, but preliminary evacuation and drainage of pus may be required. More often the acute infection subsides with antibiotics and the patient can be investigated, and operated on, in a quiescent phase.

THE CHILD WITH A MEDIASTINAL MASS

A child may present with a mediastinal mass in one of two ways:

(1) A symptomless mass demonstrated in a chest X-ray, or

(2) Symptoms caused by compression of mediastinal structures.

A symptomless mass

The thymus is large in infancy, and determining whether its appearance on chest X-ray is normal requires experience. Some radiographic techniques cause apparent enlargement.

A symptomless mediastinal mass may develop in the course of a generalized disease, for example from enlarged hilar lymph nodes in leukaemia or Hodgkin's disease, or as metastases from a known malignant disease. Paravertebral and para-aortic masses of neuroblastoma may involve the mediastinum, often as the primary site but also as metastases from tumour elsewhere, for example in the abdomen (Chapter 25).

Compression of mediastinal structures

In childhood, this is nearly always the result of a malignant mass, of which lymphosarcoma is the commonest. Congestion of the veins of the head, neck and upper limbs from obstruction of the superior vena cava, wheezing respirations, an unproductive or reverberating brassy cough and increasing dyspnoea are all ominous signs.

Lymphosarcomas usually arise in the anterior mediastinum in the region of the thymus, and X-rays usually show a large mass which extends laterally. The edges are irregular, rounded or ill-defined; the tumour may extend into the pleura and cause a pleural effusion. The histological diagnosis can be made from cytology of the cells in the pleural effusion.

A neural crest tumour (neuroblastoma or ganglioneuroma) is the usual cause of a paravertebral mass: areas of both neuroblastomas and ganglioneuromas may be present in a single tumour (Fig. 51.3). Erosion of the ribs and extension into a vertebral foramen causing spinal symptoms are seen with infiltrating mediastinal neuroblastomas.

A ganglioneuroma is a benign tumour arising in a paravertebral gutter. It often grows through a vertebral foramen into the spinal canal, resulting in two solid elements connected by a narrow isthmus in the intervertebral foramen, a 'dumb-bell' tumour.

Thymomas are much less common and are difficult to distinguish from lymphosarcomas. They tend to grow slowly, to reach an even larger size, and to have a more distinct margin in X-rays of the chest.

Teratomas in the anterior mediastinum are very rare. They are cystic or solid, only occasionally malignant and may extend laterally into one or other pleural cavity.

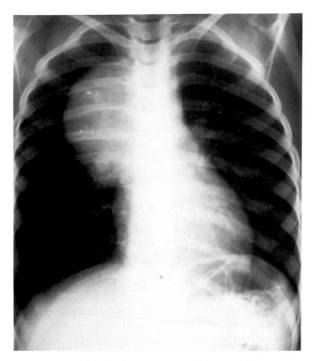

Fig. 51.3 A mediastinal mass: a neuroblastoma with calcification in the posterior mediastinum.

Bronchogenic cysts arise close to the trachea or the hilum of the lung; they usually contain air and many show a fluid level in X-rays. There may be a history suggestive of intermittent partial obstruction of one of the larger bronchi, and surgical excision is curative.

Duplication cysts of the alimentary canal occasionally arise in the thorax and form either a simple spherical cyst or a bizarre cylindrical structure, which may extend below the diaphragm into the abdomen.

Management

Management varies depending on whether the clinical presentation is symptomatic or is on an incidental X-ray.

Symptomatic lesions

Compression of the trachea and/or bronchi may cause severe respiratory distress, sometimes precipitated by a supervening virus infection. Nasotracheal intubation may be necessary as an emergency.

When a chest X-ray shows a mediastinal mass, tracheostomy is usually of no assistance, for the obstruction is below the level of the suprasternal notch. This situation is most commonly caused by a lymphosarcoma, and this presumptive diagnosis should be confirmed quickly by examination of the peripheral blood, the bone marrow or an accessible enlarged lymph node (or occasionally the mass itself). As with other malignancies, the stage of the disease will determine treatment. However, use of cytotoxic agents, even without a histological diagnosis, is justified in an emergency and brings dramatic relief. The prognosis for most types of lymphosarcoma is good.

Incidental chest X-ray presentation

Sometimes a symptomless mass is found incidentally. The investigations which should precede operation are:

(1) Examination of the peripheral blood for evidence of leukaemia

(2) Examination of the bone marrow for metastatic neuroblastoma

(3) Examination of the urine to determine the excretion of MHMA in a 24 h specimen

(4) A radiographic survey of the skeleton for metastases or sites of leukaemic infiltration

(5) A complete radiological assessment of the mediastinal mass, including oblique views, a barium swallow, tomography, myelography, computerized tomography and magnetic resonance imaging, as indicated.

In many instances, these investigations will give a good indication of the diagnosis, but in almost all cases, surgical exploration is required to obtain material for a histological diagnosis or to determine whether the mass is removable.

Surgical excision is generally curative in conditions such as teratomas, duplication ('enterogenous cysts'), bronchogenic cysts and ganglioneuromas. In the latter, both thoracotomy and laminectomy, combined or in stages, may be required to remove both components of a dumb-bell tumour.

Total removal of infiltrating primary neoplasms or extensive metastases in para-aortic lymph nodes is often impossible, but there is evidence that even incomplete removal may be of benefit in neuroblastoma, in which maturation to benign gangioneuroma can occur, particularly in those arising in the posterior mediastinum.

The operative findings, the histology and the results of the preliminary examinations will determine the need for chemotherapy and radiotherapy.

FURTHER READING

Adam A. & Hochholzer L. (1981) Ganglioneuroblastoma of the posterior mediastinum: a clinico-pathologic review of 80 cases. *Cancer* **47**: 373–381.

Buntain W. L., Isaacs H. *et al.* (1974) Lobar emphysema, cystic adenomatoid malformation, pulmonary sequestration and bronchogenic cyst in infancy and childhood. *J. Pediatr. Surg.* **9**: 85–93.

Carachi R., Campbell P. E. & Kent M. (1983) Thoracic neural crest tumours: a clinical review. *Cancer* **51**: 949–954.

De Paredes C. G., Pierce W. S. *et al.* (1970) Pulmonary sequestration in infants and children: a 20-year experience and review of the literature. *J. Pediatr. Surg.* **5**: 136–147.

Golladay E. S. & Wagner C. W. (1989) Management of empyema in children. *Amer. J. Surg.* **158**: 618–621.

Karl S. R. & Dunn J. (1985) Posterior mediastinal teratomas. *J. Pediatr. Surg.* **20**: 508–510.

Kent M. (1976) Thoracic tumours. In: Jones P. G. & Campbell P. E. (eds), *Tumours of Infancy and Childhood*, Ch. 16. Blackwell Scientific Publications, Oxford.

Kosloske A. M., Martin L. W. & Schubert W. K. (1974) Management of chylothorax in children by thoracentesis and medium chain triglyceride feedings. *J. Pediatr. Surg.* **9**: 365–371.

Phelan P. D. (1982) *Respiratory Illness in Children*. Blackwell Scientific Publications, Oxford.

Pokorny W. & Goldstein I. R. (1984) Enteric thoraco-abdominal duplications in children. *J. Thorac. Cardiovasc. Surg.* **87**: 821–824.

Thomas P. R. M., Foulkes L. A. *et al.* (1983) Primary Ewing's sarcoma of the ribs: a report from the Intergroup Ewing's Sarcoma Study. *Cancer* **51**: 1021–1027.

52

Vascular and Pigmented Naevi

VASCULAR LESIONS

Cutaneous vascular malformations are common. They may be focal (e.g. haemangioma) or regional (e.g. vascular malformations). Both haemangiomas and vascular malformations may occur as isolated pathologies or as part of a syndrome with multisystem involvement.

Haemangiomas

Haemangiomas are the most common tumours of infancy and childhood. They represent a group of 'cellularly dynamic' lesions with relatively predictable behaviour and life cycle.

Capillary haemangioma

The most common of these is the capillary haemangioma or strawberry naevus. Initially it presents shortly after birth as a pale, pink or bright red spot or patch on the skin, the so-called 'herald spot'. The hallmark of these tumours is their rapid growth in infancy which continues for 3–4 months (Fig. 52.1a). This is followed by a stable period and then gradual involution which begins at about 1 year of age. Fifty per cent of patients will show complete resolution by age 5 and 90% by age 7 (Fig. 52.1b). A small amount of redundant skin and subcutaneous tissue may remain requiring cosmetic correction. Rarely, these lesions persist and either involute later in life or require excision.

Cavernous haemangioma

Lesions with a deeper component in the subcutaneous tissues or muscle often have a more developed vasculature and are less likely to regress completely. These 'cavernous haemangiomas' are composed of blood lakes which refill slowly after compression (Fig. 52.2).

Management of these lesions consists of accurate diagnosis and careful observation. The parents need reassurance when the lesion is growing rapidly. Problems of ulceration, bleeding and (rarely) infection occur secondary to minor trauma. These are best dealt with non-operatively. Bleeding is controlled with pressure unless it is profuse or recurrent. Early surgery is indicated when there is a functional or gross cosmetic disability, and where partial or complete excision is possible. This is particularly true when the eyelid is involved as occlusion of the visual axis for even a few weeks can produce an amblyopic eye (Fig. 52.3).

Rarely, these lesions may progress rapidly with tissue destruction—the so-called 'wild fire haemangioma'. Very large haemangiomas may also lead to a consumptive coagulopathy (Kasabach-Merritt syndrome) requiring steroid therapy and blood product support.

Pyogenic granuloma

Pyogenic granuloma is the other common 'cellularly dynamic' lesion. It is a small troublesome lesion, usually found on the head and neck region, which grows rapidly, becomes ulcerated and friable and bleeds readily. It is characterized by a central feeding vessel supplying a mass of new capillaries and an associated inflammatory infiltrate.

Pyogenic granuloma is treated by excision, which should include the feeding vessel to prevent recurrence.

Vascular malformations

Regional vascular malformations, in contrast to haemangiomas, are composed of mature vascular elements

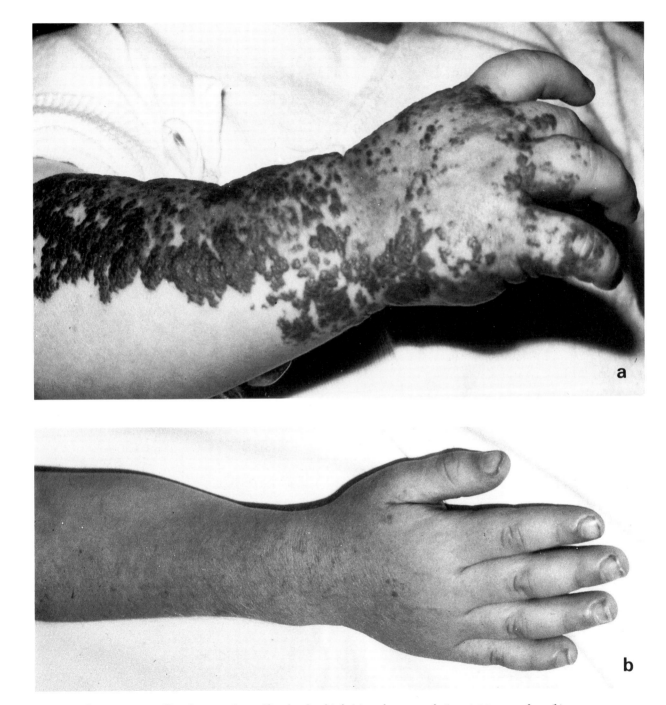

Fig. 52.1 The common capillary haemangioma. Shortly after birth (a), and near resolution at 4.5 years of age (b).

and do not regress. They may be capillary, venous, arterial, lymphatic or a combination. Those with large vascular elements (e.g. arteriovenous malformations) may produce haemodynamic instability. Fortunately, these extensive and often inoperable lesions are rare.

Naevus flammeus

Naevus flammeus is the most common vascular malformation. Naevus flammeus medialis is the 'salmon patch' or 'stork's beak mark' seen on the nape of the neck in infancy. This lesion does not change over time.

Naevus flammeus lateralis or 'port wine stain' (Fig. 52.4) is a cutaneous capillary malformation. There is a gradual darkening and hypertrophy of the lesion over a patient's lifetime. This lesion may be present as part of a syndrome in which larger vessels are involved, for example Klippel-Trenauney syndrome, or lesions involving the trigeminal nerve distributions may be associated with intracranial pathology, for example

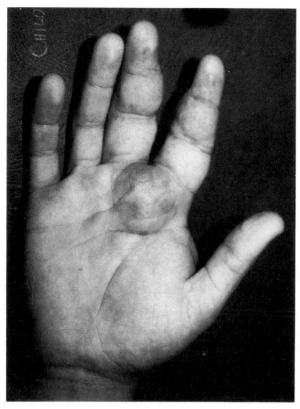

Fig. 52.2 A cavernous haemangioma.

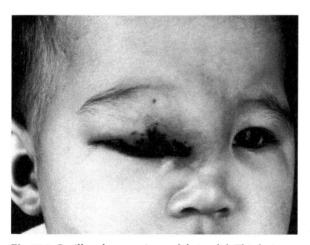

Fig. 52.3 Capillary haemangioma of the eyelid. This lesion requires frequent assessment as obstruction of the visual axis for even a few weeks will result in an amblyopic eye.

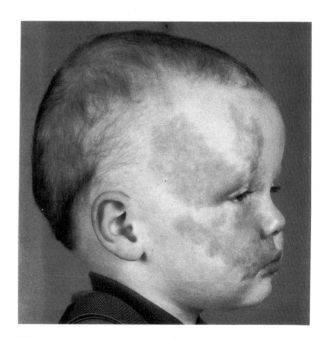

Fig. 52.4 A port wine stain in infancy.

Sturge-Weber syndrome, in which there is also a high incidence of congenital glaucoma.

Various surgical procedures have been used over the years to excise and reconstruct these lesions. Current therapy centres on the use of lasers using wavelengths which are selective for haemoglobin so as to photocoagulate the lesion while producing the least possible amount of scarring in the skin.

Naevus araneus and naevus senilis

Other lesions in this category are the naevus araneus or 'spider angioma' and the naevus senilus or 'cherry angioma' also known as the Campbell de Morgan spot.

Telangiectasia

Telangiectasias also may be congenital and may be isolated or appear as part of a syndrome, for example Rendu-Osler-Weber syndrome.

LYMPHATIC MALFORMATIONS

Malformations of the lymphatic system present a broad spectrum from small nodular lesions of lymphangioma simplex to the large cervical cystic hygromas (Chapter 16). These lesions represent malformations of various parts of the lymphatic system from the capillary lymphatics to the ducts and sacs.

Lymphangiomas have a propensity to infection, which must be treated with antibiotics. Well-defined lesions should be excised if possible. Cystic hygromas are usually located deep in the cervical and upper thoracic area and may be associated with inflammatory and infectious complications; these too should be excised where possible. Excision is rarely complete as these lesions are not encapsulated and do not respect tissue planes.

PIGMENTED NAEVI

True pigmented naevi are melanocytic in origin.

Junctional naevus

The junctional naevus is the basic type of abnormality in which there is an increase in the number of melanocytes in the basal layer of the skin. These lesions are flat brown or black spots.

They are harmless throughout childhood but junctional activity persisting after puberty is a risk for malignant melanoma. Nonetheless, this transition is so rare that excision of these naevi in childhood should not be advised solely for this reason.

Compound and intradermal naevi

A compound naevus has both junctional and intradermal components. Naevus cells bud off into the dermis where they proliferate and form a cluster of cells resulting in a raised palpable lesion. In later years the junctional activity ceases and the lesions become purely intradermal naevi. Nests and cords of cells are present in the papillary dermis while bundles of spindle-shaped cells are seen in the reticular dermis. These intradermal naevi are felt to be benign with no risk of malignant transformation. Surgical excision is for cosmetic reasons.

Spitz naevi

The juvenile or Spitz naevus is usually reddish in colour as melanin is less prominent. There is considerable junctional activity and spindle cells are present in the dermis. Although occasionally referred to as a juvenile melanoma it is a benign lesion.

Giant congenital naevi

The giant congenital naevus is present at birth and may be very large, for example bathing trunk naevus. Multiple smaller naevi may also be present in other areas. The giant naevus is largely intradermal but does have a junctional component. There is a small potential for malignant melanoma mainly after puberty and rarely sarcomas may develop in the extensive lesions. With growth the lesions tend to become more nodular and hairy (Fig. 52.5).

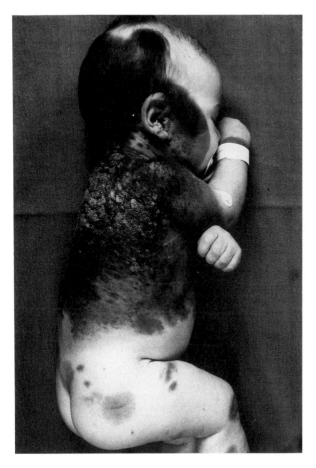

Fig. 52.5 A 'bathing trunk' giant congenital naevus.

Treatment is performed mainly for cosmetic reasons by excision and reconstruction with flaps or grafts, though in many instances complete removal is impossible. Surgery is performed early in life before the age of awareness, that is at 2 or 3 years of age.

Halo naevi

A halo naevus occurs when melanocytes disappear from the periphery of a pigmented naevus. This is felt to be an immunological phenomenon and lymphocytes are seen on histological examination. The naevus may disappear completely leaving a pale patch of skin.

Ephilis

An ephilis or freckle is a localized increase in epidermal pigmentation only.

Lentigo

A lentigo is a patch of increased pigmentation localized to the upper dermis. There is no junctional activity.

Blue naevi

A blue naevus is a dermal naevus in the deeper dermal layers. The presence of the dark pigment beneath the translucent epidermis produces the characteristic colour. The Mongolian spot is a classical example.

FURTHER READING

Fitzpatrick T. B. & Freedberg I. M. (eds) (1987) *Dermatology in General Medicine* (2 vols). McGraw-Hill, New York.

Muir I. F. K. (1987) The hamartomata. In: Muir I. F. K. (ed.), *Plastic Surgery in Paediatrics*, pp. 128–158. Lloyd-Luke (Medical Books), London.

Ryan T. J. & Cherry G. W. (eds) (1987) *Vascular Birthmarks: Pathogenesis and Management*. Oxford University Press, Oxford.

Williams H. B. (ed.) (1983) *Symposium on Vascular Malformations and Melanotic Lesions*. C. V. Mosby, Toronto.

53

Soft Tissue Lumps

There are many cutaneous and subcutaneous lesions in childhood. Some of the more common are covered in this chapter. Vascular and pigmented lesions of the skin are discussed in Chapter 52. Inguinoscrotal and head and neck lesions are discussed elsewhere.

Cutaneous lesions are classified by their cellular origin within the epidermis and its appendages. They may be solid or cystic and invariably are benign.

WARTS

These are small epidermal tumours produced in response to papillomavirus infection of the skin. They are contagious to a limited degree. Those on the soles of the feet can cause discomfort on weight-bearing.

Treatment involves removal of the entire lesion, including its 'roots', either by topical application of liquid nitrogen or a concentrated solution of salicylic acid; or, if these measures fail, by surgical curettage.

EPIDERMAL AND PILAR CYSTS

These are common benign inclusion cysts of epidermal and pilar origin respectively. Though most often seen in adults, they are not uncommon in children and are found on the face. Treatment is simple surgical excision.

NAEVUS SEBACEOUS

Naevus sebaceous is present at birth and appears as a yellowish slightly raised lesion, usually on the scalp or face. There is a 15–20% incidence of basal cell carcinoma if left untreated. These lesions are best excised electively during early childhood.

PILOMATRIXOMA

This relatively common lesion occurs on the face, neck and upper extremities of young children. It is a hard, non-tender and irregular intradermal lesion and may appear white or yellow in colour through the skin. It is characterized histologically by areas of calcification and 'ghost cells'. Excision is recommended.

DERMATOFIBROMA

This is a benign dermal tumour that may be solitary or multiple, usually on the lower extremity but also on the trunk and arms. It appears as a reddish brown firm dermal tumour (Fig. 53.1). The colour is due to haemosiderin pigment. Treatment is by excision.

DERMOID CYSTS

These are most commonly found in the head and neck. Dermoid cysts contain epithelium and adnexal structures of varying degrees of differentiation. Nasal dermoids may have a small pit or sinus with associated hair growth. External angular dermoids appear in the lateral eyebrow region (Chapter 16). Treatment is simple surgical excision, except for nasal dermoids where deep extension has to be ruled out first.

NEUROFIBROMATOSIS

Neurofibromatosis and other neurocutaneous disorders may present as soft tissue tumours. The specific diagnosis is made after a careful history and examination of the whole body has been undertaken.

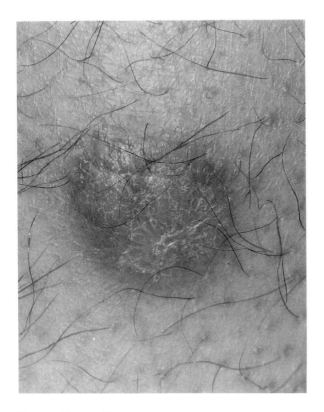

Fig. 53.1 Dermatofibroma.

LIPOMAS

These are the most common subcutaneous soft tissue tumours in adults, but are quite uncommon in children.

SOFT-TISSUE SARCOMAS

These make up 4–8% of all malignancies in childhood with rhabdomyosarcoma and fibrosarcoma being the most common.

FURTHER READING

Okun M. R. *et al.* (eds) (1988) *Gross and Microscopic Pathology of the Skin* (2 vols). Dermatology Foundation Press.

Index